ARTERIAL AND VENOUS SYSTEMS IN ESSENTIAL HYPERTENSION

DEVELOPMENTS IN CARDIOVASCULAR MEDICINE

Recent volumes

Hanrath P, Bleifeld W, Souquet, J. eds: Cardiovascular diagnosis by ultrasound. Transesophageal, computerized, contrast, Doppler echocardiography. 1982. ISBN 90-247-2692-1.

Roelandt J, ed: The practice of M-mode and two-dimensional echocardiography. 1983. ISBN 90-247-2745-6.

Meyer J, Schweizer P, Erbel R, eds: Advances in noninvasive cardiology. 1983. ISBN 0-89838-576-8.

Morganroth J, Moore EN, eds: Sudden cardiac death and congestive heart failure: Diagnosis and treatment. 1983. ISBN 0-89838-580-6.

Perry HM, ed: Lifelong management of hypertension. 1983. ISBN 0-89838-582-2.

Jaffe EA, ed: Biology of endothelial cells. 1984. ISBN 0-89838-587-3.

Surawicz B, Reddy CP, Prystowsky EN, eds: Tachycardias. 1984. ISBN 0-89838-588-1.

Spencer MP, ed: Cardiac Doppler diagnosis. 1983. ISBN 0-89838-591-1.

Villarreal H, Sambhi MP, eds: Topics in pathophysiology of hypertension. 1984. ISBN 0-89838-595-4.

Messerli FH, ed: Cardiovascular disease in the elderly. 1984. ISBN 0-89838-596-2.

Simoons ML, Reiber JHC, eds: Nuclear imaging in clinical cardiology. 1984. ISBN 0-89838-599-7.

Ter Keurs HEDJ, Schipperheyn JJ, eds: Cardiac left ventricular hypertrophy. 1983. ISBN 0-89838-612-8.

Sperelakis N, ed: Physiology and pathophysiology of the heart. 1984. ISBN 0-89838-615-2.

Messerli FH, ed: Kidney in essential hypertension. 1984. ISBN 0-89838-616-0.

Sambhi MP, ed: Fundamental fault in hypertension. 1984. ISBN 0-89838-638-1.

Marchesi C, ed: Ambulatory monitoring: Cardiovascular system and allied applications. 1984. ISBN 0-89838-642-X.

Kupper W, MacAlpin RN, Bleifeld W, eds: Coronary tone in ischemic heart disease. 1984. ISBN 0-89838-646-2.

Sperelakis N, Caulfield JB, eds: Calcium antagonists: Mechanisms of action on cardiac muscle and vascular smooth muscle. 1984. ISBN 0-89838-655-1.

Godfraind T, Herman AS, Wellens D, eds: Calcium entry blockers in cardiovascular and cerebral dysfunctions. 1984. ISBN 0-89838-658-6.

Morganroth J, Moore EN, eds: Interventions in the acute phase of myocardial infarction. 1984. ISBN 0-89838-659-4.

Abel FL, Newman WH, eds: Functional aspects of the normal, hypertrophied, and failing heart. 1984. ISBN 0-89838-665-9.

Sideman S, Beyar R, eds: Simulation and imaging of the cardiac system. 1985. ISBN 0-89838-687-X.

Van der Wall E, Lie KI, eds: Recent views on hypertrophic cardiomyopathy. 1985. ISBN 0-89838-694-2.

Beamish RE, Singal PK, Dhalla NS, eds: Stress and heart disease. 1985. ISBN 0-89838-709-4.

Beamish RE, Panagio V, Dhalla NS, eds: Pathogenesis of stress-induced heart disease. 1985. ISBN 0-89838-710-8.

Morganroth J, Moore EN, eds: Cardiac arrhythmias. 1985. ISBN 0-89838-716-7.

Mathes E, ed: Secondary prevention in coronary artery disease and myocardial infarction. 1985. ISBN 0-89838-736-1.

I owell Stone H, Weglicki WB, eds: Pathology of cardiovascular injury. 1985. ISBN 0-89838-743-4.

Meyer J, Erbel R, Rupprecht HJ, eds: Improvement of myocardial perfusion. 1985. ISBN 0-89838-748-5.

Reiber JHC, Serruys PW, Slager CJ: Quantitative coronary and left ventricular cineangiography. 1986. ISBN 0-89838-760-4.

Fagard RH, Bekaert IE, eds: Sports cardiology. 1986. ISBN 0-89838-782-5.

Reiber JHC, Serruys PW, eds: State of the art in quantitative coronary arteriography. 1986. ISBN 0-89838-804-X.

Roelandt J, ed: Color Doppler Flow Imaging. 1986. ISBN 0-89838-806-6.

Van der Wall EE, ed: Noninvasive imaging of cardiac metabolism. 1986. ISBN 0-89838-812-0.

Liebman J, Plonsey R, Rudy Y, eds: Pediatric and fundamental electrocardiography. 1986. ISBN 0-89838-815-5.

Hilger HH, Hombach V, Rashkind WJ, eds: Invasive cardiovascular therapy. 1987. ISBN 0-89838-818-X

Serruys PW, Meester GT, eds: Coronary angioplasty: a controlled model for ischemia. 1986. ISBN 0-89838-819-8.

Tooke JE, Smaje LH: Clinical investigation of the microcirculation. 1986. ISBN 0-89838-819-8.

Van Dam RTh, Van Oosterom A, eds: Electrocardiographic body surface mapping. 1986. ISBN 0-89838-834-1.

Spencer MP, ed: Ultrasonic diagnosis of cerebrovascular disease. 1987. ISBN 0-89838-836-8.

Legato MJ, ed: The stressed heart. 1987. ISBN 0-89838-849-X.

Roelandt J, ed: Digital techniques in echocardiography. 1987. ISBN 0-89838-861-9.

Sideman S, Beyar R, eds: Activation, metabolism and perfusion of the heart. 1987. ISBN 0-89838-871-6.

Safar ME et al., eds: Arterial and venous systems in essential hypertension. 1987. ISBN 0-89838-857-0.

ARTERIAL AND VENOUS SYSTEMS IN ESSENTIAL HYPERTENSION

Editor:

M.E. SAFAR
Diagnostic Center, Department of Internal Medicine
Hôpital Broussais, Paris, France

Associate Editors:

G.M. LONDON, A.CH. SIMON and Y.A. WEISS

1987 **MARTINUS NIJHOFF PUBLISHERS**
a member of the KLUWER ACADEMIC PUBLISHERS GROUP
DORDRECHT / BOSTON / LANCASTER

Distributors

for the United States and Canada: Kluwer Academic Publishers, P.O. Box 358, Accord Station, Hingham, MA 02018-0358, USA
for the UK and Ireland: Kluwer Academic Publishers, MTP Press Limited, Falcon House, Queen Square, Lancaster LA1 1RN, UK
for all other countries: Kluwer Academic Publishers Group, Distribution Center, P.O. Box 322, 3300 AH Dordrecht, The Netherlands

Library of Congress Cataloging in Publication Data

```
Arterial and venous systems in essential hypertension.

    (Developments in cardiovascular medicine)
    Includes index.
    1. Essential hypertension--Etiology.  2. Physiology,
Pathological.  3. Hemodynamics.  4. Cardiovascular
system.  I. Safar, Michel.  II. Series.  [DNLM:
1. Cardiovascular System--physiopathology.  2. Hyper-
tension--complications.  W1 DE997VME / WG 340 A7828]
RC685.A725 1987      616.1'32           86-31256
```

ISBN 978-94-010-7983-9   ISBN 978-94-009-3303-3 (eBook)
DOI 10.1007/978-94-009-3303-3

Copyright

Preface

The hemodynamic mechanisms of hypertension are often limited to the study of three dominant parameters: blood pressure, cardiac output and vascular resistance. Accordingly, the development of hypertension is usually analyzed in terms of a 'struggle' between cardiac output and vascular resistance, resulting in the classical pattern of normal cardiac output and increased vascular resistance, thus indicating a reduction in the caliber of small arteries. However, during the past years, the clinical management of hypertension has largely modified these simple views. While an adequate control of blood pressure may be obtained with antihypertensive drugs, arterial complications may occur, involving mainly the coronary circulation and suggesting that several parts of the cardiovascular system are altered in hypertension. Indeed, disturbances in the arterial and the venous system had already been noticed in animal hypertension.

The basic assumption in this book is that the overall cardiovascular system is involved in the mechanisms of the elevated blood pressure in patients with hypertension: not only the heart and small arteries, but also the large arteries and the venous system. For that reason, the following points are emphasized. First, the cardiovascular system in hypertension must be studied not only in terms of steady flow but also by taking into account the pulsatile components of the heart and the arterial systems. Second, arterial and venous compliances are altered in hypertension and probably reflect intrinsic alterations of the vascular wall. Third, such abnormalities suppose a geometrical redesign of the cardiovascular system, and the structural and the functional components are therefore critical for the understanding of hypertension. Finally, regional blood flows are more important than cardiac output itself for the description of the complications of hypertensive vascular disease.

Despite (or due to) the striking remodelling of the cardiovascular system observed in hypertension, it is important to recognize that the principal function of this system, i.e. to maintain an adequate blood flow for the metabolic needs of the tissues, is largely preserved during an important part of the life. Thus an adequate analysis of hypertension requires the description of auto-regulatory mechanisms contributing to maintain flow within normal ranges. Of course, such mechanisms are operating in untreated hypertensives, but they are also important to evaluate following antihypertensive treatment. Indeed, each antihypertensive agent is expected to be characterized by a specific mechanism of action, a prerequisite which is in opposition with the apparently non-specific geometrical redesign of the overall cardiovascular system described in patients with essential hypertension. Clearly, the relationships between antihypertensive agents and remodelling of the cardiovascular system following treatment is a key point in the future for a better understanding of cardiovascular morbidity and mortality in patients treated for hypertension.

M.E. Safar
G.M. London
A.Ch. Simon
Y.A. Weiss

Table of contents

Part I

Small arteries and the concept of resistance

Hemodynamic basis for the concept of resistance and impedance in hypertension

MICHAEL F. O'ROURKE

Hypertension is caused by increased resistance to flow in peripheral vessels. This was appreciated by Bright [1] in 1827 as the probable cause of cardiac hypertrophy in patients with chronic nephritis '. . . that it so affects the minute and capillary circulation, as to render greater action necessary to force the blood through the distant subdivisions of the vascular system.' This point of view was emphasised by Sutton and by Gull [2], who in a lecture at Guy's Hospital, London in 1872 observed 'It is always dangerous to rest in a narrow pathology; and I believe that to be a narrow pathology which is satisfied with what you now see before me on this table. In this glass you see a much hypertrophied heart and a very contracted kidney. This specimen is classical. It was, I believe, put up under Dr Bright's own direction and with a view of showing that the wasting of the kidney was the cause of the thickening of the heart. I cannot but look upon it with veneration, but not with conviction. I think, with all deference to so great an authority, that the systemic capillaries, and had it been possible, the entire man, should have been included in this vase; then we should have had, I believe, a truer view of the causation of the cardiac hypertrophy and of disease of the kidney.'

Marey in Paris [3] developed the first sphygmograph for measuring arterial pressure in man. This was refined in London by Mahomed (Fig. 1) who must be credited with the first description of the syndrome of essential hypertension [4]. 'My first contention is that high pressure is a constant condition in the circulation of some individuals and that this condition is a symptom of a certain constitution or diathesis', and further – 'These persons appear to pass through life pretty much as others do and generally do not suffer from high blood pressures, except in their petty ailments upon which it imprints itself . . . As age advances the enemy gains ascession of strength . . . the individual has now passed forty years, perhaps fifty years of age, his lungs begin to degenerate, he has a cough in the winter time, but by his pulse you will know him . . . Alternatively headache, vertigo, epistasis, a passing paralysis, a more severe apoplectic seizure and then the final blow.' Referring to etiology, Mahomed wrote 'What has been the cause in one case may be the result in the other; thus general disorder may cause high blood pressure

4

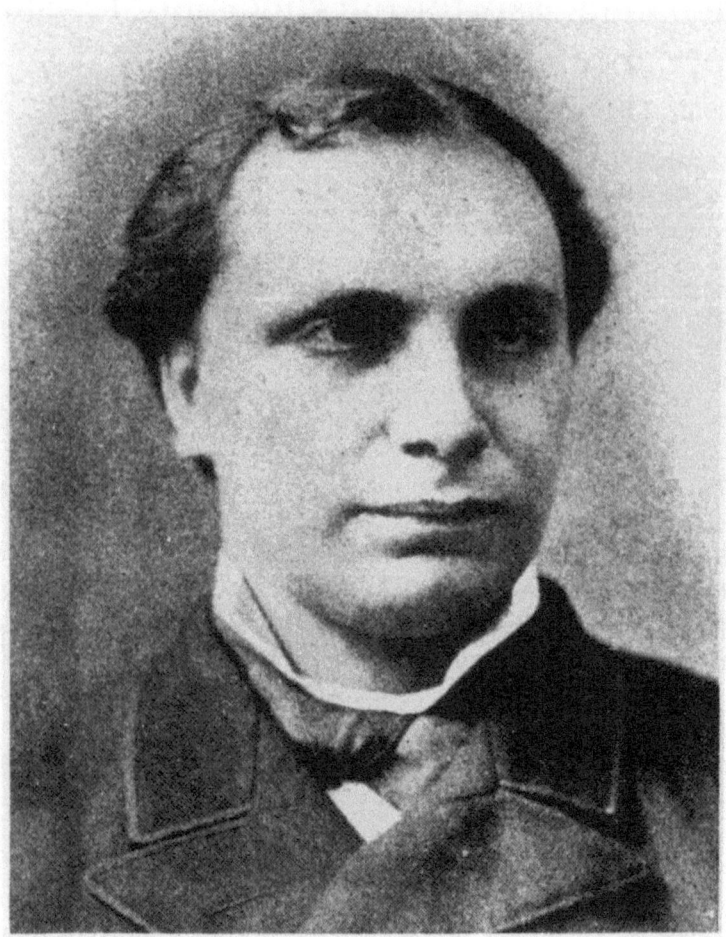

Figure 1. F. Mahomed, Circa 1874.

and this in turn kidney changes; while on the other hand kidney changes may be primary and acute and they may in their turn produce impurity of blood and thus general pressure. But whether we read the tale backwards or forward, it is the same tale in the end.'

Thus, in 1874, primary and secondary hypertension had been described and their natural history set out, and yet the sphygmomanometer as we use it now had not been described. The diagnosis of high blood pressure was made on the basis of compressibility of the radial artery and on peripheral arterial pressure pulse contour. The modern sphygmomanometric method, attributable to Riva-Rocci [5] and Korotkov [6], has focused attention on the numerical values of the systolic and the diastolic pressure in the brachial artery rather than on the parameters that

Mahomed and colleagues had determined – the mean pressure, and the amplitude and contour of the pressure wave. Clinicians have come to view the basic underlying condition in terms of systolic and diastolic pressure, and to speak of systolic hypertension and diastolic hypertension as though these were separate and distinct rather than sphygmomanometric artifices. Over-simplified interpretations of systolic and diastolic pressure levels have been responsible for the erroneous view that elevation of the former is benign and the latter only of serious concern. The views of Sir James MacKenzie have persisted for generations after 1926 when he taught 'As regards the relative importance of systolic and diastolic pressures, it may be said that the systolic pressure represents the maximum force of the heart while the diastolic pressure measures the resistance the heart has to overcome' [7]. Use of the sphygmomanometer forced on clinicians a view of cardiovascular hemodynamics that had not prevailed before the beginning of the 20th century. This was the debit side; the credit side was, of course, substantial: – arterial pressure could be measured quickly and reasonably accurately in man for the first time. The approach to be taken in this chapter will be consistent with the 19th century approach before introduction of the sphygmomanometer, but based on concepts of arterial hemodynamics derived from direct measurement of arterial pressure. This should enable sphygmomanometric measurements to be interpreted more completely, and potential and real anomalies to be recognised.

Resistance

Bright, Gull and Sutton, and Mahomed described increased arterial pressure as resulting from increased peripheral resistance due to decreased calibre of small peripheral vessels. Stephen Hales, the first man to measure arterial pressure (as mean pressure), formulated the concept of circulatory resistance as arteriovenous mean pressure gradient divided by mean flow [8]. Poiseuille [9] in 1828 developed the mercury manometer and measured mean pressure in the arterial system of experimental animals. He showed that the arteries are excellent hydraulic conduits and that there is no detectable pressure gradient below the proximal aorta and peripheral arteries, establishing a point made by Hales that most of the resistance to blood flow through the systemic circulation resides in the small peripheral vessels – that systemic resistance is 'peripheral'. Pursuing this subject, Poiseuille [10] performed his classic studies on narrow capillary tubes establishing the relationship between resistance and the fourth power of radius. The relationship between Poiseuille's constant and viscosity was clarified by Hagen so that the Poiseuille equation is expressed as

$$Q = \frac{(P_1 - P_2) \times r^4}{8\,uL}$$

where Q is volume flow, $P_1 - P_2$ is pressure gradient, r is internal diameter, u is viscosity and L is vessel length. And resistance is expressed as

$$R = \frac{8\,uL}{\pi r^4}$$

Poiseuille's equation describes a linear relationship between mean flow and pressure, and emphasises the dominance of resistance on the fourth power of vessel radius. While it can be applied in a qualitative sense to the circulation, there are a number of objections to its strict quantitative application. These problems include the anomalous viscous properties of blood – streaming of red cells in the axial stream of small vessels with apparent decrease in viscosity [11], aggregation of red cells at low rates of shear with increase in viscosity [12], non-laminar blood flow under many conditions, passive dilation of blood vessels under increased distending pressure, autoregulation in many organs, and 'critical closing pressure' [13–18]. One usually wishes to apply Poiseuille's law not to a single tube, but to a complex network of tubes such as that which makes up a vascular bed. Since in the single tube, and indeed in the network, vessel lengths remain constant and viscosity is presumed to do likewise, changes in resistance are considered to indicate changes in calibre of the small resistance vessels. Such a presumption is rarely justified. It has been shown that in a maximally dilated peripheral vascular bed, perfused with a colloid solution, there is a near linear relationship, passing through the origin between perfusion pressure and flow (Fig. 2). When such a vascular bed is perfused with blood there is usually a positive intercept on the pressure axis caused by anomalous viscous properties of blood; as flow velocity slows, and shear rate falls, the red cells tend to aggregate with marked increase in viscosity and so in resistance (Fig. 2). Fig. 3 shows another pattern of pressure flow/relationships in a peripheral vascular bed perfused with oxygenated blood; here the relationship is convex towards the pressure axis, probably caused by physical dilation of the constricted resistance vessels from increased pressure with lower resistance at high pressure. Other patterns of pressure flow relationship are seen in the heart, brain and kidney, where over the physiological range of mean pressure, flow remains relatively constant as a result of autoregulation, caused by change in arteriolar tone or from increased tissue pressure compressing blood vessels from without [12, 13]. It is clear that one cannot assume in the living organism, a constant relationship between pressure and flow in any segment of the vascular tree let alone in the whole systemic circulation. Yet, the relationship between mean arteriovenous pressure gradient and flow is usually expressed as resistance, assuming linearity and assuming zero flow is achieved at zero pressure. Changes in resistance under different conditions are usually taken to indicate changes in arteriolar calibre, and so to reflect changes in arteriolar tone. Such changes in calculated resistance must be interpreted with caution; since resistance to flow varies inversely with the

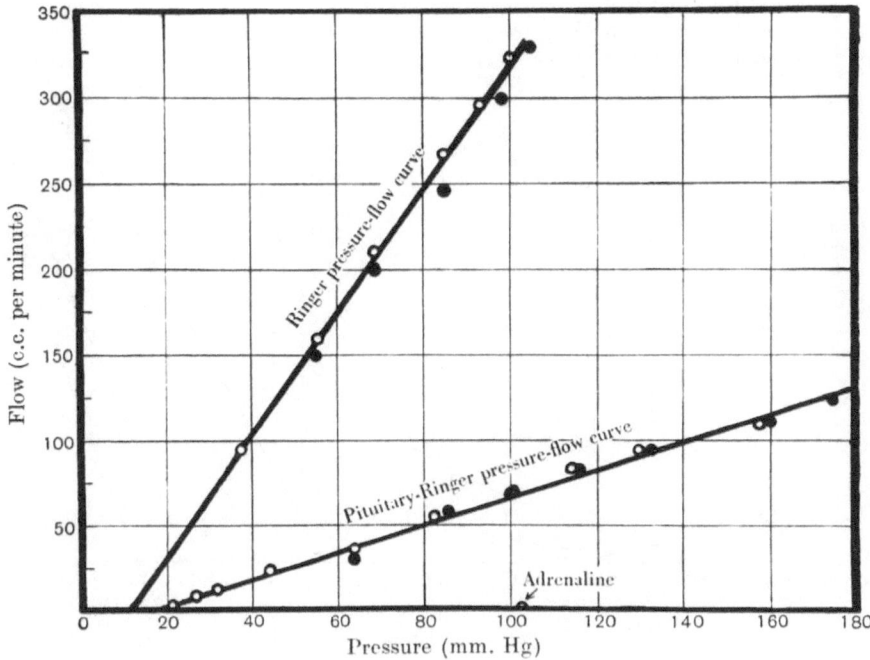

Figure 2. Relationship between pressure and flow of a cell free colloid solution, and of blood in a maximally dilated vascular bed. From Whittaker and Winton 1933 [12].

fourth power of radius, arteriolar tone and calibre will have a profound effect on calculated resistance. The other factors must, however, be borne in mind.

That peripheral resistance is elevated in essential hypertension was confirmed by Pickering [19] and by Prinzmetal and Wilson [20]. The cause of this is in most cases the arteriolar and other small vessel narrowing proposed by Bright and demonstrated by Gull and Sutton and by many others since. This subject is discussed by Folkow (p. 21ff.). But arteriolar narrowing is not the only possible cause of increased peripheral resistance. Another is microvascular rarefaction (Fig. 4). This has been demonstrated to develop in spontaneously hypertensive rats [21], in diabetic patients [22] and in human hypertensive subjects [22, 23]. MacKenzie [24] described this quite clearly in 1902 as a cause of increasing resistance and arterial pressure with age: 'There is a third factor of great importance, namely the diminution of the capillary field which occurs as an accompaniment of advancing years. This can be recognised in many ways, as for instance, the thinning and wasting of skin and subcutaneous tissues and the absence of oozing when the skin is cut e.g. in surgical operations.' The changes of arterial pressure with age are well known (Fig. 5), and have usually been interpreted in terms of systolic and diastolic pressure. It is acknowledged that cardiac output falls with age in humans [25], so that calculated peripheral resistance must

8

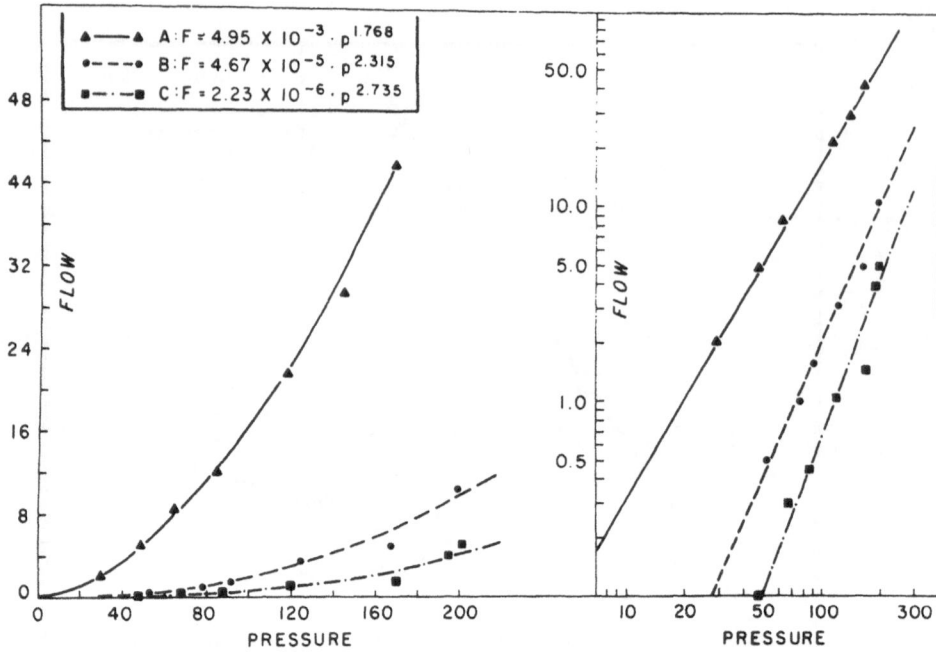

Figure 3. Plots of the arteriovenous difference pressure vs the blood flow in a cutaneous (saphenous) bed at three levels of spontaneous 'vasomotor tone'. *Left half,* plotted linearly; *right half,* plotted on log-log paper. *Triangles* represent the lowest level of vasomotor tone; *circles* represent an intermediate level and *squares,* the highest level of vasomotor tone. Flow in ml/min, pressure in mm Hg. From Green, Rapela, Conrad [13].

increase. The changes with age (i.e. marked increase in systolic with lesser increase in diastolic pressure) are attributable to just two factors: increasing resistance causing increase in mean pressure and arterial stiffening which causes increase in fluctuation around this mean pressure [26]. The degree of change in systolic and diastolic pressure in any individual would be expected to depend on the relative degree of increase in resistance and in arterial stiffness. If the former was to increase with no change in the latter, one would expect systolic and diastolic pressure to increase to the same degree; if the latter increased with no change in the former, one would predict an increase in systolic pressure but a fall in the diastolic level. The changes seen in Fig. 5 are attributable to a combination of increased resistance and decreased compliance.

Impedance

The concept of vascular impedance is an extension of resistance [11, 27]. Resistance describes the relationship between mean pressure and mean flow at the

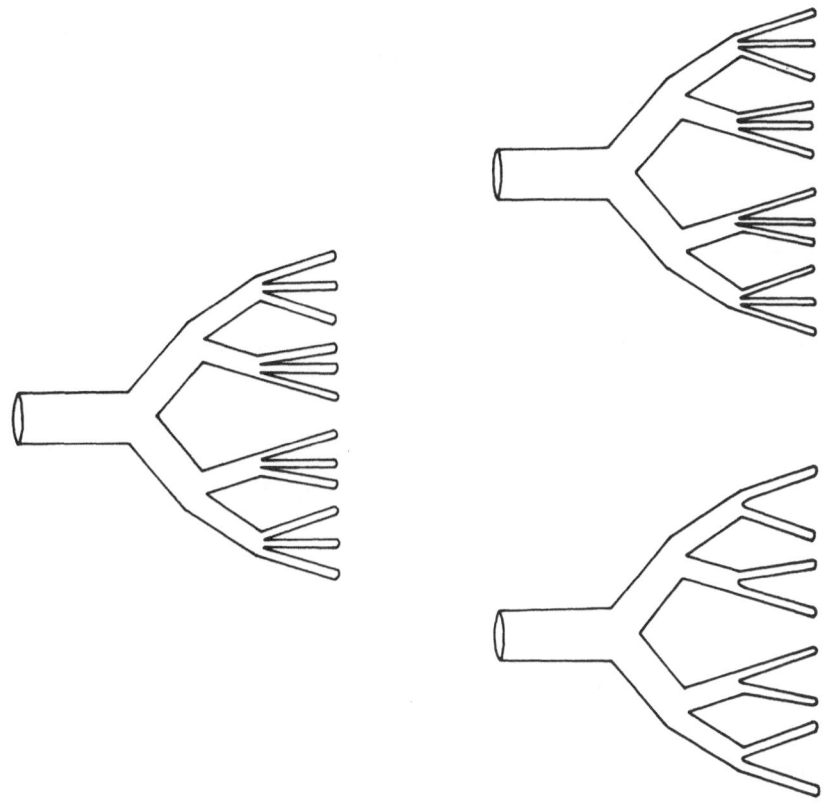

Figure 4. Increased resistance in a vascular bed caused by two mechanisms, illustrated schematically – constriction of resistance vessels, and rarefaction of resistance vessels. 'Normal' bed at left, abnormal beds at right.

input of a vascular bed (assuming venous flow to have zero pressure). Impedance describes the relationship between the pulsatile components of the pressure and flow waves from which resistance is determined. The relationship is determined by breaking down the pressure and flow waves into their component harmonics using Fourier analysis, then relating the corresponding harmonics of pressure and flow (Fig. 6). In practice one usually only uses the first 5–8 harmonics, thus with a heart rate of 90/min (1.5/sec) determining impedance up to 12 Hz. Impedance graphs take the form of modulus (amplitude of pressure ÷ amplitude of flow) and phase (delay between pressure and flow) plotted against frequency. They are similar to graphs of electrical impedance, acoustic impedance, and hydraulic impedance and can be interpreted in the same way [11, 26–30].

Merrillon and colleagues from Paris [29] have described the changes of impedance which occur in patients with hypertension (Fig. 7). These are similar to those seen in experimental animals with acute elevation in arterial pressure [26–28]. In

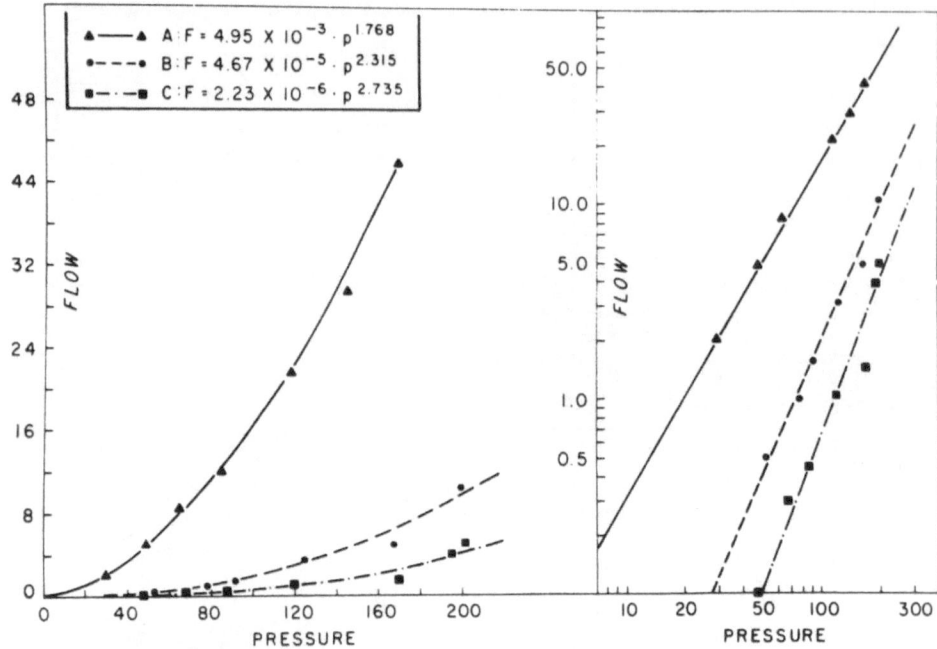

Figure 5. Change in arterial pressure with age. Pressure expressed in terms of systolic and diastolic values at left, in terms of mean and pulse pressure at right. From O'Rourke [26].

hypertension there is increase in both impedance modulus at zero frequency (the peripheral resistance) and at higher frequencies after the first minimal value (the characteristic impedance). Increase in characteristic impedance may not be apparent when as in Fig. 7, impedance is expressed in terms of volume rather than in terms of velocity flow [26]. There is also an increase in the frequency of the first minimum. These changes are shown diagrammatically in Fig. 8. Increased characteristic impedance and higher frequency of the first impedance minimum are due to the same mechanism – increased stiffness of arterial walls at higher distending pressure [26, 29]. As pressure is increased within an artery, the vessel dilates passively and tension is transferred from elastin to collagenous fibres [31]. As a consequence of increased arterial stiffness, flow fluctuations cause greater pressure fluctuations, even in the absence of reflections – hence the increase in aortic characteristic impedance. The stiffened artery also transmits pressure waves more quickly – the pulse wave velocity is increased [26]; as a consequence of this, reflected waves return earlier from peripheral sites and cause the shift in impedance minimum to higher frequencies. In chapter 10, Avolio describes further details of pulse wave velocity in hypertension.

The changes in ascending aortic impedance caused by elevated arterial pres-

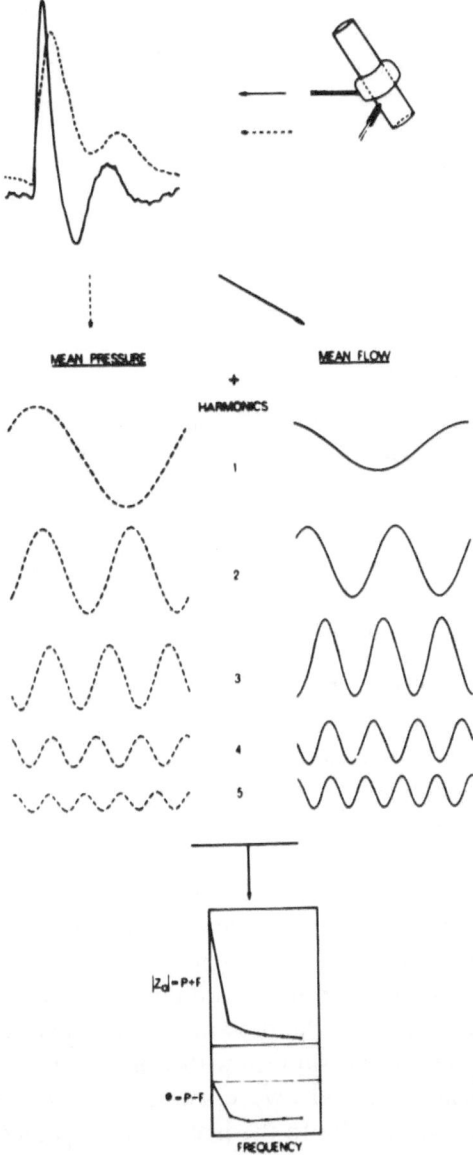

Figure 6. Pressure and flow waves (above) broken down into other harmonic components (centre) and with the mean values and corresponding components related (below) to give modulus and phase of impedance as a function of frequency.

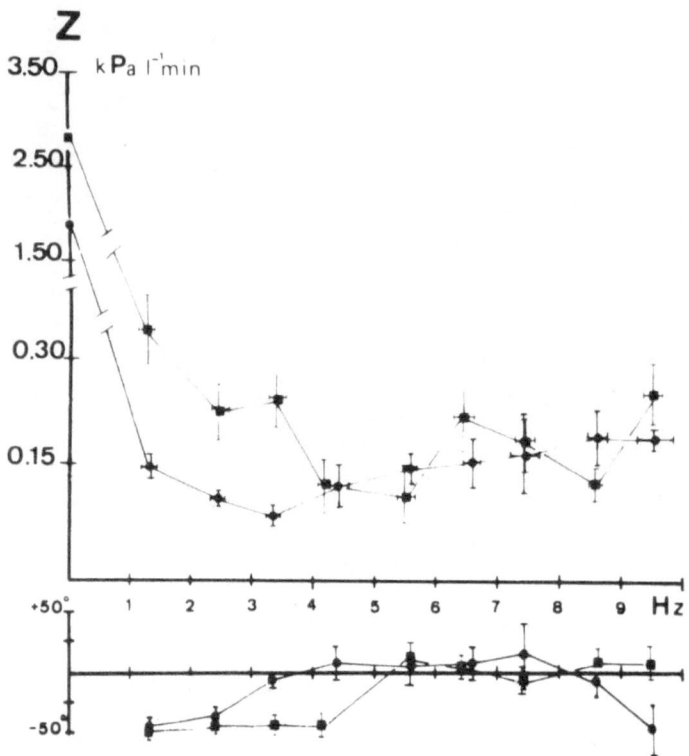

Figure 7. Modulus and phase of impedance in a group of hypertensive patients and in a group of normal subjects. In hypertension, modulus and phase plots are displaced to the right. From Merillon et al. [30].

sure in hypertension are disadvantageous to the heart. These can be discussed in terms of relationship between the impedance graph and harmonics of the ventricular ejection (flow) wave [26, 32], but are more readily and conveniently explained in terms of the change in ascending aortic pressure wave contour. Figure 9 shows diagrammatically the pressure wave generated in the ascending aorta of a young normotensive subject with normal arterial system and in a patient with hypertension. Pressure wave shapes are quite different as indeed emphasised by Mahomed in 1874. In the hypertensive subject mean pressure is higher (because peripheral resistance is increased), but pulse pressure is higher as well and the diastolic wave is lost. These two features are attributable to high characteristic impedance and increased pulse wave velocity. The former is responsible for the higher 'shoulder' on the pressure wave: – even in the absence of reflection, a given flow impulse generates a greater pressure fluctuation. The latter is responsible for the late systolic peak: – the reflected wave from peripheral sites returns so soon that it merges with the systolic part of the wave.

The characteristic aortic pressure waves of normotension and hypertension are

Effects of Hypertension

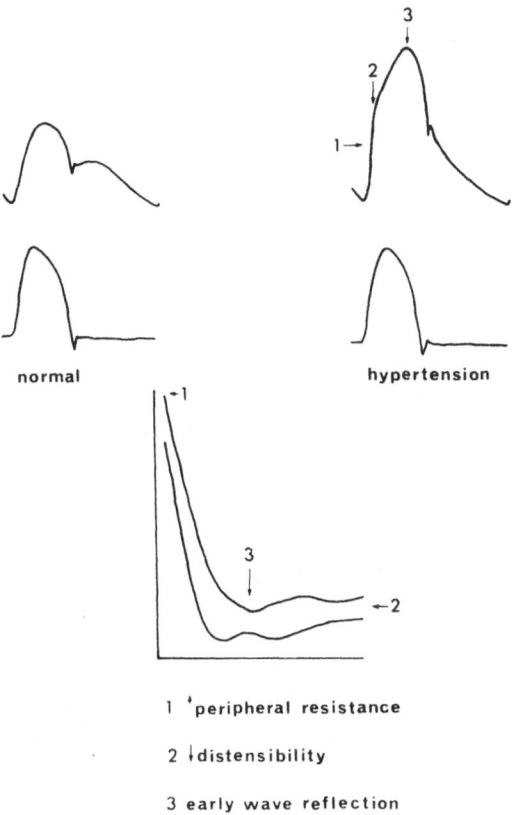

1 'peripheral resistance

2 ↓distensibility

3 early wave reflection

Figure 8. Below: Diagrammatic representation of impedance modulus under normal conditions (lower curve) and in hypertension (upper curve). Above: The pressure waves resynthesised from impedance curves using the same ventricular ejection (flow) wave. The cause of change in impedance curves and in impedance plots are identified as: 1. increased peripheral resistance, 2. decreased arterial distensibility, 3. early return of wave reflection.

shown in Fig. 9. Mean systolic pressure (M.S.P.) is markedly increased. This is due to increase in mean pressure (M.P.) and to increased characteristic impedance and earlier wave reflection as well. Increased mean systolic pressure represents greater afterload to left ventricular ejection with increased myocardial oxygen demands and constitutes a stimulus to hypertrophy as well as an impediment to optimal ventricular ejection [26]. In contrast to the increase in mean systolic pressure, mean diastolic pressure (M.D.P.) is relatively low, largely as a consequence of earlier wave reflection and absence of a positive diastolic wave. This is an impediment to optimal coronary perfusion that is normally augmented by the presence of a reflected wave during diastole [26].

14

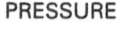

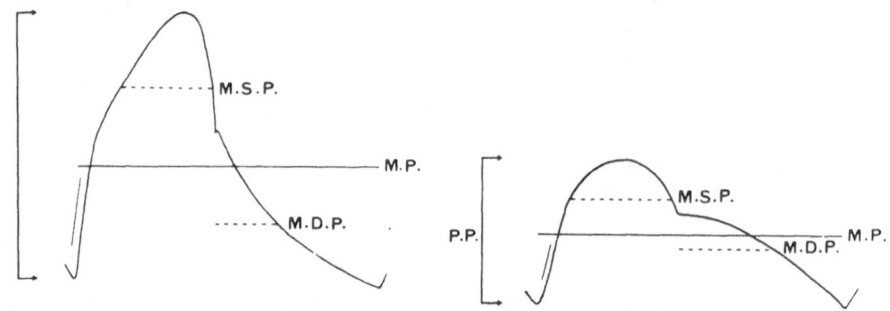

Figure 9. Characteristic contour of ascending aortic pressure waves in hypertension (left) and in a normal young subject (right). Abbreviations: see text.

With respect to cardiac load and to coronary perfusion, change in the aortic pressure wave in hypertension has adverse effects. This change also affects the arterial wall with greater pulsatile stresses on the arterial wall – greater peak stress, greater fluctuation and greater rate of change of stress. It is argued elsewhere according to established principles of mechanical engineering and material fatigue that such pulsatile change is likely to accelerate arterial degeneration and predispose to development of atheroma, arterial dilation, aneurysm formation and ultimately rupture [26, 29, 33] (Fig. 10).

Changes in contour of the arterial pressure pulse in hypertension can be explained on the basis of change in vascular impedance. Such change in pulse contour was first noted by Mahomed [4] and used by him in the diagnosis of high blood pressure: 'by his pulse you will know him'. It is a tribute to the clinical skills of 19th century physicians that such information could be obtained from examination of the pulse, and a reflection on our own lack thereof that such a clinical sign should be overlooked today.

Pressure wave transmission

Conventional descriptions of arterial pressure are of the systolic and the diastolic pressures as though they were the same everywhere in all major arteries and at the aortic root, and capable of measurement with a sphygmomanometer on the brachial artery. This is not the case [16, 26]. The pressure wave generated in the ascending aorta by ventricular ejection is altered by peripheral wave reflection – with, as previously described, systolic pressure augmented if arterial wave velocity is fast, and pressure during diastole augmented if wave velocity is normal. The pressure wave itself is altered in transmission to the peripheral arteries, with the systolic peak increased and diastolic pressure slightly decreased (Fig. 11). Amplitude of the pressure pulse is increased by up to 50% in normal young individuals between the ascending aorta and brachial artery [26]. In patients with

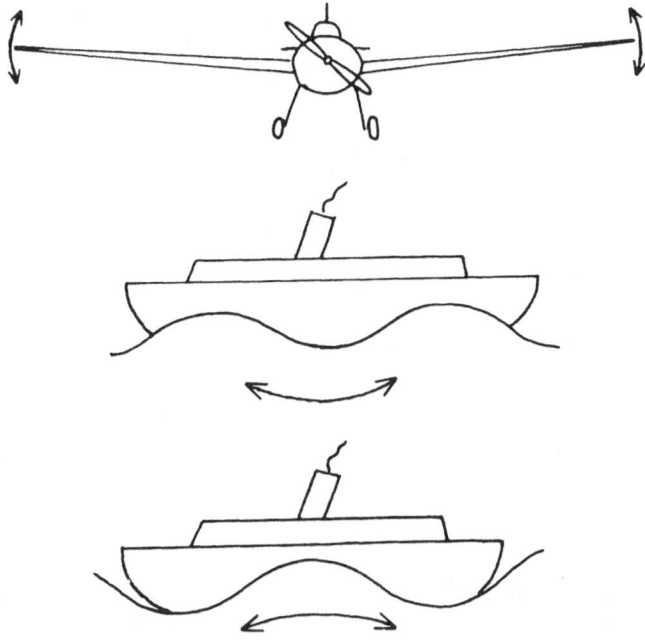

Figure 10. Cyclic stress on the wings of an aeroplane and the hull of a ship; the stresses cause material fatigue and ultimately, fracture. After Sandor [41].

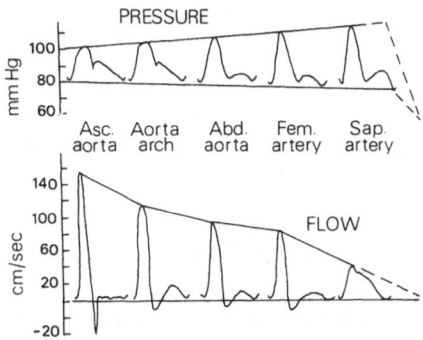

Figure 11. Amplification of the arterial pressure wave between the ascending aorta and peripheral arteries; this is associated with decrease in amplitude of pulsatile flow. After McDonald [16].

established hypertension such amplification is probably much lower [34] so that brachial artery systolic and diastolic pressures are reasonably close to those in the ascending aorta. Under different conditions, as in low output heart failure [26], shock (Fig. 12) or during exercise [36], brachial artery systolic and diastolic pressure may be considerably different to systolic and diastolic pressure in the ascending aorta. It is important that amplification of the peripheral pressure pulse

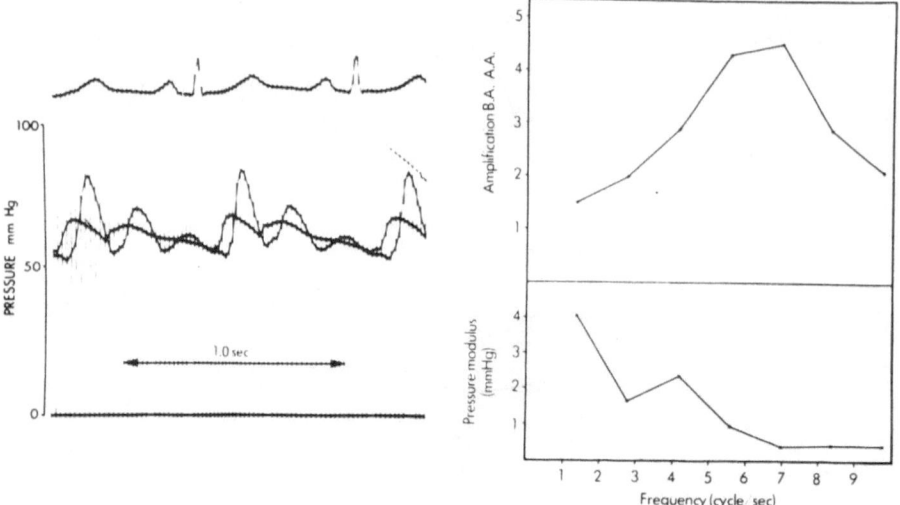

Figure 12. (Left) – Simultaneous recordings of pressure in the brachial artery and aortic arch of a patient with hypotension and clinical features of peripheral vasoconstriction. (Right) – Ratio of corresponding harmonics of the brachial and aortic pressure waves (above), and the modulus of the harmonics of the aortic pressure waves (below).

be considered when interpreting brachial artery pressure recordings under different conditions. Calculations of left ventricular stroke work during exercise are likely to be erroneously high if brachial artery systolic pressure is considered analogous to ascending aortic and left ventricular peak pressure. The changes in brachial artery pulse pressure with age probably underestimate the increase in ascending aortic pulse pressure with age, owing to the greater amplification of the peripheral pulse in the young, and the lesser amplification in the elderly [26].

Accuracy of sphygmomanometric recordings

When the sphygmomanometer was first introduced by Riva-Rocci in 1895 there was considerable controversy as to the accuracy of the technique, and on how precisely pressure applied to the outside of the arm was applied to blood in the brachial artery. Oliver [37] pointed out the difference, especially in systolic pressure, that was found in elderly persons when the Korotkov/Riva-Rocci technique was compared with his own tonometer. Oliver believed that the conventional sphygmomanometric technique overestimated systolic (and to a lesser degree, diastolic) pressure in elderly subjects. This subject has been addressed again in recent years under the title of 'pseudohypertension' [38]. It has been shown (Fig. 13) that there is a substantial difference between sphygmomanometrically determined and directly recorded pressure in the brachial artery

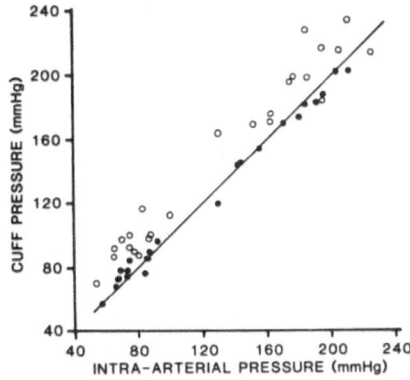

Figure 13. Relationship between sphygmomanometrically-recorded, and directly measured arterial pressure in patients with (open circles) and without (closed circles) a palpable radial artery. Messerli [38].

in subjects with evidence of arteriosclerosis, as evidenced by a palpable radial artery or increased brachial arterial pulse wave velocity. 'Pseudohypertension' is probably quite common, especially in the elderly and is attributable to the thickened, stiffened brachial artery resisting the compression force applied from without. It is almost certainly not due to atheroma [39] but to the generalised sclerosis that is an accompaniment of age even in communities with very low prevalence of atherosclerosis (see p. 133ff.). A suspicion of pseudohypertension may warrant direct arterial puncture [40] so that inappropriately strong therapy is not administered.

Summary and conclusion

Hypertension is caused by elevated peripheral resistance. This may be due to increased arteriolar tone or to rarefaction of blood vessels in bodily tissues. There is normally a complex and non-linear relationship between mean pressure and flow in different vascular beds and in the whole systemic circulation, so that changes in resistance cannot always be attributed to like changes in arteriolar tone. Changes of vascular impedance in hypertension are attributable to arterial stiffening, caused by the rise in arterial pressure *per se* and by accelerated arterial degeneration. Changes in impedance explain the characteristic contour of the arterial pressure pulse in hypertension, altered wave transmission to peripheral arteries, unfavourable vascular/ventricular interaction and accelerated arterial degeneration. Consideration of the pressure pulse in terms of separate mean and pulsatile components as in the determination of resistance and impedance aids in interpreting the changes seen under different conditions. 'Pseudohypertension' is

18

a real and long-recognised problem, warranting direct arterial puncture under certain circumstances.

References

1. Bright R (1827): Reports of medical cases selected with a view of illustrating the symptoms and cure of diseases by a reference to morbid anatomy. London, Longmans.
2. Gull WW (1872): Chronic Bright's disease with contracted kidney (arteriocapillary fibrosis). British Med J 673.
3. Marey E (1863): Physiologic medicale de la circulation du sang . . . Paris, Delahaye.
4. Mahomed F (1874): The aetiology of Bright's disease and the prealbumineric stage. Med Chir Trans 57: 197–228.
5. Riva-Rocci S (1956): A new sphygmomanometer. In: Ruskin A (ed) Classics in arterial hypertension. Springfield Thomas 104–125.
6. Korotkov NS (1956): A contribution to the problem of methods for the determination of blood pressure. In: Ruskin A (ed) Classics in arterial hypertension. Springfield Thomas 127–133.
7. MacKenzie J (1926): Principles of diagnosis and treatment in heart affections. London, Oxford.
8. Hales S (1769): Statical essays; Vol 2, containing haemostatics. London, Innys and Manby.
9. Poiseuille JLM (1840): Recherches experimentales sur le mouvement des liquides dans les tube de très petits diamètres. Comptes Rendu Hebdomadaires des séances de L'Academie des Sciences 11: 961–967, 1041–1048.
10. Poiseuille JLM (1956): Recherches sur la force du coeur aortique. In: Ruskin A (ed) Classics in arterial hypertension. Springfield Thomas 31–59.
11. Fahraeus R, Lindquist T (1931): Viscosity of blood in narrow capillary tubes. Amer J Physiol 96: 562–568.
12. Whittaker SRF, Winton FR (1933): Apparent viscosity of blood flowing in the isolated vessel of the dog and its variation with corpuscular concentration. J Physiology London, 78: 339–369.
13. Green HD, Rapela CE, Conrad MC (1965): Resistance (conductance) and capacitance phenomena in terminal vascular beds. In: Hamilton W (ed) Handbook of Physiology Circulation, Section 2, Vol 2, 935–960. Am Physiol Soc, Washington DC.
14. Mellander S, Johansson B (1968): Control of resistance, exchange and capacitance functions in the peripheral circulation. Pharmacol Rev 20: 117–196.
15. Whitmore RL (1968): Rheology of the circulation. Pergamon London.
16. McDonald DA (1974): Blood flow in arteries. London, Arnold 2nd ed.
17. Gow BS (1980): Circulatory corretatis: vascular impedance, resistance and capacity. In: Bohr DF, Somlyo AP, Sparks HV (eds) Handbook of Physiology, Section 2, Vol 2, American Physiological Society, Bethesda 353–408.
18. Burton AC (1962): Physical principles of circulatory phenomena. Handbook of Physiology, America Physiological Society, Washington DC, Vol 2. Circulation No 1: 85–106.
19. Pickering GW (1936): The peripheral resistance in persistent arterial hypertension. Clinical Science 2: 209–235.
20. Prinzmetal M, Friedman B (1936): The nature of the peripheral resistance in arterial hypertension with special reference to the vasomotor system. J Clin Invest 15: 63–68.
21. Prewitt RL, Chen IIH, Dowell R (1982): Development of microvascular rarefaction in the spontaneously hypertensive rat. Clin J Physiol 243: H243–H251.
22. Bohlen HG (1982): Pathological expression in the microcirculation: hypertension and diabetes. The Physiologist 25: 391–395.
23. Harper RN, Moore MA, Marr MC, Watts LE, Hutchings PM (1978): Arteriolar rarefaction in the conjunction of human essential hypertensives. Microvasc Res 16: 369–372.

24. Pickering G (1968): High Blood Pressure. London, Churchill.
25. Dittmer DS, Grebe RM (1959): Handbook of Circulation. Saunders, Philadelphia.
26. O'Rourke MF (1982): Arterial function in health and disease. Churchill Edinburgh.
27. O'Rourke MF, Taylor MG (1966): Vascular impedance of the femoral bed. Circulation Res 18: 126–139.
28. O'Rourke MF (1970): Arterial hemodynamics in hypertension. Circ Res 26, Suppl 123–133.
29. O'Rourke MF (1976): Pulsatile arterial hemodynamics in hypertension. Aust NZ J Med Suppl 2: 40–48.
30. Merrillon JP, Fontenier GJ, Lerallut JF et al. (1982): Aortic input impedance in normal man and arterial hypertension: its modification during changes in arterial pressure. Cardiovascular Res 16: 646–656.
31. Roach MR (1977): Biophysical analysis of blood pressure walls and blood flow. Annual Rev Physiol 39: 51–71.
32. O'Rourke MF, Yaginuma T, Avolio AP (1984): Physiological and pathophysiological implications of ventricular/vascular coupling. Annals Biomed Eng 12: 119–134.
33. Kaplan NM (1982): Clinical Hypertension. 3rd ed. Baltmore, Williams & Wilkins.
34. O'Rourke MF, Blazek JV, Morreels CL, Krovetz LJ (1968): Pressure wave transmission along the human aorta; changes with age and in arterial degenerative disease. Circ Res 23: 567–579.
35. O'Rourke MF (1970): Influence of ventricular ejection on the relationship between central aortic and brachial pressure pulse in man. Cardiovasc Res 4: 291–300.
36. Rowell LB, Brengelmann GL, Blackmon JR, Bruce RA, Murray JA (1968): Disparity between aortic and peripheral pulse pressures induced by upright exercise and vasomotor changes in man. Circulation 37: 954–964.
37. Oliver G (1908): Studies in blood pressure: physiological and clinical. Lewis London.
38. Messerli FH, Ventura HO, Amoded C (1985): Osler's manouver and pseudohypertension. N England J Med 312: 1548–1551.
39. O'Rourke MF, Kelly R (1985): 'Osler's manouver' and pseudohypertension. N Engl J Med 313: 1300.
40. Breit SN, O'Rourke MF (1974): Comparisons of direct and indirect arterial pressure measurements in hospitalised patients. Aust NZ J Med 4: 485–491.
41. Sandor B (1972): Fundamentals of cyclic stress and strain. University of Wisconsin, Madison, p 3.

Structural component of vascular resistance in hypertension

BJÖRN FOLKOW

A. Introduction

All biologic tissues are able to adapt their design, though in their own characteristic way, whenever sustained changes of activity or/and load occur, a process often modified also by 'trophic' influences as by local and blood-borne humoral agents and nerve transmitters. For example, it is well known that the design of the skeletal muscle system, being basically genetically determined as expressed in 'leptosomic' or 'mesomorphic' constitutions, is considerably affected not only by the duration, frequency and intensity of imposed physical training but also by trophic influences, as shown by the effects of anabolic steroids when abused in modern athletics. It is also well known that relative inactivity soon leads to regression of muscle hypertrophy and, when severe, even to atrophy.

In these respects the cardiovascular system is certainly no exception, which the following particularly obvious examples amply illustrate: during wound healing new microvessels grow within days; veins used as arterial bypasses have within few weeks closely approached the design of arteries, and the uterine vessels undergo dramatic design changes under the cyclic influence of female sex hormones. This article deals specifically with *the situation in hypertension,* concerning the ways and extent to which the cardiovascular system then adapts its structural design, with particular emphasis on *the systemic resistance vessels* [1, 2, 3]. It is then obvious that such adaptation is of true relevance only to the extent that it alters the hemodynamic characteristics of the resistance vessels, i.e. concerning their responses to local and remote functional adjustments. Reference to the by now extensive literature is given mainly by way of some recent survey articles, with addition of a limited number of experimental studies that illustrate certain aspects of this topic particularly well.

B. Methodological aspects

It should in this context be remembered that even modest changes of inner radius (r_i), wall thickness (w) and their relationship (w/r_i) in the various parts of the cardiovascular system can considerably influence overall hemodynamics. For example, concerning the heart the structural w and r_i dimensions of the cardiac ventricles set the upper limits for contractile force, diastolic filling and stroke volume, and here volume changes with the *third* power of r_i. Concerning the resistance vessels, maximal capacity of flow (and minimal resistance; Rmin) varies directly (inversely) with the *fourth* power of their average structural r_i value (Poiseuille's law). Further, concerning venous capacitance function, which is critical for cardiac priming and output, it varies with the *second* power of the average venous r_i. In any estimations of cardiovascular structural adaptation it is therefore paramount to use methods that really can reveal even minor changes of average design, and in precisely those cardiovascular sections that really are of hemodynamic importance, which calls for some methodological considerations.

Because of the immense architectural complexity of the cardiovascular system, it is, for example, very difficult to adequately 'sample' the resistance compartment, concerning its hemodynamic characteristics when *direct morphometric* analyses are attempted. The reason is that this compartment encompasses many consecutive sections of a given vascular circuit, varying both in degree of branching, bore and w/r_i relationships. Further, all blood vessels are distensible, where r_i and w vary in *opposite* directions during both distension-recoil and contraction-relaxation. This fact easily introduces considerable errors in direct measurements, and particularly so concerning w/r_i [1, 2, 3]. Finally, as resistance varies inversely to the *fourth* power of r_i, it is obvious that direct morphometric estimations of the precise degree of structural 'resetting' of the resistance function are exceedingly difficult to perform. No doubt, at first sight this 'direct' approach appears to be the most natural one, and many such studies dealing with hypertension have been performed starting with the pioneer studies by George Johnson in 1868 [1, 2] but, not surprisingly, often with conflicting results. However, in recent years improved techniques for standardizing luminal distension and media activity have been developed, providing increasingly accurate morphometric estimations of r_i, w and w/r_i [1, 2]. Nevertheless, the difficulties to select representative vascular 'samples' remain, as does the inherent problem that resistance varies inversely to the fourth power of r_i.

Therefore, other approaches are badly needed and have, indeed, been much utilized, applying the same principles as those used in engineering when the average dimensional characteristics of complex tube systems (or electric circuits) are determined by way of Poiseuille's law (or Ohm's law) [1, 2]. As both pressure (P) and flow (Q) can usually be precisely estimated, and complete vascular relaxation can often be readily induced also in vivo, exact deductions of the structurally determined resistance at maximal vasodilatation (Rmin) can be performed, and also related to the resistance level at 'resting' steady state vascular tone (Rr), as well as to the resistance levels reached by induced degrees of vasoconstriction. For example, the ratio Rr/Rmin will closely reflect the average level of smooth muscle tonic activity in the resistance vascular section, as present in the resting steady state. Further, if accentuations of regional smooth muscle tone are induced via neurogenic influences or constrictor agents, such values can together with the Rmin and Rr values be used to plot more or less complete 'resistance curves', even in man [1, 2, 4]. Such curves can provide detailed insight into alterations of geometric design of the resistance vessels, both via the observed changes of Rmin and via the slope of the resistance curve, which latter is a consequence of a geometrically (via the w/r_i relationship) determined shift in 'vascular' reactivity'. A selective alteration of smooth muscle sensitivity-reactivity will merely shift the resistance curve in a parallel fashion, without changing either Rmin or the curve slope.

This hemodynamic test principle, which has been utilized both in vivo and particularly in vitro in artificially perfused vascular systems, as experimentally illustrated in Fig. 1, is actually the same as that widely used in physiologic and pharmacologic estimations of the degree of muscle activity in e.g. isolated vascular strips in vitro, by means of relating the active and resting lengths (or tensions) to each other under well-defined experimental conditions. However, resistance measurements here have the great advantage that they amplify to at least the fourth power (thanks to the Poiseuille relationship between r_i and R) any changes of average vascular smooth-muscle length, or/and any differences in r_i at full relaxation which, of course, markedly improves the accuracy of the estimations. Further, the hemodynamic approach automatically averages the design and responses of the myriad of otherwise poorly accessible microvascular sections, which together constitute the resistance compartment, and does so precisely in proportion to their relative contributions to resistance. Moreover, when the perfusion pressure corresponds to the normal one in vivo, the measurements are always performed at the appropriate level of transmural pressure, and, hence, degree of distension for individual sections. Finally, only the hemodynamic approach can be applied to man in vivo, and also be used for repeated estimations of Rmin and Rr to follow e.g. the development, or regression, of adaptive vascular structural changes. It is true, it does not allow for any distinction between the consecutive vascular sections, except at the capillary exchange level by using a modified 'isogravimetric' technique. However, as thereby the resistance vessels can be separated into the pre- and postcapillary sections [1, 6] this is for most purposes enough, simply because significant fluid transfer along a vascular circuit occurs only at the capillary level.

This by no means denies that it is often of great interest to know also to what extent e.g. the consecutive precapillary resistance subsections differ in structural adaptation, because they are both structurally and functionally to some extent differentiated [1, 2, 3]. Thus, the vasoconstrictor fibres seem to mainly command

24

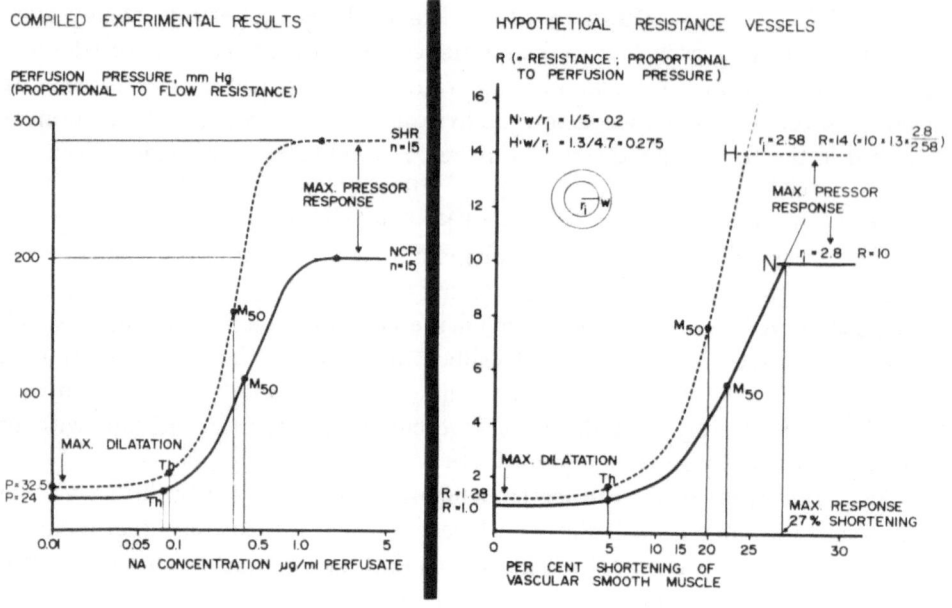

Figure 1. Left part: Average 'resistance curves' to increasing noradrenaline (NA) concentrations, derived from the results of 15 paired constant-flow perfusions of the hindquarter vascular beds from spontaneously hypertensive rats (SHR) and normotensive control rats (NCR). *Right part:* Mathematically deduced 'resistance curves' for two hypothetical resistance vessels, H and N; H differs from N only by a 30% increase of media thickness (w; 1→1.3), which reduces the inner radius (r_i) at maximal relaxation from 5 to 4.7.

Note the striking similarities between the relationships of the two sets of 'resistance curves' concerning 1. *Resistance at maximal relaxation* (Rmin). 2. *'Threshold' (Th) of NA effect.* 3. *Steepness of curves,* 4. *50 per cent of the maximal pressor (resistance) response* (M_{50}; which approximately corresponds to ED_{50}, though increases of w/r_i tend to displace M_{50} to the left, as evident from the right part). and 5. *Maximal constriction (pressor, resistance) response.* (For details see [5]; With kind permission of the Editor of Acta Physiol Scand).

the proximal sections and local-chemical mechanisms mainly the distal ones. Here direct morphometric analyses of the individual sections are indispensible and, in general, the 'hemodynamic' and 'morphometric' approaches are both badly needed, and they complement each other whenever there is a demand for exact analyses of vascular structural adaptation. Estimations of structural adaptation of the heart may seem to be more straightforward, but as both w and r_i of the cardiac chambers can be, in part, *independently* altered by structural adaptation (section C), it is necessary to measure both the diastolic pressure-volume (P/V) relationships of e.g. the ventricles (which in a way corresponds to Rmin for the resistance vessels) and the, at least in animals, more easily available ventricular wall mass. From such data r_i and w can then be calculated, also at various levels of distending diastolic pressure [7, 8, 9]. It is, however, technically quite difficult to perform exact pressure-volume estimations on an otherwise intact heart [8, 9] making such evaluations of cardiac geometric design fairly cumbersome.

C. General principles of cardiovascular structural adaptation

Before going into the particular situation for the resistance vessels in hypertension, it is worthwhile to outline some general principles governing the process of structural adaptation both in heart and vessels. It is, for example, important to realize that the structural changes of lumen (r_i) and of wall thickness (w) can to some extent be independent of each other, and are then related to different types of sustained hemodynamic change. However, it is usually also the case that alteration of either of them soon leads to adaptation of the other one as well, and in such a way as to keep their relationship (w/r_i) reasonably well balanced to the prevailing pressure load [1, 3]. It is further typical of these local structural adaptations of both heart and vessels that they can occur quite rapidly if the onset of the appropriate stimulus is prompt. Thus, in rats they can then be largely completed in 10–15 days [1, 2, 3, 8] and in man, because of a 5–6-fold lower metabolic rate, in perhaps a few months. They may be looked upon as a 'second line of defence', which at e.g. increases of load serves to relieve the more prompt but also more easily fatigued functional adjustments, once the increased load becomes more sustained.

1. Heart

Concerning cardiac design, prolonged elevations of *'preload'* (filling), and hence of cardiac output (as occurs in endurance exercise training, pregnancy, increased basal metabolism, etc) trigger a luminal (r_i) outgrowth, as evident by a rightward shift of the entire ventricular diastolic pressure-volume curve [7, 8, 9]. It is usually associated with a secondary w increase, thereby keeping wall tension per unit layer (T) for the given systolic afterload (P) largely constant (Laplace's law, T = P × r/w) (excentric hypertrophy). – Selective 'afterload' (arterial pressure) elevations, on the other hand, soon lead to largely proportional w increases, usually at little or no r_i change (concentric hypertrophy). In many pathophysiological situations combinations of excentric and concentric hypertrophy are, however, seen because pre- and afterload increases are then often associated [7]. – The reverse structural cardiac adaptations are seen upon sustained pre- and afterload reductions.

What happens if pre- and afterloads are changed in *opposite* directions? This is illustrated by the cardiac structural adaptation elicited when a pharmacologically induced systemic vasodilatation in hypertension lowers arterial pressure but increases venous return and cardiac output. This hemodynamic situation leads to wall regression in association with a luminal growth of the left ventricle [9], so balanced as to adjust w/r_i both to the reduced arterial pressure and to the increased lumen, again keeping T relatively unchanged. Total heart weight may then remain almost unchanged, at first sight giving the impression that cardiac design may have remained unaltered. However, cardiac *geometry* is, of course, now entirely altered in terms of both r_i and w, adjusting cardiac performance towards an increased stroke volume capacity, but to be delivered at a lowered afterload level. Clearly, measurements of only heart weight cannot reveal such complexities of cardiac structural adaptation.

2. Blood vessels

Sustained elevations of tissue nutritional demands induce a luminal (r_i) outgrowth of the corresponding resistance vessels, increasing maximal blood flow capacity and decreasing resistance at maximal dilatation (Rmin) correspondingly [1, 3]. This is associated with capillary 'sprouting' which increases the density of capillary networks [1, 10], both types of vascular growth being probably caused by local chemical changes. Similarly, upon tissue hypertrophy, as when the remaining kidney increases its mass after unilateral nephrectomy, the renal vascular bed becomes correspondingly enlarged in terms of maximal flow capacity, but maintains the same w/r_i relationships and also the same balance between the pre- and postglomerular resistances, provided that arterial pressure is not altered as well [1, 11]. Thus, at such adaptive r_i increases w also seems to increase somewhat, presumably mainly by means of a secondary media growth whereby w/r_i, and wall tension per unit wall layer (T), are kept well balanced to the regional pressure (P).

When P is elevated at unchanged tissue metabolism w increases, mainly by way of media hypertrophy. This is in the precapillary resistance section associated with some structural r_i reduction, whereby Rmin is raised more or less proportionally to the pressure elevation so that maximal flow capacity remains almost unchanged despite the raised pressure head [1, 2, 3, 4]. In principle, the reverse changes of resistance vessel design occur upon sustained arterial pressure reductions, as shown e.g. for rat hindquarter vessels when aortic obstruction has caused regional hypotension [12]. As the average w/r_i is in this way kept more or less balanced to the prevailing transmural pressure, wall tension per unit wall layer, T, remains largely unchanged (Laplace's law) in the resistance vessels.

Such locally induced 'upward' or 'downward' structural adaptations of the precapillary resistance vessels deserve to be called *'structural autoregulation'*. Thus, like the prompt precapillary smooth muscle adjustments to acute pressure changes ('functional autoregulation'), they serve to maintain regional blood flow and capillary pressure about the same upon pressure alterations, though now by means of an altered vascular design. For the *individual* vascular bed and tissue this rapidly established structural autoregulation is entirely appropriate, as it not only resets the range of functional flow changes to suit sustained arterial pressure alterations, but also offers long-term protection against undue pressure increases for the important capillary exchange section, as exemplified by the cerebral circulation in hypertension [3, 13]. However, when this per se 'normal' local structural response of the resistance vessels afflicts *all* systemic circuits, as in hypertension, it can have dangerous consequences as outlined in section D.

What happens if e.g. a prolonged arterial pressure elevation becomes associated with increased tissue demands? This is, for example, the situation for the coronary and skeletal muscle circuits during prolonged exercise training in hypertensive organisms, and it appears that r_i and w then adapt appropriately to *both* these altered demands [1, 14]. The raised Rmin, consequent to the high-pressure state, then becomes to some extent reduced in the muscle vascular bed, as a long-term response to the exercise-induced local chemical changes. However, w/r_i remains well adapted to the hypertensive state, which must imply some secondary, additional w increase to match the exercise-induced average r_i increase.

Also the walls of the aorta and the major conduit arteries (the 'Windkessel vessels') respond similarly to sustained pressure changes [2, 3, 15], as do the venous capacitance vessels. Concerning the latter type of vessels w and w/r_i are kept closely adapted to the regional transmural pressure levels in the *upright* body position, as seen in human dependent veins [2, 3, 16], even though a good part of each day is spent in the reclining position.

Even though these adaptive growth processes are primarily induced by sustained changes of local pressure and/or chemical environment, they are as mentioned often modified by various extrinsic 'trophic' influences of hormonal or/and nervous (transmitter-cotransmitter) nature. For example, angiotensin and catecholamines seem to facilitate the development of cardiac hypertrophy [13, 17] and the adrenergic nerve activity reinforces vascular media hypertrophy-hyperplasia [2, 3, 13, 18], presumably at least in part by way of trophic effects by the released transmitters-cotransmitters.

D. The systemic resistance vessels in hypertension

1. General aspects

Even before arterial pressure was estimated in man for the first time, more than 100 years ago, it had been observed that heart, arteries and arterioles, though hardly veins, showed thickened walls in hypertension [2, 3, 13]. As, however, little was known either about hemodynamics or about physiology-biophysics of cardiovascular muscle, and because these structural changes were at that time usually thought to represent late, irreversible complications, little or no attention was paid to the possibility that they might be of importance even for the very induction of chronic high-pressure states. Nevertheless, it is surprising that it should take almost another century before it was realized that this type of cardiovascular structural adaptation profoundly affects overall hemodynamics [19] and that it occurs early, sometimes evidently representing even one of the genetically reinforced elements in primary hypertension [1, 2, 19, 20].

To indicate the proper role of the *structural factor* in the multifactorial induction of primary (essential) hypertension, Fig. 2 may be useful, showing three major causative elements which are also more or less interdependent of each other [2, 3]. Here the polygenetically linked predisposition represents the *sine qua non,* where its various cardiovascular expressions are derived from the fact that some macromolecules, like membrane components, enzymes, carriers or transmitters deviate from the average in such a way as to affect overall hemodynamics in some way or other. Even though each of these genetic deviations may well represent per se 'normal' variants rather than genetic 'lesions', they can in certain constellations so affect the cardiovascular system as to cause a gradual pressure elevation. In case heart and vessels had for *other* genetic reasons been able in the long run to 'take' the increased load without harm, as in the giraffe who spends a giraffe's lifespan with an arterial pressure at heart level around 250–300 mm Hg [3], primary hypertension might well have been looked upon as a harmless 'normal' variant, like long feet, a choleric temperament, etc. Unfortunately, however, in most species and individuals chronic high-pressure states do accelerate cardiovascular aging and invite to degenerative-lesional alterations, though also in these respects individuals may differ considerably and presumably in part for genetic reasons.

It has for decades been almost taken for granted that the predisposing genetic elements should express themselves mainly as *functional* changes, but obviously they may as well have mainly *structural* consequences. For example, key enzymatic or membrane links of importance for muscle protein synthesis might be more efficient, so that their actions tend to reinforce the normal process of structural adaptation of cardiovascular muscle cells whenever they are exposed to elevations of functional load [1, 2, 3, 20]. In such a case this process, which basically represents a 'secondary' response, even though it is so rapid as to be largely intertwined with functional excitatory elements [3], would in primary hypertension also be one of the genetically endowed, *truly 'primary' factors* (section D:3).

2. Principal structural changes

Established primary hypertension is well-known to be characterized mainly by the elevated systemic resistance to flow, being the key phenomenon of hemodynamic alteration. It is therefore justified to devote an article like this mainly to the structural changes, and their hemodynamic consequences, for the *systemic resistance vessels* and then mainly for their precapillary section, even though

---

PRIMARY   HYPERTENSION

I. POLYGENETICALLY TRANSFERRED PREDISPOSITION, in man of individually varying
balance; in hypertensive rat
strains uniformized though
differing between strains

II. ENVIRONMENTAL FACTORS, influencing and reinforcing I:

    a. Excitatory psychoemotional influences —— relative importance varies
    b. Increased salt intake   with the balance of I

III. SECONDARY ADJUSTMENTS influencing I + II and very early initiated:

    a. Of reinforcing nature   (introduction of positive feedback)
    b. Of stabilizing nature   Structural adaptation (resetting of negative feedbacks)
    c. Of counteracting nature   (largely unaffected negative feedbacks)

PRINCIPLE: Chronic hypertensive state initiated and maintained by interactions between
I + II + II a, b, where the balance differs between individuals but where III a, b
increasingly dominates, while III c tends to counteract the development. Also III a, b
may sometimes be genetically 'reinforced'.

Figure 2. Outline of principal causative elements in primary hypertension illustrating its multifactorial nature, as well as the relationship of the 'structural factor' (IIIa, b) to other elements. In case the process of structural adaptation of heart and vessels is genetically reinforced (see section D"3), it also forms one of the truly 'primary' elements. (From [2] with kind permission of the Editor of Clin Sci.)

almost all other cardiovascular parts are also structurally altered with often quite important consequences [3, 13]. Far from being any sluggish, late 'complications' in primary hypertension these structural adaptive changes develop, as mentioned, very early and can in rats be almost fully completed in 10 days or so, and in man perhaps in a few months [1, 2, 3]. Actually, morphometric microvascular analyses by Mulvany's group [21] have revealed how considerable w/r_i increases have been developed already after short periods of human preeclampsia hypertension. It follows that the 'structural factor' can certainly *not* be the rate-limiting factor which explains why human (and often rat) primary hypertension usually shows an almost insiduous rate of development.

An increasing amount of hemodynamic as well as morphometric studies of e.g. forearm, hand, calf and renal vascular beds in hypertensive humans are now available, like a great number of more detailed analyses of the hindquarter, coronary, cerebral, renal mesenteric circuits, etc., in the various types of rat strains with primary hypertension, mainly then in the Okamoto-Aoki spontaneously hypertensive rats (SHR) [1, 2, 3, 13]. They all indicate that w and w/r_i are increased and r_i reduced, on an average, in the precapillary resistance vessels, *and* almost always to an extent as to largely balance off the raised arterial pressure. These structural changes prove to be particularly pronounced in the proximal sections and taper off gradually towards the capillary level, presumably because the distal sections are little exposed to any pressure rise thanks to the high upstream resistance [2, 22].

As Rmin, i.e. the resistance to flow at complete smooth muscle relaxation, is in many circuits raised almost in proportion to the rise in pressure, when studied in human primary hypertension during resting conditions, it follows that the ratio between Rr and Rmin is here largely the same as in normotensive individuals [3, 4, 13, 20]. From this fact it follows that there is, indeed, usually *little or no sign* of any raised smooth muscle activity in the resting steady state. Actually, it must often be even *sub*normal, as in the human skeletal muscle vascular bed, because blood flow is here often slightly above that in normotensive controls [3]. Thus, the systemic precapillary resistance vessels are in primary hypertension structurally redesigned to function at a higher pressure range, and can therefore maintain a higher resistance, and pressure, also at normal tonic smooth muscle activity, as schematically illustrated in Fig. 3 when curve H is compared with curve N.

The precapillary resistance vessels are not only somewhat narrowed and more thick-walled but are, as a result of this, also stronger, more 'reactive' and less distensible than normotensive resistance vessels, which is shown by the experimental data in Fig. 4. Here the complex relationships between design, distensibility, transmural pressure and degree of smooth muscle contraction are analysed in terms of their hemodynamic consequences, comparing pair-perfused SHR and WKY hindquarter resistance vessels, under circumstances where possible differences in smooth muscle *sensitivity* were ruled out. This comparison illustrates particularly well how a geometric w/r_i increase leads to '*vascular hyperreactivity*'; i.e., steeper resistance increases ensue from given smooth muscle shortenings, and do so despite the higher distending pressure in SHR. This is clear from the 'resistance response curves' in the right part of Fig. 4, which are directly deduced from the experimental data shown in the left part of this Figure.

Thus, the structural w and w/r_i increases act as a 'structural amplifier' to produce this vascular hyperreactivity [2, 3, 24], and together with the r_i reduction they result in an upward resetting of the entire range of resistance adjustments which may even be widened (cf. Fig. 4, right part). For the individual circuit, and its control, this process is from most points of view entirely appropriate, but it becomes dangerous when generalized to *all* systemic circuits, because a positive feedback interaction is then established between this 'structural amplifier' effect and functional pressor influences, as indicated in Fig. 3. Moreover, a raised systemic resistance can thereby, as mentioned, be maintained *even when tonic vascular smooth muscle activity is entirely normal* – a fact which is certainly disturbing for the common, sometimes almost dogmatic assumption that smooth muscle activity of the resistance vessels 'should' be increased in primary hypertension. However, any closer analysis of the hemodynamic events, occurring when a structural w/r_i increase of the resistance vessels is at hand, shows that resistance *must* be higher for a given smooth muscle activity, compared with normotensive resistance vessels. Neglect of this, after all, fairly simple hemodynamic consequence of a per se 'nomal' structural adaptive process has for decades led hypertensive research astray.

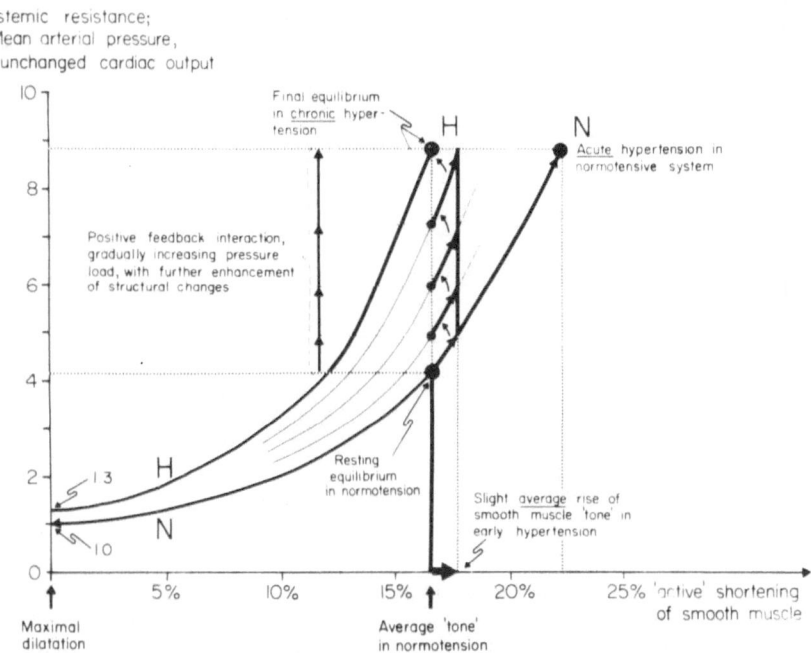

Figure 3. A diagrammatic illustration of the changed relationship between degree of smooth muscle shortening and increase of flow resistance when media hypertrophy increases average wall thickness (w) in association with a structural reduction of inner radius (r_i) in the precapillary resistance vessels; both being local responses to increases of average pressure ('structural autoregulation'). Resistance curve *N* represents normotensive resistance vessels with w/r_i around 0.2 at full relaxation while curve *H* represents the 'structurally autoregulated' vessels in established hypertension, r_i being reduced some 7% and w increased some 35%. Note how any elevation of pressure load, whether caused by marginal increases in average smooth muscle activity and/or in cardiac output, may introduce a *positive feedback interaction* between such functional excitatory influences and the process of structural autoregulation. Thus, both tend to reinforce each other with respect to the pressor effects, causing a gradual transfer towards steeper and steeper resistance curves as the structural adaptation becomes more pronounced. (From [2] with kind permission of the Editor of Clin Sci.)

The fact that arterial pressure does not rise even more rapidly than is commonly the case in primary hypertension, thanks to the presence of the mentioned positive feedback interaction, is presumably due to the influence of some powerful negative feedbacks in the cardiovascular system that are evidently still poorly understood. Actually, the negative feedbacks based on the baro- and volume-receptor reflexes and also that inherent in the renal 'barostat function' [2, 3, 13], seem to be fairly readily reset in hypertension. At least partly this seems to be due to the same type of structural adaptation, by causing a thickening and stiffening of aortic and left cardiac walls while in the renal vascular bed it tends to cause a structurally based increase of the pre/postglomerular resistance ratio [1, 2, 3, 13]. Thereby a higher pressure is needed for giving the same wall deformation and, in

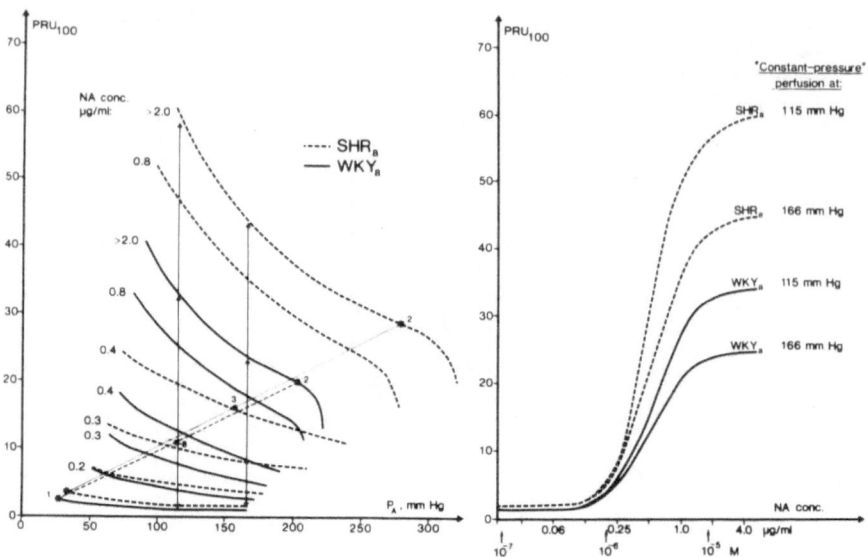

Figure 4. Left panel: Relationships ('resistance lines') between mean arterial distending pressure (P_A) and resistance to flow (PRU units; i.e. mm Hg/flow in ml/min per 100 g tissue) for adult SHR and WKY hindquarter vascular beds. Each of the 'resistance lines' represents a *steady* constriction level, exposed to various distending pressures. The different constriction levels are evenly spread along the entire noradrenaline dose-response curve, as obtained during constant-flow perfusion and ranging from maximal vascular relaxation up to maximal vascular constriction (cf. Fig. 1). When plotted into this diagram these 'resistance curves' are represented by the slanting straight lines with maximal dilatation at '1', maximal constriction at '2' and ED_{50} at '3'. The vertical straight lines represent the mean arterial pressures in vivo of the WKY and SHR groups. – This hemodynamic analysis reveals how the 'structurally autoregulated' SHR resistance vessels are 'hyperreactive', as well as stiffer and stronger than the normotensive WKY ones, when compared at equal levels of smooth muscle activity. *Right panel:* Derived from the intercepts between the vertical pressure lines and the 'resistance lines' in the left panel. By plotting these intercepts the average *'constant-pressure resistance curves'* are also obtained, as they would appear if the SHR and WKY vascular beds had instead been perfused at their respective mean arterial pressures in vivo *and* at equal degrees of increasing smooth muscle activation up to maximal constriction. Note the considerable 'vascular hyperreactivity' in SHR despite the higher arterial distending pressure, a difference that is markedly accentuated if SHR and WKY are instead compared at *equal* pressures. (Modified from [23] with kind permission of the Editor of Acta Physiol Scand.)

the kidneys, for maintaining glomerular filtration even if renal vascular smooth activity should be the same as in normotension. It is not impossible that the renomedullary depressor lipids of Muirhead *et al.* [25, 26], and perhaps also the unmyelinated baroafferents, which seem to be less completely reset in hypertension than the myelinated ones [27, 28], represent increasingly important negative feedbacks as primary hypertension develops and hence serve to counteract the positive feedback influence of the 'structural amplifier'.

Even though some structural wall thickening usually occurs also on the venous 'low-pressure side', it hardly acts here as a significant 'structural amplifier', simply because the w/r_i ratio is here, anyhow, so low as to largely nullify the geometric impact of the increased w. However, the w thickening leads to a *reduced venous compliance,* which, for any level of smooth muscle activity, tends to 'centralize' the normally slightly reduced total blood volume in established primary hypertension with consequences for cardiac diastolic filling as discussed in other chapters of this book and in some of the present references [3, 13, 17].

3. Genetic reinforcement of the structural-adaptive process

As reviewed elsewhere [3, 29] there is increasingly strong evidence that a genetic reinforcement of the 'structural factor' is present in at least some genetic types of primary hypertension (e.g. in SHR and perhaps also in human variants). While no single study provides unequivocal proof, the combined experimental evidence from various approaches lends strong support for this view, and perhaps stronger than for any other mechanism thought to be genetically reinforced in primary hypertension [29].

The following types of studies have been used: (*a*) comparisons of primary and secondary hypertension in rats suggest that the structural adaptation is stronger in primary hypertension for any given pressure level. This may be so also in man, because the line relating mean arterial pressure to Rmin in primary hypertension is placed modestly above that for normotension-secondary hypertension [19, 20], as shown in Fig. 5; (*b*) in early SHR, and perhaps also in early human primary hypertension, the structural cardiovascular changes may even *precede* the pressure elevation, according to several studies [29]; (*c*) it usually seems to be more difficult to prevent structural cardiovascular changes, or to cause regression if already established, in primary hypertension by pharmacological antihypertensive treatment when compared with secondary hypertension [29]; finally (*d*), tissue culture growth of vascular smooth muscle is more pronounced in SHR than in WKY, also when in the same medium. Thus, some 'intrinsic' smooth muscle characteristic, like some key enzyme involved in protein synthesis and/or some membrane transport mechanism, might be genetically 'reinforced' in SHR [30]. In addition, catecholamines further reinforce growth [29, 31], and sympathetic activity seems to be genetically increased in SHR, and evidently also in man in some common variants [3]. Thus, such findings suggest that genetically linked influences that are both 'intrinsic' and 'extrinsic' to cardiovascular muscle cells might reinforce their growth, at least in SHR. When taken together, such in vivo and in vitro findings strongly suggest that the process of cardiovascular structural adaptation may be in various ways genetically reinforced, both in man and in rats.

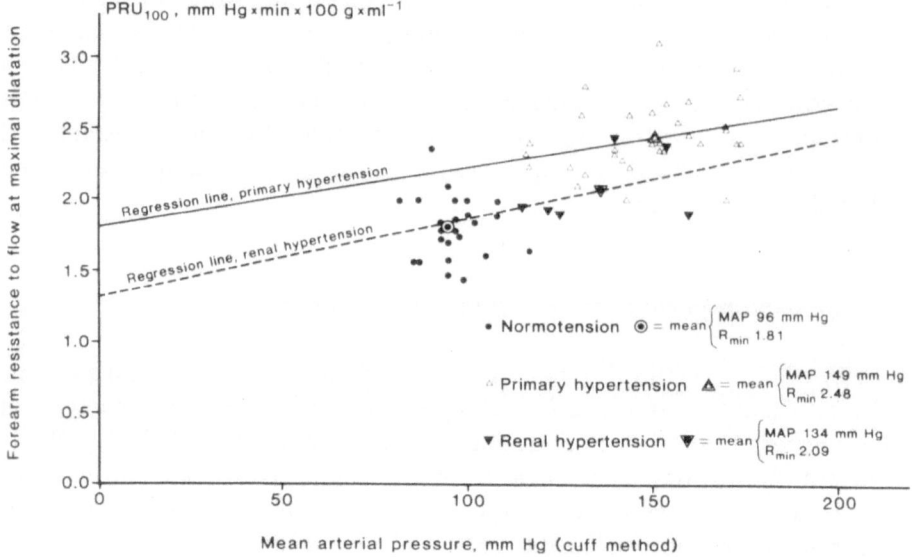

Figure 5. Relationship between mean arterial pressure and flow resistance in human forearm vascular beds at maximal vasodilatation (Rmin; given as PRU units). Three groups of subjects are studied: Normotensives, patients with primary hypertension and a small group of patients with secondary renal hypertension. Note how the controls form a homogeneous group, while Rmin increases with the MAP elevation in the hypertensive groups, where the regression line for the group of primary hypertensives is placed *above* that for secondary hypertension and *above* the mean value for the normotensive controls. This may reflect some genetic reinforcement of the 'normal' process of structural cardiovascular adaptation in human primary hypertension. (Modified from [19, 20].)

4. Therapeutic regression of structural cardiovascular adaptation

It has already been mentioned that reduced load causes regression of wall thickness and somewhat increases r_i in the resistance vessels. For example, regional hypotension [12], or reversal of shortlasting renal hypertension in rats [13, 32] lead to such changes, and this regression can be fully completed in a few weeks. However, the more longlasting the hypertensive state, the slower and less complete the regression [13, 33]. Further, it is, as mentioned, more difficult to induce structural regression in e.g. SHR primary hypertension than in genetically normotensive rats with induced secondary hypertension [29].

It is further important to realize that acute pharmacological normalization of arterial pressure in chronic hypertension implies that a *sub*normal smooth muscle and/or cardiac activity is imposed on a cardiovascular system that is structurally adapted for operation at higher pressure [3, 13, 34]. As a result most control mechanisms are also reset, and consequently tend to *counteract* the pharmacological pressure lowering, which greatly contributes to the disturbing side-effects experienced when too rapid and extensive pressure reductions are attempted in man.

For such reasons structural regression can be expected to occur only gradually in man, being slower and less complete the less pronounced the pharmacological pressure reduction, the longer the high-pressure state has lasted, and/or the more genetically reinforced the 'structural factor' happens to be. It should then be remembered that a true hemodynamic normalization is possible only when a largely complete regression is at hand [13, 34] and still the genetic reinforcing elements always remain in the background in primary hypertension and tend to raise the pressure level again. These circumstances have recently been interestingly illustrated in experimental studies on human primary hypertension by Korner et al. [35].

References

1. Folkow B (1983): 'Structural autoregulation' – the local adaptation of vascular beds to chronic changes in pressure. In Development of the vascular system. Ciba Foundation Symp. London: Pitman Books 100: 56–79.

2. Folkow B (1978): The Fourth Volhard Lecture. Cardiovascular structural adaptation; its role in the initiation and maintenance of primary hypertension. Clin Sci Mol Med 55: 3s–22s.

3. Folkow B (1982): Physiological aspects of primary hypertension. Physiol Rev 62: 347–504.

4. Sivertsson R (1970): The hemodynamic importance of structural vascular changes in essential hypertension. Acta Physiol Scand, Suppl. 343: 1–56.

5. Folkow B, Hallbäck M, Lundgren Y, Weiss L (1970): Background of increased flow resistance and vascular reactivity in spontaneously hypertensive rats. Acta Physiol Scand 80: 93–106.

6. Folkow B, Hallbäck M, Jones JV, Sutter M (1977): Dependence on external calcium for the noradrenaline contractility of the resistance vessels in spontaneously hypertensive and renal hypertensive rats, as compared with normotensive controls. Acta Physiol Scand 101: 84–97.

7. Mirsky I (1979): Elastic properties of the myocardium: a quantitative approach with physiological and clinical applications. In Handbook of Physiology, Chapter 14, section 2, vol 1: 497–531.

8. Friberg P, Folkow B, Nordlander M (1985): Structural adaptation of the rat left ventricle in response to changes in pressure and volume loads. Acta Physiol Scand 125: 67–79.

9. Friberg P, Folkow B, Nordlander M (1986): Cardiac dimensions in spontaneously hypertensive rats following different modes of blood pressure reduction by antihypertensive treatment. J Hypertension 4: 165–173.

10. Myrhage R, Hudlicka O (1978): Capillary growth in chronically stimulated adult skeletal muscle. Microvasc Res 16: 73–90.

11. Göthberg G, Hallbäck-Nordlander M, Karlström G, Ricksten S-E, Folkow B (1983): Structurally based changes of renal vascular reactivity in spontaneously hypertensive and two-kidney, one-clip renal hypertensive rats, as compared with kidneys from uninephrectomized and intact normotensive rats. Acta Physiol Scand 118: 61–67.

12. Folkow B, Gurévich M, Hallbäck M, Lundgren Y, Weiss L (1971): The hemodynamic consequences of regional hypotension in spontaneously hypertensive and normotensive rats. Acta Physiol Scand 83: 532–541.

13. Folkow B, Nordlander M, Strauer B-E, Wikstrand J (eds) (1984): Pathophysiology and clinical implications of early structural changes. Hypertension 6, Suppl. III: III-1–III-187.

14. Weiss L (1978): Adaptive cardiovascular changes to physical training in spontaneously hyperten-

sive and normotensive rats. Cardiovasc Res 12, no 6: 329–333.

15. Safar ME, Simon AC, Levenson JA (1984): Structural changes of large arteries in sustained essential hypertension. Hypertension 6, Suppl. III: III-117–III-121.
16. Kügelgen A von (1955): Uber das Verhältnis von Ringmuskulatur und Innendruck in menschlichen grossen Venen. Z Zellforsch Mitrosk Anat 43: 168–183.
17. Tarazi RC (1982): The role of the heart in hypertension. Clin Sci 63, Suppl 8: 347s–358s.
18. Bevan RD (1984): Trophic effects of peripheral adrenergic nerves on vascular structure. Hypertension 6, Suppl. III: III-119–III-126.
19. Folkow B (1956): Structural, myogenic, humoral and nervous factors controlling peripheral resistance. In Hypotensive Drugs, edited by Harington M, London: Pergamon, pp 163–174.
20. Folkow B, Grimby G, Thulesius O (1958): Adaptive stuctural changes of the vascular walls in hypertension and their relation to the control of the peripheral resistance. Acta Physiol Scand 44: 255–272.
21. Aalkjaer C, Danielsen H, Johannesen P, Pedersen EB, Rasmussen A, Mulvany MJ (1985): Abnormal vascular function and morphology in preeclampsia: a study of isolated resistance vessels. Clin Sci 69: 477–482.
22. Folkow B (1979): Relationships between vessel design and hemodynamics along the precapillary resistance compartment in normo- and hypertension. Blood Vessels 16: 277–280.
23. Folkow B, Karlström G (1984): Age- and pressure-dependent changes of systemic resistance vessels concerning the relationships between geometric design, wall distensibility, vascular reactivity and smooth muscle sensitivity. Acta Physiol Scand 122: 17–33.
24. Korner PI (1982): The Sixth Volhard Lecture. Causal and homeostatic factors in hypertension. Clin Sci 63: 5s–26s.
25. Muirhead EE, Pitcock JA, Nasjletti A, Brown P, Brooks B (1985): The antihypertensive function of the kidney. Its elucidaion by captopril plus unclipping. Hypertension 7, Suppl I: I-127–I-135.
26. Masugi F, Ogihara T, Saeki S, Otsuka A, Kumahara Y (1985): Role of acetyl glyceryl ether phosphorylcholine in blood pressure regulation in rats. Hypertension 7: 742–746.
27. Jones JV, Thorén PN (1977): Characteristics of aortic baroreceptors with non-medullated afferents arising from the aortic arch of rabbits with chronic renovascular hypertension. Acta Physiol Scand 101: 286–293.
28. Thorén P, Andresen MC, Brown AM (1983): Resetting of aortic baroreceptors with non-myelinated afferent fibres in spontaneously hypertensive rats. Acta Physiol Scand 117: 91–97.
29. Folkow B (1986): The structural cardiovascular factor in primary hypertension – pressure dependence and genetic reinforcement. J Hypertension 4 (Suppl. 3): S51–S56.
30. Kanbe T, Nara Y, Tagami M, Yamori Y (1983): Studies of hypertension-induced vascular hypertrophy in cultured smooth muscle cells from spontaneously hypertensive rats. Hypertension 5: 887–892.
31. Yamori Y, Igawa T, Tagami M, Kanbe T, Nara Y, Kihara M, Horie R (1984): Humoral trophic influence on cardiovascular structural changes in hypertension. Hypertension 6, Suppl III: III-27–III-32.
32. Lundgren Y, Hallbäck M, Weiss L, Folkow B (1974): Rate and extent of adaptive cardiovascuar changes in rats during experimental renal hypertension. Acta Physiol Scand 91: 103–115.
33. Lundgren Y, Weiss L (1979): Cardiovascular design after 'reversal' of longstanding renal hypertension in rats. Clin Sci 57: 19–21.
34. Folkow B (1985): Vascular changes in hypertension. Therapeutic implications. Drugs 29, Suppl 2: 1–8.
35. Korner PI, Jennings GL, Esler MD (1986): Pathogenesis of human primary hypertension: a new approach to the identification of causal factors and to therapy. J Hypertension 4 (Suppl. 3): S149–S154).

Baroreflex mechanisms and the high pressure system in hypertension

EDUARDO KRIEGER

Introduction

The most important mechanism for maintaining the blood pressure stable within a narrow range under different physiological conditions is the baroreceptor reflex. It is activated by the carotid and aortic baroreceptors and regulates heart rate, myocardial contractility, cardiac output, regional vasoactivity and blood flow distribution. However, this mechanism cannot counteract a permanent increase in pressure because the baroreceptors automatically reset to operate at the new hypertensive level exhibited by the individual. The development of resetting during permanent change in blood pressure and the mechanisms involved in the resetting process will be discussed in this chapter. Major emphasis will be placed on resetting itself, and this review will not cover the sensitivity of the baroreceptor reflex and its implications in the pathogenesis of hypertension [1, 2] nor the 'central resetting', responsible for the set point of the baroreceptor reflex [3].

1. Resetting in chronic hypertension

Evidence that the baroreceptors are able to respond to further excitation in addition to that caused by the existing hypertension was provided by Kezdi and Hilker [4] in experiments with hypertensive patients and by Matton [5] in renal hypertensive dogs, by local injection of norepinephrine into the adventia of the carotid sinuses. However, the first demonstration that the carotid and aortic baroreceptors indeed are reset in chronic hypertension was reported by McCubbin, Green and Page [6] who used electroneurographic techniques to record the baroreceptor activity in renal hypertensive dogs. Additional evidence for the displacement of the pressure threshold and pressure range for baroreceptor activation in hypertension has been obtained in experiments using chronic hypertensive rats [7], chronic renal hypertensive rabbits [8] and SHR [9]. Therefore, resetting of the baroreceptors in chronic hypertensives is well documented and is now a universally accepted phenomenon [for references see 1, 10, 11]. However, it is yet not clear how rapid and how complete the process of resetting is during the development of sustained hypertension nor what are the exact mechanisms of resetting in acute or chronic hypertension.

2. Acute resetting of the baroreceptors

The concept that the resetting of the baroreceptors lags behind the pressure rise was already stressed in 1956 by McCubbin, Green and Page [6]. Accordingly when the time required for complete resetting of the baroreceptors to a new level of hypertension is analysed, the time for the blood pressure to reach this level must be considered. If the hypertensives stimuli are applied progressively, rather than in a single step, the process would be expected to be completed only after the hypertension has attained a stable level. Using the technique of subdiaphragmatic aortic constriction which produces in the rat an immediate and maintained hypertension in the upper half of the body, where the aortic baroreceptors are located, a partial resetting of 39% (percent increase of baroreceptor pressure threshold over the total increase in pressure) was observed after 6 hours of hypertension [11, 12]. When the time course for complete resetting in hypotension was studied in rats, a partial resetting of 21% was observed even after 15 minutes [11, 13]. More recently the acute or rapid resetting observed after a short-lasting change in pressure (hypo- or hypertension) was studied in detail.

Maximal resetting is usually observed as rapidly as 5 to 15 minutes after the pressure alteration is initiated and it remains stable for the first hours with no change in the baroreceptor gain. However, the acute resetting is incomplete because the displacement of the pressure threshold for baroreceptor activation is only a fraction of the total change produced in arterial pressure. The extent of acute resetting was described as 28, 40 and 23%, respectively, in dogs [14], rabbits [15] and rats [16]. The detailed mechanism of acute resetting has not yet been established. It has been attributed to viscoelastic relaxation or 'creep' of the arterial wall [17], to ionic alteration [18] or to a change in the receptor ending itself [19]. Thus, there is a rapid or acute resetting that develops within the first 5 to 15 minutes of hypertension and changes little within the first few hours. Acute resetting is partial and only becomes complete if the pressure change is held permanently.

3. Complete resetting of the baroreceptor

The full range of aortic baroreceptor activation, from threshold to maximum discharge, can be demonstrated in the rat when the whole-nerve activity is recorded during rapid (10–15 seconds) changes in pressure produced by bleeding and reinjection of blood. The best single index for monitoring the process of resetting during hypertension is the relationship of the systolic threshold pressure (SPth) that initiates baroreceptor firing and the control diastolic pressure (CDP) measured in freely moving rats, before the animals are anesthetized to record baroreceptor activity. As shown in Fig. 1 there is an exact coincidence between the SPth and CDP in the control normotensive rats. Six hours after the onset of hypertension produced by subdiaphragmatic aortic constriction, a partial resetting of the baroreceptors of 39% (percent change of SPth over total CDP) was observed. The extent of the average resetting was 57% after 24 hours and 88% after 2 days of hypertension, when 9 out of the 10 rats studied had complete resetting (the average resetting would be 100% if all rats had exhibited complete resetting). Therefore, for the majority of rats, complete resetting of the aortic baroreceptors occurred within the first 2 days after the pressure had been permanently elevated. The reflex bradycardia observed during the development of hypertension in the same model (aortic constriction) also takes 2 days to normalize [20], thus providing indirect confirmation of the time-course taken by the baroreceptors to complete the resetting process. Moreover, resetting is permanent since after 2 months of renal hypertension [21] SPth was similar to the CDP (149 ± 4 vs 141 ± 5 mm/Hg). The sequence of baroreceptor resetting in hypotension in rats [11, 13] was quite similar to that observed in hypertension: a partial resetting within the first 6 hours (44% in hypotension vs 39% in hypertension) and complete resetting within the first 2 days. Thus, resetting of the baroreceptors occurs whenever there is a permanent change in arterial pressure to hypertensive or to hypotensive levels and the process is completed in approximately 2 days as shown in rat aortic baroreceptors studies [10, 11].

4. Reversibility of the baroreceptor resetting

The resetting process compromises the efficiency of the baroreceptors to counteract any mechanism trying to elevate blood pressure permanently. On the other hand, resetting can be considered to be helpful because it enables the baroreceptors to function very effectively in regulating blood pressure within a narrow range, independently of the pressure permanently exhibited by the individual. However, the effectiveness of the baroreceptor reflex would be very limited if the resetting process were not reversible. Indeed reversal of baroreceptor resetting from hypertension and hypotension was demonstrated, and shown to be a faster process than that of complete resetting itself (approximately 6 hours versus 2 days). As shown in Fig. 2, for rats with chronic renal hypertension of 2 months duration, the complete (100%) reversal of the resetting to normal was observed within 6 hours after the normalization of the arterial pressure [21]. A partial reversal of 46% was already demonstrable 1 hour after removing the clip from the

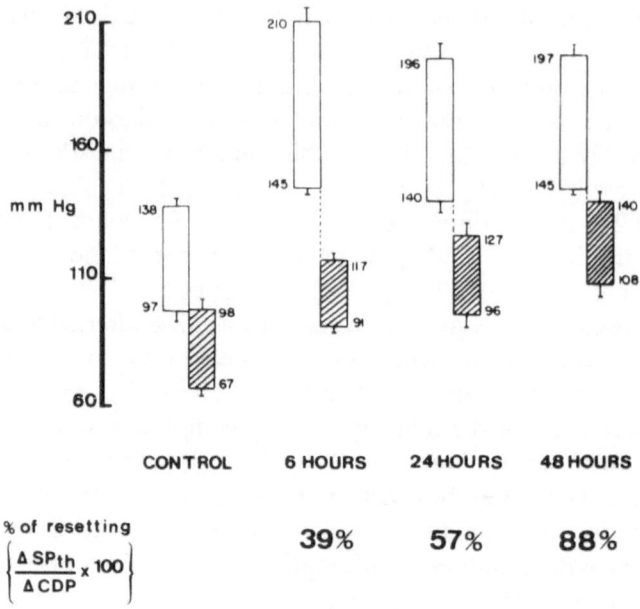

Figure 1. Time course for complete resetting of the aortic baroreceptors during the development of a sustained hypertension produced by subdiaphragmatic aortic constriction in rats. The extent of the resetting process was calculated as the percent change of systolic threshold pressure (SPth from shaded bars) over the total change of control diastolic pressure (CDP from open bars), studied in different groups of rats (n = 10) 6, 24 and 48 hours after onset of hypertension. After 48 hours the average resetting was 88% when 9 of the 10 rats showed complete resetting. (Adapted from Krieger [12] by permission of the American Journal of Physiology.)

renal artery of the rats. The reversal of baroreceptor resetting from hypotension is also a much more rapid process than the resetting to hypotension [22].

5. Mechanisms of complete resetting

The mechanism responsible for resetting of the baroreceptors in chronic hypertension is not yet clear. Apparently resetting is not caused by selective destruction of low threshold receptors, and it can develop in the absence of reduced arterial wall distensibility [for reference see 10, 11]. The structural relationship between wall deformation and deformation of the receptors seems to play an important role in baroreceptor activation. As shown by Brown's group in a series of experiments using an vitro aortic arch-aortic nerve preparation, the baroreceptor sensitivity to strain somehow tries to compensate for alterations in the mechanical properties of the vessel produced by hypertension and growth, in order to maintain normal baroreceptor function [23–26]. However, it is suprising that only a few studies provide the information really necessary to evaluate the alternations

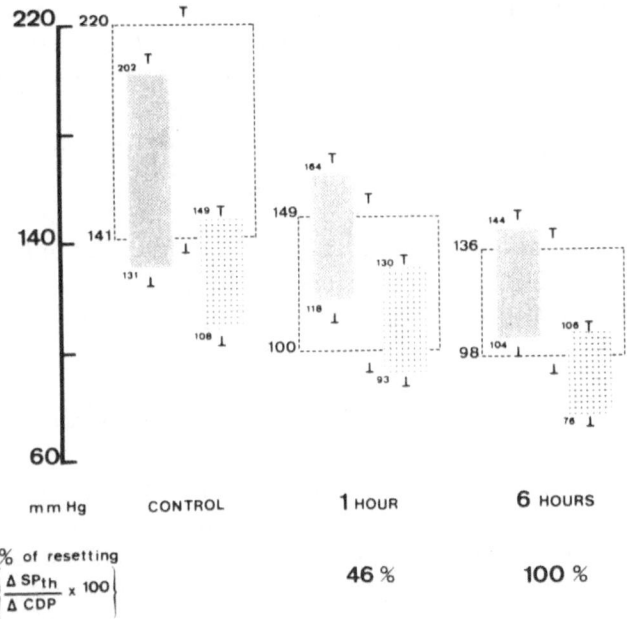

Figure 2. Downward displacement in the range of aortic baroreceptor activation indicates the reversal of the resetting following 1 and 6 hours of pressure normalization in rats with chronic renal hypertension of 2 months duration. The interrupted rectangles indicate the pressure exhibited by the 13 rats: the control pressure was measured in the conscious state and the pressure 1 and 6 hours after unclipping was measured under pentobarbital anesthesia during the session to record the baroreceptor activity. The extent of the resetting was calculated as the percent change of systolic threshold pressure (SPth from reticulated bars) over the total change of control diastolic pressure (CDP from the interrupted rectangles). The pressures necessary to produce 'normal' firing are indicated by shaded bars. (From Salgado and Krieger [21] modified with permission of Clinical Science.)

in the degree of stretch produced in the arterial wall by the pulse pressure in intact hypertensive animals. Also, little information is available to correlate the sequence followed by the resetting during the development of hypertension and the actual alterations produced by the increased pressure on the caliber and pulsation of the arteries, where baroreceptors are located.

5.1 Sequence of aortic changes in hypertension

The development of an electrolytic strain gauge of high sensitivity and stability permits the continuous measurement of the circumference of the aorta in freely moving rats for up to 20 days [27]. The device was used to analyse the changes in aortic caliber of conscious rats during onset and development of hypertensive produced by subdiaphragmatic aortic constriction, the same model of hypertension in which the sequence of resetting was studied. While the increase in pressure was immediate and remained constant after aortic constriction, the mean aortic dilated gradually: 1.2, 3.4, and 6.8% after 6, 24 and 48 hours respectively (Fig. 3). No further dilation was observed for up to 5 days of hypertension. It is remarkable that the time-course for the aortic caliber to achieve maximal dilation during onset and maintenance of hypertension closely coincides with the time taken by the baroreceptors to complete the resetting process. Analysis of the data of individual animals further emphasizes the temporal relationship between the two phenomena. Whereas complete resetting was observed in 1 of 10, 5 of 10 and 9 of 10 rats [12], maximal dilation was observed in 1 of 10, 2 of 10 and 9 of 10 rats studied [28, 29] 6, 24 and 48 hours after the onset of hypertension.

5.2 Diastolic caliber versus pulsation changes in hypertension

As shown in Fig. 3, during the development of hypertension the aortic pulsation increases (60, 90 and 100% after 6, 24 and 48 hours, respectively) but changes less from 6 to 48 hours than the mean aortic caliber, which exhibited a gradual dilation (1.2, 3.4 and 6.8% after 6, 24 and 48 hours, respectively). When the absolute values of systolic and diastolic calibers are considered it can be seen (Fig. 4) that of the total displacement of 6.8% of the mean aortic caliber (0.457 mm) the diastolic caliber accounted for 95%, whereas the increase in pulsation, which was double that of the control period, accounted for only 5%. The small dilation observed after 6 hours of hypertension was also achieved mainly by the permanent displacement of the resting diastolic caliber (83%). Therefore, there is a striking parallelism between the time for complete resetting of the aortic baroreceptors and the time required for the diastolic caliber to achieve a new resting position. In the new state of equilibrium the sustained diastolic pressure no longer stimulates the receptors which are distorted only when the resting caliber is again momentarily increased by the pulse pressure.

5.3 Transient changes in aortic calibers

The changes in diastolic caliber assume a major role not only during development of a sustained hypertension but also during transient increases in pressure. The diastolic caliber displacement, rather than the increase in aortic pulsation, accounts for most of the change observed in the mean aortic caliber [30]. As shown in Fig. 5 a 40 mm Hg increase in pressure produces increases of only 19% and 20%, respectively, in the pulsation of normotensive and hypertensive rats, whereas the increase in diastolic caliber accounts for 81% and 80%, respectively, of the total differences in systolic caliber. The predominance of diastolic caliber changes over the pulsation changes is also observed when sudden pressure alterations are produced in conscious rats in a pressure range of −40 to +40

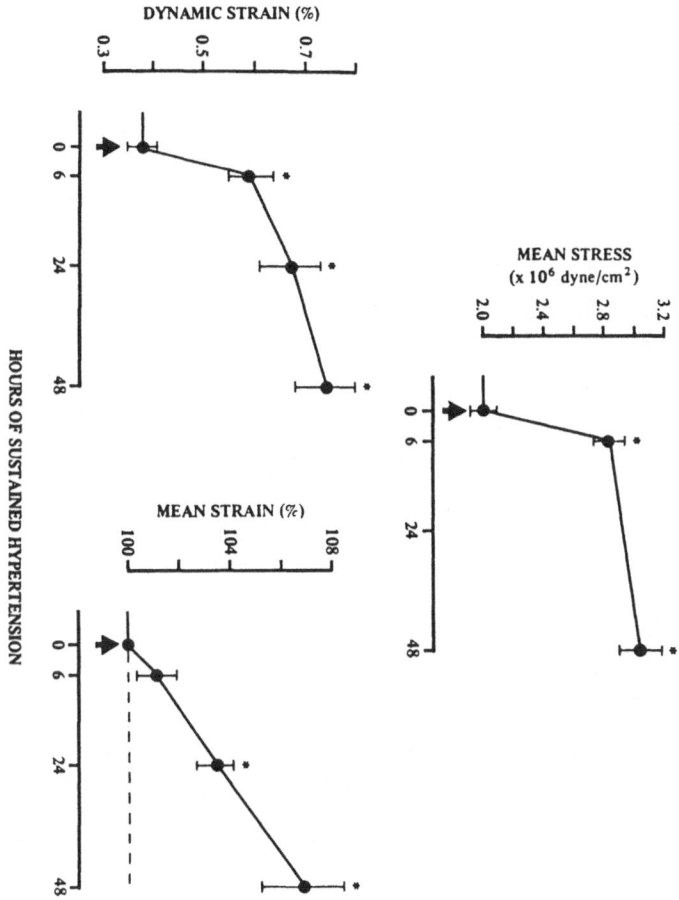

Figure 3. Sequence of aortic pulsation and mean aortic caliber changes during the development of a sustained hypertension (subdiaphragmatic aortic constriction) in rats. Pulsation is expressed as dynamic strain (pulsation over diastolic caliber ×100) and mean caliber as mean strain (percent change of mean caliber over the control mean caliber). The dynamic strain increases 60, 90 and 100% after 6, 24 and 48 hours of onset of hypertension, whereas the mean caliber increases more gradually: 1.2, 3.4 and 6.8%, respectively. (From Michelini and Krieger [28], with permission of the American Journal of Physiology.)

mm Hg [30]. Therefore, the sustained distension of the diastolic caliber rather than vessel pulsation is the major determinant of baroreceptor distortion during rapid changes in pressure.

5.4 Percent change of diastolic caliber

As shown in Fig. 6 (upper panel B) aortic pulsation of chronic hypertensive rats is

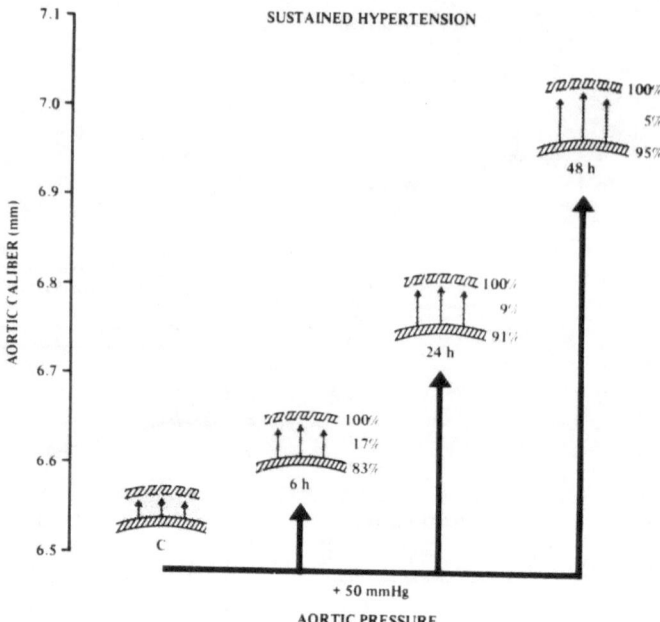

Figure 4. Sequential increase of aortic pulsation and resting diastolic caliber during the development of hypertension produced by subdiaphragmatic aortic constriction in rats. The doubled pulsation observed after 48 hours of hypertension accounted for only 5% of the total dilation of the systolic caliber (0.457 mm), the displacement of the resting diastolic caliber (95%) being the most important factor. (Adapted from Michelini and Kreiger [28] with permission of the American Journal of Physiology.)

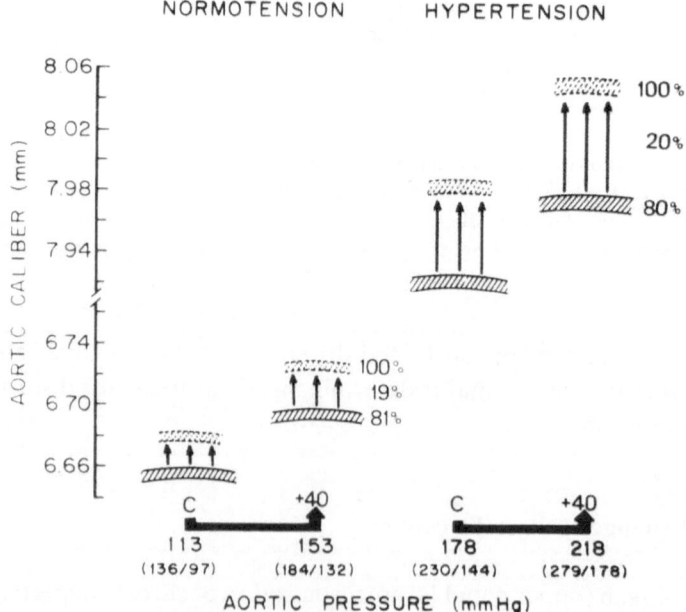

45

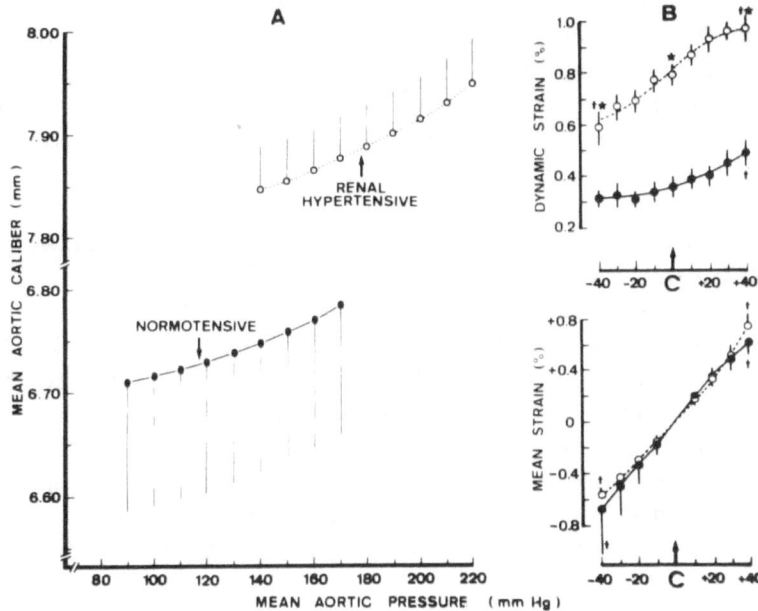

Figure 6. Aortic behavior during sudden pressure changes (−40 to +40 mm Hg) of normotensive and renal hypertensive rats. A. Actual values of mean aortic caliber at different pressures. B. Dynamic strain calculated as percent of the pulsation over the control diastolic caliber and mean as the percent change of the mean caliber over the control mean caliber. Note that the mean strain during transient pressure changes remains constant in spite of the fact that the aorta of hypertensive rats was 20% larger (adapted from Michelini and Krieger [30] with permission of Hypertension).

larger and increases more in response to transient pressure elevation than that of the normotensive rats. However, the mean strain (percent displacement of mean caliber over control caliber) behaved exactly the same as in the normotensive rats, because in hypertension the aorta had a larger response to pressure which was proportional to the larger caliber (Fig. 6, lower panel b). This means that the ratio of diastolic displacement (which accounted for more than 80% of the mean aortic displacement) remained unchanged during rapid pressure change in hypertensive rats, in spite of the 20% dilation of the vessel. More recently it was also shown in rats that developed from 3 to 21 months of age and which had large increase in aortic caliber [31], that the percent change in the diastolic caliber in relation to control caliber remained essentially the same when the rats were

◄——

Figure 5. Relative increase in aortic pulsation and aortic diastolic caliber during a 40 mm Hg transient increase in pressure observed in normotensive and chronic renal hypertensive rats. From the total increase in the systolic caliber (100%) the relative (percentage) contribution of the diastolic caliber is much greater than that of aortic pulsation (indicated by arrows) for both normotensive and hypertensive rats (adapted from Michelini and Krieger [30] with permission of Hypertension).

submitted to rapid and progressive changes in pressure of -40 to $+40$ mm Hg (Sumitami, Michelini and Krieger, unpublished results). Therefore, the aortas of different calibers, produced by aging or hypertension, have a common characteristic when studied in freely moving rats: i.e. the percent change of the resting diastolic caliber during transient pressure changes remained relatively constant. Since the change of the diastolic caliber, rather than aortic pulsation, is the major determinant of the distortion of the aortic baroreceptors during rapid pressure changes, the fact that the percent change of the resting diastolic caliber remained relatively constant seems to be relevant for explaining the process of resetting. Because the absolute strain of the aortic wall produced by the pulse pressure in freely moving rats is increased during growth and chronic hypertension, (also the absolute displacement of the diastolic caliber during rapid pressure changes is greater in these animals) a decreased sensitivity of the baroreceptors to strain should be postulated to explain the normal excitation of the baroreceptors under these circumstances. With the use of an in vitro aortic arc-aortic preparation the increased distensibility of the aorta of rats during growth was shown to be matched by a proportional decrease in the strain sensitivity of the baroreceptors [23–26].

Concluding comments

1. During development of sustained hypertension there is a rapid or acute resetting of the baroreceptors which attains a maximum within the first 5–15 minutes and changes little within the first few hours. It is only a partial resetting because the pressure threshold for baroreceptor activation increases approximately 40% of the total pressure increase. For complete resetting, when the increase in pressure threshold matches the increase in pressure, hypertension must be sustained for a longer time. In the rat complete resetting usually occurs within the first 2 days after the pressure has been permanently elevated.

2. The time course for complete resetting of the aortic baroreceptors in hypertension closely parallels the time taken by the aorta to achieve maximal dilation, when the resting diastolic caliber attains a new operational level. Even when pulsation is doubled, it is the displacement of the diastolic caliber which accounts for 95% of the total aortic dilation. At the new state of equilibrium the increased diastolic caliber compensates for the increased stress and the baroreceptors again are only stimulated by the pulse pressure and not by the increased diastolic pressure.

3. The large increase in aortic caliber observed in freely moving rats during growth or chronic renal hypertension is caused primarily by the permanent displacement of the resting diastolic caliber and to a much less extent by the increase in aortic pulsation (even when pulsation can be twice the values seen in normotensive or younger rats).

4. The aortas of increased caliber produced by growth or chronic hypertension maintain a common behavior: the relative change of the diastolic caliber, in relation to control caliber, remains relatively constant during transient pressure changes (-40 to $+40$ mm Hg) produced in freely moving rats. This fact may be important for the process of resetting since the sustained distension of the resting diastolic caliber (which accounts for approximately 80% of the total systolic caliber displacement), rather than aortic pulsation, should be considered to be the major determinant for baroreceptor distortion during transient pressure changes. Therefore, the normal function of the baroreceptors in aortas of different calibers suggests that the receptors also participate in the adaptive process within the arterial wall.

5. Two findings derived from electroneuro-graphic studies of aortic baroreceptors in rats emphasize that complete resetting is somehow related to achievement of a new operational level for the resting diastolic caliber. First, the lowest systolic pressure threshold for activation of the aortic baroreceptors is the same as the control diastolic pressure, suggesting that below resting diastolic caliber, strain of the aortic wall is not effective to stimulate the receptors in intact rats. Second, whenever pressure is permanently changed to hyper- or hypotensive levels, complete resetting occurs when the baroreceptors again begin to fire at a systolic pressure threshold similar to the new control diastolic pressure.

Acknowledgments

The experiments were supported by grants from FINEP (Financiadora de Estudos e Projetos, FAPESP (Fundação de Amparo à Pesquisa do Estado de São Paulo) and CNP_q (Conselho Nacional de Desenvolvimento Científico e Technológico). The experiments were performed with the technical assistance of Mr. Edson Dias Moreira.

References

1. Ferrario CM, Takeshita S (1983): Baroreceptor reflexes and hypertension. In: Genest J, Kuchel O, Hamet P, Cantin M (eds.) Hypertension – Physiopathology and Treatment. Montreal: McGrow-Hill Book Company, 161–170.
2. Brody MJ, Barron KW, Berecek KH, Faber JE, Lappe RW (1983): Nervous system and hypertension. In: Genest J, Kuchel O, Hamet P and Cantin M (eds.) Hypertension – Physiopathology and Treatment. Montreal: McGrow-Hill Book Company, 117–140.
3. Korner PI (1979): Central nervous control and autonomic cardiovascular function. In: Berne RM (ed.) Handbook of Physiology, Section 2, The Cardiovascular System, Vol. I, pp. 691–739. American Phisiological Society, Bethesda, Maryland.
4. Kezdi P, Hilker RRJ (1955): Local application of epinephrine to carotid sinus. Arch Int Med 95: 720–726.
5. Matton G (1954): Carotid sinus and neurogenic and renal hypertension. J Physiol (Lond.) 126: 13P–14P.

48

6. McCubbin JW, Green JH, Page IH (1956): Baroreceptor function in chronic renal hypertension. Circ Res 4: 205–210.
7. Krieger EM, Marseillan RF (1966): Neural control in experimental hypertension: The role of baroreceptors and splanchnic fibers. Acta Physiol Lat Am 16: 343–352.
8. Aars H (1968): Aortic baroreceptor activity in normal and hypertensive rabbits. Acta Physiol Scand 72: 298–309.
9. Nosaka S, Okamoto K (1970): Modified characteristics of the aortic baroreceptor activities in the spontaneously hypertensive rat. Jpn Circ J 34: 685–693.
10. Krieger EM, Salgado HC, Michelini LC (1982): Resetting of the baroreceptors. In: Guyton AC, Hall JE (eds.) Cardiovascular physiology IV (International review of physiology, Vol. 26). Baltimore: University Park Press. pp. 119–146.
11. Krieger EM (1986): Neurogenic mechanism in hypertension: Resetting of the baroreceptors. Hypertension 8 (Suppl I): I-7–I-14.
12. Krieger EM (1970): Time course of baroreceptor resetting in acute hypertension. Am J Physiol 218: 486–490.
13. Salgado HC, Krieger EM (1978): Time course of baroreceptor resetting in short-term hypotension in the rat. Am J Physiol 234: H552–H556.
14. Coleridge HM, Coleridge JCG, Kaufman MP, Dangel A (1981): Operational sensitivity and acute resetting of aortic baroreceptors in dogs. Circ Res 48: 676–684.
15. Dorward PK, Andresen MC, Burke SL, Oliver JR, Korner PI (1982): Rapid resetting of the aortic baroreceptors in the rabbit and its implications for short-term and longer-term reflex control. Circ Res 50: 428–439.
16. Munch PA, Andersen MC, Brown AM (1983): Rapid resetting of aortic baroreceptors in vitro. Am J Physiol 244: H672–H680.
17. Coleridge HM, Coleridge JCG, Poore ER, Roberts AM, Schultz HD (1984): Aortic wall properties and baroreceptor behaviour at normal arterial pressure and in acute hypertensive resetting in dogs. J Physiol Lond 350: 309–326.
18. Heesch CM, Abboud FM, Thames MD (1984): Acute resetting of carotid sinus baroreceptors: II Possible involvement of electrogenic Na^+ pump. Am J Physiol 247: H833–H839.
19. Munch PA, Brown AM (1985): Role of vessel wall in acute resetting of aortic baroreceptors. Am J Physiol 248 (Heart Circ Physiol 17): H843–H852.
20. Soato GG, Krieger EM (1974): Heart rats after acute hypertension in the rat. Am J Physiol 227: 1389–1393.
21. Salgado HC, Krieger EM (1973): Reversibility of baroreceptor adaptation in chronic hypertension. Clin Sci Mol Med 45: 123s–126s.
22. Salgado HC, Krieger EM (1981): Barorecepor resetting during pressure recovery from hypotension. Hypertension 3 (Suppl II): II-151–II-154.
23. Andresen MC, Krauhs JM, Brown AM (1978): Relationship of aortic wall and baroreceptors properties during development in normotensive and spontaneously hypertensive rats. Circ Res 43: 728–738.
24. Andresen MC, Kuraoka S, Brown AM (1980): Baroreceptor function and changes in strain sensitivity in normontensive and spontaneously hypertensive rats. Circ Res 47: 821–828.
25. Brown AM (1980): Receptors under pressure: An update on baroreceptors. Circ Res 46: 1–10.
26. Andresen MC (1984): Short and long term determinants of baroreceptor function in aged normontensive and spontenously hypertensive rats. Circ Res 54: 750–759.
27. Michelini LC, Leite JVP, Krieger EM (1979): A new electrolytic strain-gauge to study changes in aortic caliber produced by hypertension. In: Prophylatic Approach to Hypertensive Diseases, edited by Y. Yamori, W. Lovenberg and E.D. Freis. New York: Raven Press, Vol. 4, p. 249–257 (Perspectives Cardiovasc. Res. Ser.).
28. Michelini LC, Krieger EM (1986): Aortic caliber changes during developments of hypertension in freely moving rats. Am J Physiol 250: H662–H671.

29. Michelini LC, Krieger EM (1984): Importance of the timecourse of aortic diastolic caliber dilation for baroreceptor resetting in acute hypertension. J Hypert 2 (Suppl. 3): 387–389.
30. Michelini LC, Krieger EM (1981): Mechanoelastic properties of the aorta in chronically hypertensive conscious rats. Hypertension. 3 (Suppl. II): II-177–II-182.
31. Sumitami M, Michelini LC, Krieger EM (1986): Long-term analysis of aortic dynamics in growing conscious rats. Hypertension 8 (Suppl. I): I-200–I-204.

Part II

Low pressure system and the concept of venous distensibility

Venous compliance in essential hypertension

G.M. LONDON and M.E. SAFAR

Introduction

The function of intravascular volume is to ensure the adequacy of the circulation, i.e. a cardiac output adapted to the metabolic needs of the tissues. The adequacy of the circulation depends on its filling pressure, especially on the filling pressure of the heart [1, 2]. For the overall circulatory system, a well-defined relationship must exist between changes in blood volume and changes in circulatory filling pressure [1]. The slope of the relationship between intravascular volume and pressure defines vascular compliance, which reflects the inherent elasticity of the vascular system [1, 2]. Changes in vascular compliance are of primary importance in the control of cardiovascular function and extracellular fluid volume regulation [1, 2, 3].

In hypertension, complex hemodynamic abnormalities with derangements of various cardiovascular and fluid volume control mechanisms have been described [4, 5, 6, 7, 8], resulting in a decrease in total vascular compliance, mainly in its venous compartment [9, 10, 11, 12]. While numerous reviews have dealt with the control and function of veins in animal hypertension [13, 14, 15], little research has been done in hypertension in man. The purpose of this report is to evaluate the importance of venous abnormalities and their hemodynamic correlates in hypertensive humans. Only the systemic capacitance function of the whole circulation will be considered. Studies on local segments of venous system will be included only when data on the total systemic venous bed are not available. This review will comprise information derived from a larger number of patients with untreated and uncomplicated essential hypertension in which total vascular compliance (TVC) was measured in addition to measurements of cardiac output, total and cardiopulmonary blood volumes, and filling pressure of the heart. The methods used have been described in detail elsewhere [9, 16]. No reference will be made to the relationship of the veins to kidney function and interstitial fluid volume.

Definition of the pressure volume relationship in arteries and veins

Blood vessels are elastic structures with the capacity to offer resistance to stretching force and to return to their resting length after this force is removed. The relationship between the stretching force and the length changes is defined by Hooke's law:

$$T = E \Delta L / L \tag{1}$$

In this equation, T is the tension developed by stretching an elastic element by a force (F) per cross-sectional area (S) (T = F/S). L is the initial length and ΔL is the stretch-induced change in length. The quantity E is termed Young's modulus and defines the elasticity of the stretched structure. Hooke's law is applicable to longitudinal elements and is difficult to apply to anatomical structures which are rather like sacs (e.g. lungs) or cylinders (e.g. blood vessels). For this reason, physiologists have proposed quantifying the elasticity of anatomic structures by measuring the volume changes resulting from the changes in pressure which are able to distend these anatomical structures [17]. The distending pressure should be considered as the transmural pressure (difference between inside and outside pressures).

The slope of the curve relating volume (abcissa) and pressure (ordinate) is termed elastance (E'). Elastance is analogous to Young's modulus used in Hooke's law (E' = $\Delta P / \Delta V$), where ΔP is the change in pressure and ΔV the change in volume. E' is quantitative evaluation of the elasticity of anatomical structures. Nevertheless, most physiologists define elastic behavior in terms of compliance (C), which is the reciprocal of elastance:

$$C = \Delta V / \Delta P \tag{2}$$

However, in most anatomical structures, the pressure-volume relationship cannot be extrapolated toward zero, and intercept of the curve must be defined so that:

$$C = (V - Vo) / P - 0 \tag{3}$$

In this equation, Vo is the unstressed volume, i.e. the volume contained within the compliant structure when the transmural pressure (P) is zero (O); V is the volume contained in the structure when the transmural pressure is P. Units for measuring compliance are expressed in ml/mm Hg or in ml/kg/mm Hg. In such conditions, it is clear that compliance expresses the inherent elasticity of anatomical structures.

Compliance of the overall vascular system in animal experiments

In cardiovascular physiology, vascular compliances must be defined by the relationship between changes in intravascular volume and changes in intravascular pressure. Over a wide range of pressure and volume changes the relationship is non-linear. However, for a limited range of pressure and volume changes, linearized curve may be approximated to define compliance [18]. In a lumped model of the circulation, vascular compliance represents total vascular compliance, which is the sum of the compliances of all vascular segments from arteries to central veins [17, 18]. Total vascular compliance is obtained in experimental animals from determination of Mean Circulatory Filling Pressure (MCFP)-blood volume curves. MCFP refers to the pressure level that would occur throughout the entire circulation if the heart is stopped suddenly and intravascular volume redistributed in the overall vascular system according to the capacity of the vessels [2, 19]. Compliance is thus defined as the change in blood volume divided by the change in MCFP. From equation [3], it appears that total vascular compliance (TVC) is:

$$TVC = (V - Vo)/(MCFP - 0) \qquad (4)$$
$$\text{or } TVC = \triangle V/\triangle MCFP \qquad (5)$$

where V is blood volume, Vo is unstressed blood volume, i.e. the blood volume contained in the vascular system when MCFP equals zero.

From this definition, it is clear that the functional capacity of the circulatory system is determined by vascular compliance and unstressed volume. It is important to distinguish between these two parameters. When a given change in blood volume or cardiac output passively dilates or shrinks the vascular system, the resulting changes in pressure are determined by compliance. When the vascular tone is modified, the pressure resulting from volume changes is dependent on both unstressed volume and on compliance [18, 19, 20].

Classical estimation of MCFP requires that the systemic flow be stopped. To obviate this methodological constraint, different methods have been developed to measure compliance. Instead of MCFP, measurement of the pressure in central veins has been proposed [9, 18, 20, 21]. Under such conditions, it has been shown that the values for TVC are very close whatever the pressure studied. In dogs, values from 1.4 to 4.2 ml/kg/mm Hg were observed with an average of 2.57 mg/kg/mm Hg [2, 17, 18, 21, 22, 23]. Independent measurements of arterial compliance in dogs have revealed values of 0.067 ml/kg/mm Hg [20], which is a very small portion (1–3%) of the total vascular compliance. Total vascular compliance can be therefore approximated to the compliance of the venous system [17]. Total vascular compliance is then itself considered as the sum of the compliance of systemic veins and cardiopulmonary vessels. The compliance of the intrathoracic vascular system is lower than the compliance of systemic vessels.

In dogs, values are between 0.213 and 0.627 ml/kg/mm Hg [24, 25]. Since veins are able to hold large volumes of blood for small pressure changes, they are usually called capacitance vessels. They are considered as a reservoir connected in series with the heart pump. The characteristic pressure in this reservoir is MCFP which is defined according to equation [6] as:

$$MCFP = (V - Vo)/TVC \tag{6}$$

Thus MCFP is the upstream pressure for venous return, which depends on the two dominant characteristics of the capacitance system: the compliance and the intravascular volume.

Total effective compliance in normal and hypertensive humans

Mean circulatory filling pressure cannot be measured in humans and an alternative index of capacitance function has to be defined. For this purpose another circulatory pressure than MCFP must be recorded. Studies in animals and humans have shown that similar correlations are observed when the circulation is not interrupted between blood volume changes and pressures measured in different parts of the venous system [18, 20]. The pressures are usually recorded in the central veins or in the right atrium [9, 18, 20]. The slope of the correlation between central venous pressure (CVP) and blood volume ($\triangle V/\triangle CVP$ ratio) has the dimension of compliance (ml/mm Hg). To differentiate the $\triangle V/\triangle CVP$ ratio from the 'true' compliance measured from MCFP, the ratio is called 'effective' total vascular compliance [21].

This differentiation is necessary since CVP does not depend exclusively on vascular volume and the elastic properties of the vascular bed. The right atrial pressure is both function of venous return and of the pumping ability of the heart [2]. CVP would reflect the blood volume or compliance modifications only when the heart function as a pump is normal. Changes in cardiac output induced by volume expansion have only a minor effect on right atrial pressure and compliance estimation [2, 18, 21]. Changes in blood volume per se also do not influence compliance estimation, unless they induce humoral or neural modifications on venous tone [18, 20]. Time-dependent variations in compliance must be excluded so that the measurement should be done in the shortest interval possible [20]. Even under such conditions, CVP does not reflect MCFP completely. MCFP may be computed as the CVP plus flow-related pressure drop along the veins due to a finite (although low) resistance of the veins to blood flow. During blood volume changes, the pressures at various sites of the venous system vary in parallel [18, 21], but it seems that the gradient for venous returns changes at the same time [21, 23]. CVP should therefore be corrected for changes in pressure drop [14]. Finally, modifications in CVP induce activations of various reflexes which might influence the mechanical properties of the vessels and possibly the compliance estimation [20, 21]. For all these reasons, only 'effective' compliance may be measured in man.

Total 'effective' vascular compliance is easily determined in man by simultaneous recording of right atrial presssure (CVP) changes induced by transfusions or bleeding [9, 21]. Several studies have shown that 'effective' total vascular compliance in normal man has the character of a biological constant with values ranging from 2.1 to 2.7 ml/kg [9, 21, 24, 25, 26]. Total effective vascular compliance is the sum of compliances of the arterial system, which is very low in man [27] (0.034 ml/mm Hg/kg, i.e. 1–3% of the total compliance), and the venous system, which accounts for 97–98% of the total compliance. Compliance of the cardiopulmonary circulation was estimated as being between 0.9 to 1.2 ml/kg/mm Hg in normal man, i.e. between 42 to 55% of total compliance. More direct evaluation of the intrathoracic circulatory compliance gave a value 0.45 ml/kg/mm Hg [28], i.e. about 20% of total compliance. These values are closer to those observed experimentally in animals [24, 25].

In patients with uncomplicated sustained essential hypertension, total effective vascular compliance is reduced in comparison with normal subjects of the similar age and sex [9, 16] (Table 1): For the same volume expansion as in normotensive controls, central venous pressure is significantly higher in hypertensives. The reduction in compliance is related to a decrease in the systemic vessels and not in the cardiopulmonary circulation [28]. As in animals [29, 30], these findings reflect a reduced distensibility of the peripheral (nonintrathoracic) venous system in hypertensive humans [10].

Table 1. Different values of compliance in controls and hypertensive men. Normalization of left ventricular compliance could not be obtained in the literature [46].

	Controls	Sustained essential hypertensive patients	Reference
Total effective vascular compliance (ml/mm Hg/kg)	2.08 ± 0.09	1.49 ± 0.06***	10
Cardiopulmonary effective vascular compliance (ml/mm Hg/kg)	0.45 ± 0.03	0.45 ± 0.06	28
Arterial compliance (ml/mm Hg/kg)	0.044 ± 0.004	0.025 ± 0.0019***	27
Left ventricular compliance (ml/mm Hg · 10)	0.07 ± 0.16	0.04 ± 0.10***	46

± 1 standard error of the mean.
*** $p < 0.001$.

Due to the difficulties in methodology when considering central venous pressure instead of MCFP, the finding of decreased 'effective' vascular compliance in hypertensive men as a reflection of decreased venous compliance may be questionable. However, this interpretation is corroborated by two important observations. First, total effective vascular compliance is strongly and positively correlated with venous compliance measured by plethysmography. Second, using an original mathematical method [4], the data of rapid volume expansion measured in man have been introduced into cardiovascular models of the circulation. Adequate mathematical analysis of the model has been performed and could rule out that the higher central venous pressure observed after volume expansion in hypertensives could not be related to a dominant cardiac factor such as congestive heart failure or cardiac hypertrophy (see also below in this report). On the other hand, it was shown that modifications in unstressed blood volume had no influence on the results observed. Finally, the higher central venous pressure observed after volume expansion in hypertensives was predominantly due to a decrease in the compliance of the venous system. Thus, the use of cardiovascular models taking into account both CVP and MCFP for the interpretation of clinical data clearly demonstrated that compliance of the overall venous system was reduced in patients with sustained essential hypertension.

Venous compliance and intravascular volume in hypertensive humans

Since the capacitance system holds about 80% of the intravascular volume [15, 21] estimation of intravascular blood volume serves to approximate the volume contained within the capacitance vessels. Indeed, the blood volume is distributed between systemic and intrathoracic vascular beds according to the distensibility of these compartments and an estimation of total and intrathoracic blood volume is a prerequisite for understanding the complex relationship between vascular compliance and intravascular volume in hypertension.

Table 2 shows the values of total blood volume in normal subjects and in patients with essential hypertension. Plasma or blood volumes are never increased in hypertension. Most investigators have found the intravascular volume to be significantly reduced [31]. Discrepancies result from methodological problems. When comparing blood or plasma volume of two distinct populations such as normal people and patients with sustained essential hypertension, two technical points should be considered. The first is the necessity of serial blood samplings. Indeed there is an increased escape rate of markers (i.e. radio iodinated albumin or Evan's blue) from circulation in hypertensives [32, 33], leading to overestimation of plasma volume in this group when the single sample method is used [31]. The second methodological problem concerns the choice of an adequate frame of reference. When intravascular volume is expressed in ml/cm of body height, increased values can be found since blood volume in ml/cm is highly correlated with body weight [31] and obesity is a characteristic feature of patients with essential hypertension [34]. On the other hand, when volume is expressed in ml/kg, the decrease in intravascular volume could be overestimated. Using a new mathematical approach, Chau *et al.* [35] have shown that the best reference parameter was body surface area. However, taking into consideration all these criticisms for the blood volume estimation, it appears clear that intravascular volume is significantly reduced in men with essential hypertension, even in patients with obesity [31].

While total blood volume (TBV) is reduced in sustained essential hypertension, cardiopulmonary blood volume (CPBV) is constantly normal (Table 3), resulting in a slight increase in the CPBV/TBV ratio [9, 36, 37]. Such a situation may favor cardiopulmonary mechanoreceptor stimulation during acute volume load. Indeed during acute volume expansion, cardiopulmonary blood volume increases more in hypertensive patients than in controls, resulting in a higher stretch of cardiac mechanoreceptors [38].

Control mechanisms for intravascular volume do not maintain a rigid fixed volume. On the contrary, their role is rather to control blood volume relative to the holding capacity of vascular space. For a long time, the finding of an inverse correlation between blood (or plasma volume) and blood pressure (or total peripheral resistance) (TPR) was considered to reflect this consideration and was used in an attempt to differentiate essential hypertensives into subgroups with 'hypovolemia' or 'hypervolemia' [5, 12, 39, 40]. From a pathophysiological point of view, such a correlation cannot provide an acceptable basis for the appreciation of the circulatory 'fullness', i.e. the control of blood volume relative to the holding capacity of vascular space. Arterial pressure and TPR are hemodynamic

Table 2. Blood volume characteristics in normal subjects and hypertensive patients (personal data). All subjects are men.

Group	Normal	Hypertensive
Number of subjects	50	150
Age	35 ± 10	37 ± 10
BW (kg)	67 ± 10	$75 \pm 9**$
BH (cm)	173 ± 5	173 ± 6
SAP (mm Hg)	124 ± 15	$184 \pm 28***$
DAP (mm Hg)	68 ± 9	$107 \pm 15***$
BV (ml)	5284 ± 551	5213 ± 692
BV/BW (ml/kg)	79.6 ± 8.3	$70 \pm 7.9***$
BV/BH (ml/cm)	30.6 ± 3.2	30.1 ± 3.8
BV/BSA (ml/m)	2953 ± 228	$2774 \pm 297***$

Abbreviations: $\pm$ standard deviation.
* = $p<0.05$, ** = $p<0.01$, *** $p = 0.001$.
BW = body weight, BH = body height, SAP = systolic arterial blood pressure, DAP = diastolic arterial pressure, BV = blood volume, BSA = body surface area.

parameters related to the 'high-pressure' system whose function is almost entirely 'resistive'. The compliance of this system is low and its capacitative role small [2, 17, 21]. The circulatory 'reservoir' function is that of the low-pressure, post-capillary venous system [2, 17, 21]. Therefore, for classification of hypertensive patients, the relationship of blood volume to mechanical properties of the capacitance low-pressure system is more appropriate. Thus blood volume must be analyzed as a function of the compliance of the vascular system. In normal people, a positive correlation is observed between intravascular volume and TVC. Subjects with high vascular compliance have a tendency to have higher blood volume and vice versa [10, 37]. This tendency is less marked in patients with essential hypertension, but when normal people and hypertensive patients are studied together, the whole population shows the same trend (Fig. 1): blood volume and TVC are positively related according to only one regression and hypertensive patients are neither 'hypervolemic' nor 'hypovolemic'. Intravascular volume is reduced in patients with essential hypertension but, from a 'hemodynamic' viewpoint, the circulatory fullness is normal or even more than normal, as further detailed below.

Filling pressure of the heart, venous compliance and cardiac ouput control in hypertensive men

In human studies, the pressure which is considered as the most representative for the circulatory filling is the right atrial pressure (central venous pressure). In patients with sustained essential hypertension, all reports in the literature have shown that right atrial pressure is slightly but significantly increased, even in the absence of congestive heart failure [37, 38, 41]. In parallel to the elevation of atrial pressure, there is also an increase in pulmonary arterial and wedge pressures [38, 41]. The pressure gradient across the pulmonary circulation is identical to that of normal subjects and the total resistance of the pulmonary circuit is also similar to normotensive controls [38, 41]. Furthermore, all circulatory pressures (arterial, right atrial, pulmonary and pulmonary wedge pressures) are positively correlated with each other [38, 41].

The right atrial pressure is influenced by parameters regulating both venous return and the pumping ability of the right ventricle [2]. Theoretically, an elevated CVP in hypertension could result from three possibilities: a decreased or modified pumping function of the heart, a decreased vascular compliance, or an increased blood volume.

The basic mechanism adjusting the stroke volume to blood inflow is described as the Frank-Starling law of the heart and expressed in terms of cardiac function curves, by plotting stroke volume or cardiac output against right atrial pressure [2]. In patients with essential hypertension, compared to normal people, right cardiac function curves exhibit a rightward shift of otherwise normally shaped

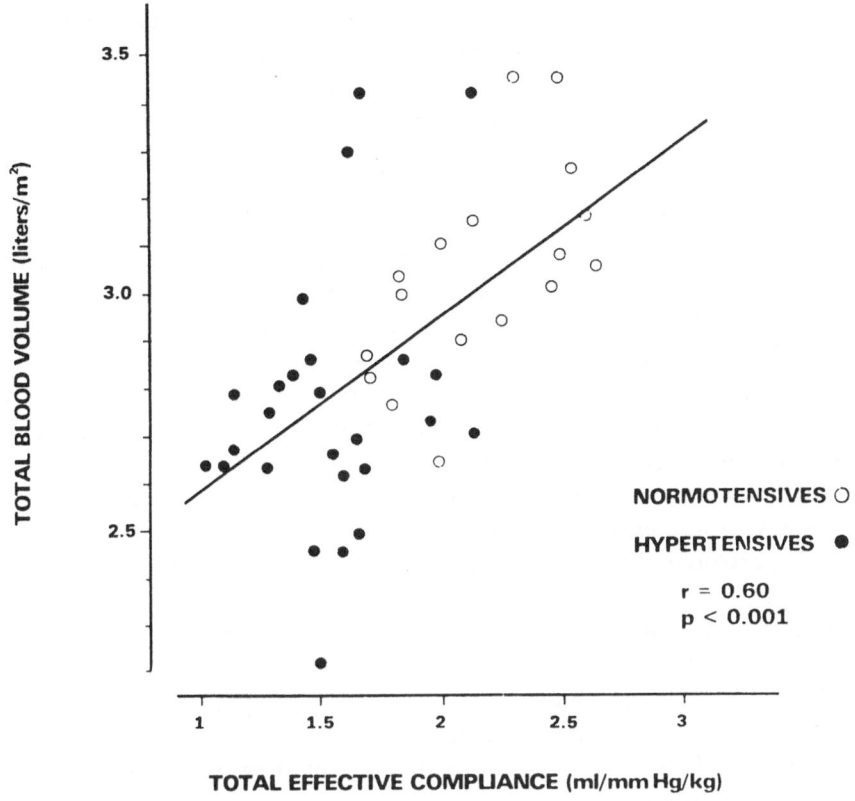

Figure 1. Steady-state relationship between total effective vascular compliance and total blood volume (personal data).

curves [10, 28]. The 'pump' operates normally but at a higher 'basic pressure level'. The increased basic pressure level might theoretically be a passive consequence of heart hypertrophy and result from a backward effect of elevated arterial pressure [41]. However, such a 'passive' mechanism cannot be the principal factor accounting for an elevated central venous pressure in hypertension. Cardiopulmonary and low pressure systems are compliant and, as such, they increase their volume, when they are submitted to an increased pressure. Nevertheless, an elevated CVP is observed in patients with essential hypertension but cardiopulmonary blood volume and total blood volume are normal and decreased respectively. Thus only a decrease of venous compliance could satisfactorily explain the changes in right atrial pressure. Several findings support this interpretation in clinical investigations. In normal and hypertensive populations, a negative correlation is observed between central venous pressure and blood volume [37] and also between central venous pressure and total vascular compliance [37]. In other words, in essential hypertension, the slight increase in central venous pressure is obtained through a reduction of total vascular compliance and this in the presence of blood volume reduction.

In patients with essential hypertension, the contribution of vascular capacitance to the regulation of cardiac output is especially important in view of the three characteristic hemodynamic features of the heart in hypertension: normal cardiac output, decreased intravascular volume and cardiac hypertrophy without congestive heart failure. Indeed, it is well accepted that the normal cardiac output in the presence of increased afterload is achieved through cardiac hypertrophy which causes a decrease in left ventricular compliance [7, 8, 12]. In such conditions, the presence of established cardiac hypertrophy would lead to a reduction in stroke volume without adequate compensation. Such compensation could be found in the form of increased cardiac filling pressure of the left and right ventricles. In patients with essential hypertension, an increase in capillary wedge pressure is observed, indirectly reflecting an increase in left atrial pressure [38, 41]. Right atrial pressure is also increased [38, 41]. This, in turn could call for decreased venous compliance in order to produce an adequate driving pressure for the hypertrophied heart. During an isotonic saline intravenous volume load, Ulrych et al. [42] showed that the increase in cardiac output was enhanced in hypertensives and suggested that a reduction in peripheral vascular capacity was responsible for this finding. More direct evidence is provided by the observation of a negative correlation observed between cardiac output or stroke volume and effective vascular compliance in patients with essential hypertension (Fig. 2): the more reduced the compliance, the higher the cardiac output level [9]. Thus, despite cardiac hypertrophy and decreased intravascular volume, a normal cardiac output in sustained essential hypertension is achieved by a reduction in venous compliance [43].

Conclusion

On the basis of animal experiments, it has been suggested during recent years that a decrease in venous compliance could be an initiating factor in hypertension, causing an increase in cardiac output with resulting autoregulatory mechanisms leading to the elevation of total peripheral resistance. Since most of the data presented in this review are based on cross-sectional analysis, clinical findings clearly do not delineate any argument in favor of this hypothesis. However, observations in man strongly suggest that reduced venous compliance plays an important role in the maintenance of normal cardiac output in essential hypertension and therefore metabolic needs of the tissues. As reported elsewhere [38], such mechanisms also involve the cardiac mechanoreceptor stimulation in the low-pressure system and the renal control of fluid volumes.

For a long time, venous abnormalities in hypertension have been interpreted as

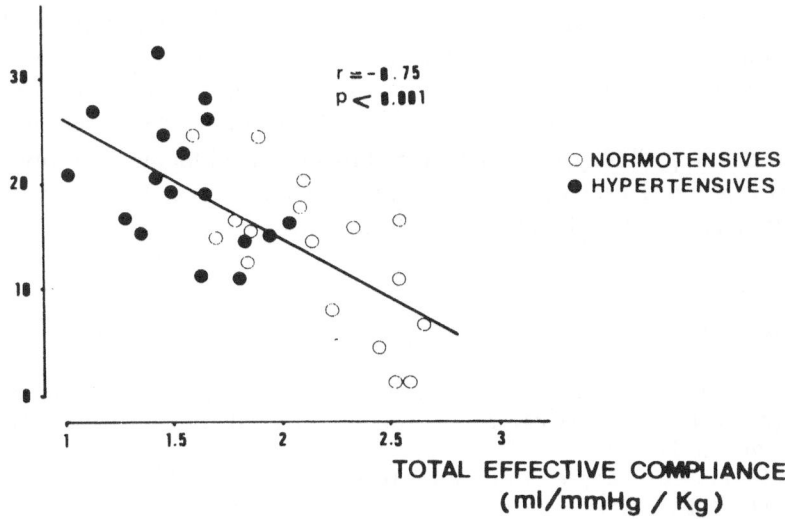

Figure 2. Relationship between total effective vascular compliance and the change in stroke volume during rapid Dextran infusion [43] (with permission).

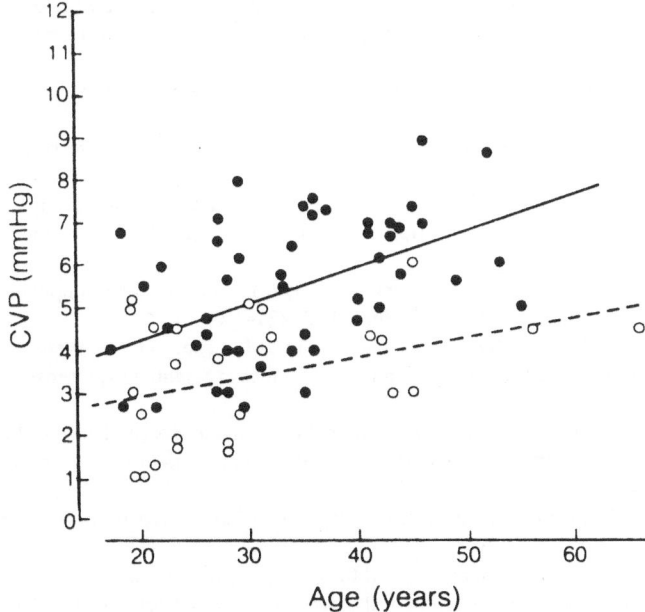

Figure 3. Relationship between age and central venous pressure (CVP). Notice the steeper slope in hypertensives (●) (r = 0.49; p<0.001) than in normotensives (○) (r = 0.39; p<0.05) [16] (with permission).

64

secondary effects of arterial and cardiac changes. Recent studies have shown that, as arterial blood pressure and resistance increase with age, venous compliance also decreases with aging, with a steeper slope of the curve in hypertensives. Similar results are observed for central venous pressure [16, 44–45] (Fig. 3). In other words, there are possibilities that modifications of the venous system in hypertension may have the same influence as the alterations of the arterial system in the course of the disease. The lack of basic knowledge about venous abnormalities is probably related to the difficulty in obtaining appropriate clinical methods for investigations of the venous system in man. This important problem remains to be solved and requires further investigations.

References

1. Gauer OH, Henry JP (1976): Neurohumoral control of plasma volume. In: Guyton AC, Cowley AW (eds.) Intern Rev Physiol Cardiovascular Physiol II, Vol. 9, Baltimore, University Park Press, pp 145–190.
2. Guyton AC, Coleman TG, Granger HJ (1982): Circulation: Overall Regulation. Annu Rev Physiol 1972, 34: 13.
3. Seely JF, Levy M (1981): Control of extracellular fluid volume. In: Brenner BM, Rector FC (eds.) The Kidney, Philadelphia, Saunders, pp 371–407.
4. Chau NP, Coleman TG, London GM, Safar ME (1982): Meaning of the cardiac output-blood volume relationship in essential hypertension. American Journal of Physiology 243: R318–R328.
5. Safar ME, Chau NP, Weiss YA, London GM, Simon AC, Milliez PL (1976): The pressure-volume relationship in normotensive and permanent essential hypertensive patients. Clin Sci Mol Med 50: 207–212.
6. Tarazi RC, Dustan HP, Frohlich ED (1968): Plasma volume in men with essential hypertension. New Engl J Med 762: 278–284.
7. Tarazi RC, Dustan HP, Frohlich ED (1969): Relation of plasma to interstitial fluid volume in essential hypertension. Circulation 40: 357–364.
8. Ulrych M, Frohlich ED, Tarazi RC, Dustan HP, Page IH (1969): Cardiac output and distribution of blood volume in central and peripheral circulations in hypertensive and normotensive man. Brit Heart J 570: 31–42.
9. London GM, Safar ME, Weiss YA, Simon AC (1978): Total effective compliance of the vascular bed in essential hypertension. Amer Heart J 95: 325–330.
10. London GM, Safar ME, Simon AC, Alexandre JM, Levenson JA, Weiss YA (1978): Total effective compliance, cardiac output and fluid volumes in essential hypertension. Circulation 57: 995–1000.
11. London GM, Safar ME, Levenson JA, Simon AC, Temmar MA (1981): Renal filtration fraction, effective vascular compliance and partition of fluid volumes and sustained essential hypertension. Kidney Int 20: 97–103.
12. Tarazi RC (1976): Hemodynamic role of extracellular fluid in hypertension. Circ Res (Suppl. II) 73: 38–47.
13. Cooper KE (1981): Functional aspects of the venous system. In: Schwartz CJ, Werthessen NT, Wolf S (eds.) Structure and function of the circulation. New York, Plenum, Vol. 2, pp 457–485.
14. Rothe CF (1983): The venous system. The physiology of the capacitance vessels. In: Shelpherd JT, Abboud FM (eds.) Handbook of physiology. The cardiovascular system. Peripheral circulation and organ blood flow. Vol. III, sect. 2, Bethesda, Am Physiol Soc, pp 397–452.

15. Shepherd JT, Vanhoutte PM (1975): Veins and their control. Philadelphia, Saunders, Vol. 1, p 269.
16. London GM, Safar ME, Safar AL, Simon ACh (1985): Blood pressure in the 'low-pressure system' and cardiac performance in essential hypertension. J Hypertension 3: 337–342.
17. Green JF (1977): Mechanical concepts in cardiovascular and pulmonary physiology. Philadelphia, Lea & Fibiger, p 166.
18. Shoukas AA, Sagawa K (1971): Total systemic vascular compliance measured as incremental volume-pressure ratio. Circ Res 277: 28–37.
19. Guyton AC (1963): Mean circulatory pressure, mean systemic pressure and mean pulmonary pressure and their effect on venous return. In: Circulating Physiology. Cardiac output and its regulation. Philadelphia, Saunders, pp 193–208.
20. Shoukas AA, Sagawa K (1973): Control of total systemic vascular capacity by the carotid sinus baroreceptor reflex. Circ Res 32: 33–39.
21. Echt M, Duweling J, Gauer OH, Lange L (1974): Effective compliance of the total vascular bed and the intrathoracic compartment derived from changes in central venous pressure induced by volume changes in man. Circ Res 34: 61–72.
22. Drees JA, Rothe CF (1974): Reflex venoconstriction and capacity vessels pressure-volume relationships in dog. Circ Res 360: 34–44.
23. Harlan JC, Smith EE, Richardson TQ (1967): Pressure volume curves of systemic and pulmonary circuit. Am J Physiol 1499: 213–219.
24. Engelberg J, Dubois AB (1959): Mechanisms of pulmonary circulation in isolated rabbit lungs. Am J Physiol 401: 196–208.
25. Maseri A, Caldini P, Horward P, Josmi RC, Permutt S, Zierler KL (1972): Determinants of pulmonary vascular volume recruitment versus distensibility. Circ Res 218: 31–38.
26. Gauer OH (1978): Mechanoreceptors in the intrathoracic circulation and plasma volume control. In: Epstein M (ed.), The Kidney in liver disease. Vol. 1, New York, Elsevier, pp 3–17.
27. Simon AC, Safar ME, Levenson JA, London JM, Levy BI, Chau NP (1979): An evaluation of large arteries compliance in man. Am J Physiology 235 (5): H550–554.
28. London GM, Safar ME, Payen DM, Gitelman RC, Guerin AM (1982): Total peripheral and intrathoracic effective compliances of the vascular bed in normotensive and hypertensive patients. In: Brod J (ed.) Contribution to nephrology, Basel, Karger, pp. 144–153.
29. Ricksten SE, Yao T, Thoren P (1981): Peripheral and central Vascular compliances in conscious normotensive and spontaneously hypertensive rats. Acta Physiol Scand 112: 167–169.
30. Trippodo NC, Yamamoto J, Frohlich ED (1981): Whole-body venous capacity and effective total tissue compliance in SHR. Hypertension 3: 104–111.
31. Safar ME, London GM Simon AC, Chau NP (1983): Volume factors, total exchangeable sodium and potassium in hypertension disease. In: Genest J, Kuchel O, Hamet P, Cantin M (eds), Hypertension Physiopathology and treatment. New York, McGraw Hill, pp 42–54.
32. Parving MH, Gyntelberg F (1973): Transcapillary escape rate of albumin and plasma volume in essential hypertension. Circ Res 643: 32–39.
33. Ulrych M (1973): Plasma volume decrease and elevated Evans blue disappearance rate in essential hypertension. Clin Sci Mol Med 173: 45–52.
34. Messerli FH, Christie B, DeCarvalho JGR, Aristimuno GG, Suarez DH, Dreslinski GR, Frohlich ED (1981): Obesity and essential hypertension. Arch Int Med 141: 81–86.
35. Chau NP, Tarazi RC, Fouad FM, Safar ME, Birkenhager WH, De Leeuw PW (1982): Index for normalization of blood volume. Clin Sci 63: 375S–377S.
36. Julius S, Pascual AV, Reilly K, London R (1971): Abnormalities of plasma volume in borderline hypertension. Arch Intern Med 127: 116–119.
37. London GM, Levenson JA, London AM, Simon AC, Safar ME (1984): Systemic compliance, renal hemodynamics and sodium excretion in hypertension. Kidney Int 26: 342–350.
38. London GM, Levenson JA, Safar ME, Simon AC, Guerin AP, Payen D (1983): Hemodynamic

effects of head-down tilt in normal subjects and sustained hypertensive patients. Am J Physiol 245 (Heart Circ Physiol 14): H194–H202.

39. London GM, Safar ME, Weiss YA, Corvol PL, Lehner JP, Menard JM, Simon AC, Milliez PL (1977): Volume-dependent parameters in essential hypertension. Kidney International 11: 204–208.

40. Safar ME, London GM, Weiss YA, Milliez PL (1975): Altered blood volume regulation in sustained essential hypertension. A hemodynamic study. Kidney International 8: 42–47.

41. Ferlinz J (1980): Right ventricular performance in essential hypertension. Circulation 61: 156–162.

42. Ulrych M, Hofman J, Hejl Z (1964): Cardiac and renal hyperresponsiveness to acute plasma volume expansion in hypertension. Am Heart J 68: 193–199.

43. Safar ME, London GM, Levenson JA, Simon AC, Chau NP (1979): Rapid dextran infusion in essential hypertension. Hypertension 1: 615.

44. Safar ME, London GM (1985): Venous system in essential hypertension. Clinical Science 69: 497–504.

45. London GM, Safar ME, Sassard J, Levenson JA, Simon AC (1984): Renal and systemic hemodynamics in sustained essential hypertension. Hypertension 6: 743–754.

46. Merillon JP, Motte G, Masquet C, Azancot I, Curien ND, Guiomard A, Gourgon R (1982): Inter relation entre les propriétés physiques du système artériel et la performance ventriculaire gauche lors du vieillissement et dans l'hypertension artérielle. In: l'Hypertrophie Ventriculaire Gauche, pp 95–104. Ed. Brutsaert DL, Masson, Paris.

Functional and structural components of reduced forearm venous distensibility in human hypertension

GEZA SIMON

To the hypertensinologist, the veins are of interest for two reasons. First, the veins contribute both passively and actively to the distribution of blood volume between the peripheral and pulmonary vascular beds, thereby influencing cardiac filling and regulating cardiac output. Second, the veins may serve as an experimental model for the study of vascular smooth muscle which is not exposed to the increased intraluminal pressure associated with arterial hypertension. Although subtle elevation of venous pressure in uncomplicated hypertension cannot be ruled out, alterations in venous function and composition are more likely to be the result of chronic neural or humoral influences than of increased intraluminal pressure. For our purposes, the veins constitute an experimental model for the study of pressure-independent vascular changes in hypertension.

Anatomy and function of veins

Veins are composed of the same passive and active components as are arteries, but with some important quantitative differences [1]. Also, the composition of veins is more variable than that of arteries [2]. The large veins contain a high percentage of collagen fibers. In the smaller veins and in the veins of the lower extremities which are subject to a large hydrostatic pressure, the muscular mass exceeds that of collagen fibers. The inferior mesenteric vein of humans, for instance, is made up primarily of collagen and elastin (>90%), while the skin veins of the foot are 50–60% smooth muscle [2]. Veins lack the heavy elastic investment of the media of arteries. The elastic modulus defined as $\triangle P/\triangle V/V$, (where $\triangle P$ is pressure in dynes/cm^2 and V is volume in ml) of the various vascular wall elements is as follows: collagen: 300×10^6 dynes/cm^2; elastin: 6×10^6; smooth muscle and endothelium: 0.1×10^6 [3]. On this basis, collagen fibers are 3000 times stiffer (or less distensible) than smooth muscle fibers. Any consideration of vascular distensibility has to take into account the contribution of collagen fibers, especially in the higher pressure ranges, along the rapidly rising portion of the pressure-volume curve (see below), where the connective tissue elements of the vessel wall are being stretched.

There are other important differences between veins and arteries [1, 2]. The veins are more securely embedded in the surrounding tissues than arteries. Changes in *in situ* venous distensibility could be due in part to changes in interstitial tissue compliance. Veins receive nutrients through the vasa venarum which extend to the intima but do not penetrate it for venous drainage. Oxygen and nutrients do not pass in significant amounts from lumen into the surrounding tissue of the vein wall. As a result, the humoral environment of venous smooth muscle is similar to that of small arteries. Although veins are innervated, the degree of innervation is much less than that of resistance vessels. The innervation of veins is sympathetic in nature, consisting exclusively of constrictor fibers. The superficial, subcutaneous and iliac veins have less innervation than the veins of the viscera or the saphenous or cephalic veins. Because of the great variability in the anatomy and, therefore, function of veins, generalizations are difficult. This is especially true in human studies, which are restricted to the veins of the extremities.

In the physiologic pressure ranges, veins are more compliant than arteries [1]. As a result, some 70 percent of intravascular blood volume resides in the venous system, with 50–60 percent in veins greater than 1 mm in diameter [1, 4]. Volume shifts in and out of this reservoir are determined by its compliance. Compliance is a property of the vascular wall arising from its distensibility. Each component of the vessel wall, smooth muscle, elastin, collagen and groud substance contribute to compliance. Compliance is expressed in terms of blood volume in the vascular segment and the attending pressure differences across the vascular wall. It is estimated by measurements of pressure-volume relationship within the vascular segment. Mathematically, it is the slope of the pressure-volume relationship at a specified point on the curve. To facilitate comparisons, compliance may be 'normalized' to a unit body weight or organ volume of the subject or animal. Ideally, one should measure venous pressure-volume relationships over the entire physiologic volume range, from unstressed volume (volume at atmospheric transmural pressure) to volumes which result in transmural pressures of 40–50 mm Hg. Assuming that the initial unstressed volume in two groups of subjects is the same, a shift of the pressure-volume curve in one group versus the other will indicate a difference in compliance over some if not all volume ranges.

In vitro and *in vivo* study of veins revealed two types of pressure-volume (compliance) curves [1]. One was described as curvilinear with convexity toward the volume axis, the other sigmoid in character (Fig. 1). The latter is observed when the veins are in spasm or constricted by neural or humoral stimuli. When the state of contraction is eliminated by warming, venodilator agents or metabolic inhibitors, the curvilinear pressure-volume curve is observed. The sigmoidal curve has been interpreted as a manifestation of the resistance to stretch of venous smooth muscle. The curvilinear curve with convexity toward the volume

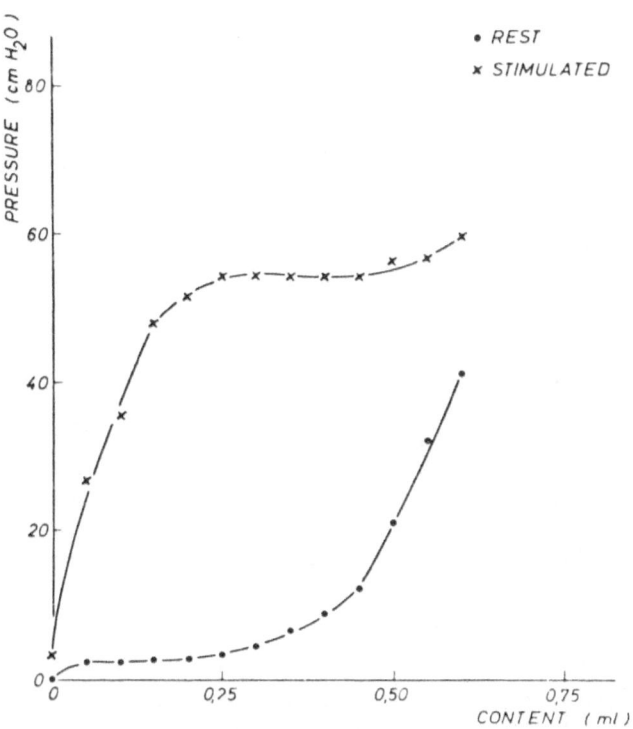

Figure 1. Pressure-volume relationships in an isolated segment of dog's saphenous vein before (solid circles) and during electrical stimulation (15 Hz) (crosses). (From Shepherd JT, Vanhoutte PM, ref. 5. By permission.)

axis represents primarily the resistance to stretch of the connective tissue elements of the venous wall, the smooth muscle elements being in a state of relaxation.

Another feature of vascular distensibility or compliance is the marked time dependency in elastic behavior, sometimes referred to as 'elastic hysteresis', 'delayed compliance', or 'stress relaxation', the latter implying that pressure dissipates following sudden distention to a constant volume [1]. As a result, pressure-volume curves observed on injection or filling and pressure-volume curves on withdrawal of fluid or emptying form a loop (Fig. 2). The width of this loop demonstrates time dependency, in that it becomes narrower at very fast and very slow rates of injection and withdrawal of fluid. The initial state of vasoconstriction or vasodilatation has a greater influence on the pressure-volume curve observed during injection than during emptying. The latter curve is more reproducible than the former, being subject to fewer stimuli (Fig. 2). Stretch relaxation also implies that a second stretch curve differs greatly from an initial stretch unless sufficient time is allowed between measurements for a complete restoration of the resting distensibility state (Fig. 2). Studies have shown that this

70

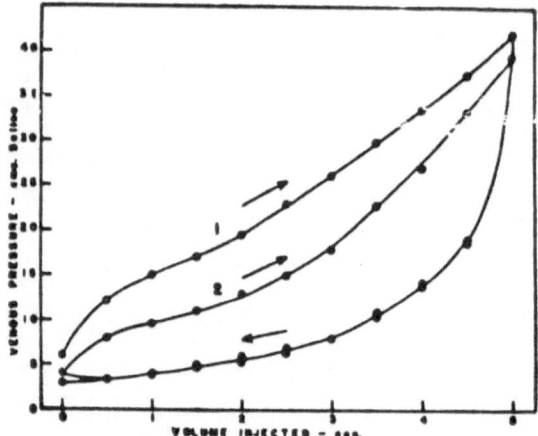

Figure 2. Pressure changes accompanying the injection and withdrawal of 5 ml of blood at 1 ml/sec into the venous end of an isolated intestinal loop with inflow and outflow occluded. (1) indicates initial cycle of injection and (2) second cycle immediately following the first. Arrow pointing to the left indicates withdrawal. (From Alexander RS *et al.*, 1953. Circ Res 1: 271–277. By permission.)

critical time period is between 20–30 minutes for veins [1].

From the experimental point of view, especially, when one is trying to compare pressure-volume data from different groups of subjects, these characteristics of vascular distensibility have important practical implications. An attempt has to be made to measure or define the initial unstressed volume. Identical rates and magnitudes of distension and emptying should be used. The time interval between subsequent pressure-volume determinations should be set. Waiting for 20–30 minutes for the complete restoration of the resting distensibility state may not be necessary as long as the pressure-volume measurements are performed at regular interval throughout the studies. If possible, entire pressure-volume curves, from unstressed volume to the physiologic upper limits of pressure, should be compared.

Methods for study of venous system in man

Studies of veins in human subjects have been restricted to the limbs. Two approaches have been used to measure venous pressure changes at constant volume [5]. In the first, a small catheter or needle is introduced into a collateral-free segment (3–5 cm) of a cutaneous vein, usually in the forearm, for pressure monitoring. The segment is isolated from the remainder of the circulation by means of two wedges placed over the arm. Because blood flow is arrested changes in intraluminal pressure represent changes in venomotor tone. Pressure-volume relationships in the occluded segment can be obtained by the infusion of saline and continuous pressure measurements through a T-tube arrangement. Because of the great variability of the size of cutaneous veins among individuals, intergroup comparisons of cutaneous vein pressure-volume relationships by this method are difficult if not impossible due to the tremendous scatter of data points (G. Simon, unpublished observations).

In the second approach, arterial inflow to a segment of the limb is occluded by means of a pneumatic cuff inflated to suprasystolic pressure, and the pressure within one of the large veins in the limb is measured. After 15–45 seconds, venous pressure comes to an equilibrium, defined as intrinsic pressure. There is one report of increased intrinsic pressure, measured in this way, in hypertensive subjects, but others could not confirm this finding [6, 7]. Because initial vascular volume is not defined, and infusion of fluid would require arterial catheterization, the method is not readily adapted for pressure-volume measurements. Venous pressure measurements at constant blood volume are useful for the study of rapidly occurring reflex changes in venomotor tone but not for estimation of venous compliance.

To measure or estimate venous compliance of the limb, changes in volume that accompany stepwise changes in venous pressure are recorded. The forearm has been studied most frequently, followed by the digits, the calf, and the hand. Changes in volume are detected by plethysmography [8, 9]. For direct measurement of volume changes, a water plethysmograph is used. The method is somewhat cumbersome and has the additional drawback of exposing the limb to an external pressure of 10–25 cm of water, depending on the water level in the plethysmograph. This will cause collapse of veins initially, some of which may not be reopened by arterial inflow as long as the limb is under water. Non-uniform filling of veins may result during stepwise venous congestion. The majority of investigators in the field have used an indirect method for the measurement of volume changes, termed electrocapacitance or mercury-in-rubber strain gauge plethysmography, whereby changes in the electrical conductance of an elastic tubing encircling the limb are translated through calibration procedures into volume changes [9]. For calibration an electrical calibrator with known volume equivalent or cylindrical formers of known circumference are used. To produce volume changes, a congesting cuff is positioned proximal to the elbow or knee for studies of the forearm or calf, at the wrist for studies of the hand, or over the proximal portion of the digit. The congesting cuff is inflated to known pressures, which after a short period of equilibrium results in equivalent pressure changes in the limb veins. Various maneuvers have been used to 'standardize' the initial limb volume. In the water plethysmograph, the level of water can be adjusted to give rise to a transmural or effective venous pressure of 1 to 2 mm Hg. For indirect plethysmography, the limb to be studied used to be elevated above heart level to achieve low initial venous pressure and volume. This maneuver like the introduction of water into the water plethysmograph will result in the collapse of some veins. The preferred method is to determine directly the minimal occluding pressure in the congesting cuff that causes a measurable increase in limb volume, and to use it as the initial pressure (and volume) (Fig. 3). At minimal occluding pressure the veins are uniformly filled with blood and cylindrical in shape. Any additional increase in venous pressure will result in distention of veins rather than being dissipated in opening up collapsed veins. Estimation of minimal occluding pressure by extrapolation of the pressure-volume curve through zero volume change is based on the assumption that the curve is linear in the low pressure ranges when it is not (Fig. 4). Direct measurement of minimal occluding pressure is, therefore, the preferred method. Venous pressure-volume curves are derived by stepwise increases of venous pressure to 30–40 mm Hg by inflating the congesting cuff. Alternatively, venous pressure-volume curves can be obtained during deflation by first inflating the cuff to 30 mm Hg above minimal occluding pressure, allowing the volume curve to reach a plateau (3 to 5 minutes), then deflating the cuff in a stepwise fashion and recording volume at each step (Fig. 3). In the forearm, due to non-uniform filling of superficial and deep veins, pressure-volume measurements during inflation phase have been shown to be poorly reproducible [10]. Non-uniform filling of forearm veins is especially troublesome when the hand is excluded from the measurements by inflation of a wrist cuff to suprasystolic pressure. Consequently, investigators have often resorted to measurements of pressure-volume relationships during deflation. These measurements may take up to 5 minutes to complete during which capillary filtration may contribute measurably to the volume changes observed. When different groups of subjects are being compared, the assumption is made that capillary filtration rate in the groups is the same. This may not always be the case, and, ideally, capillary filtration rate should be measured by maintaining congesting pressure above capillary pressure and recording the slow shift of the volume curve to higher values over several minutes (Fig. 3). As in the case of *in vitro* studies, in each subject identical rates and magnitudes of inflation and deflation should be used, and the time interval between repeat measurements should also be the same.

Reduced forearm venous distensibility in human hypertension

Early studies did not reveal a difference in forearm venous distensibility between normotensive and hypertensive subjects [11, 12]. Abramson and Fierst used water plethysmography to measure forearm (and calf) venous distensibility during inflation phase in a large group of normotensive and hypertensive subjects. The lack of difference in venous distensibility between the two groups of subjects in this study may have been due to methodological problems. The authors did not measure minimal occluding pressure; therefore, initial venous pressure and volume could have varied greatly among subjects. In normotensive subjects, the initial 20 mm Hg occluding pressure resulted in a volume increment of only 0.10 ml/100 ml forearm volume (mean), and the maximum volume increment at

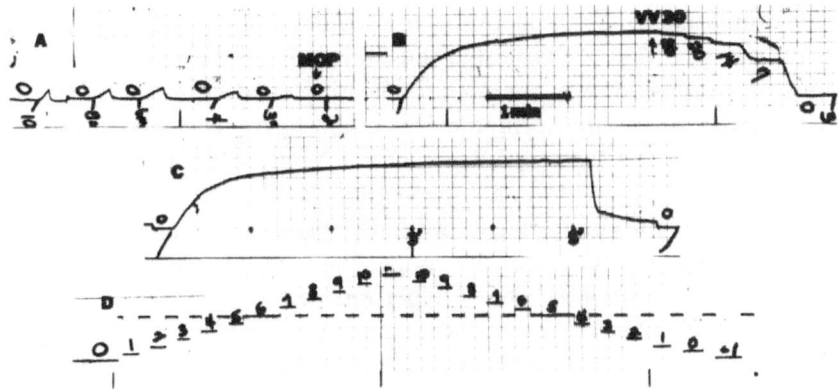

Figure 3. Recording of forearm plethysmographic measurements: A. Minimal occluding pressure (2 cm H_2O); B. Venous distensibility at 30 cm H_2O effective distending pressure (VV 30) and venous pressure-volume curve (deflation phase); C. Slope of forearm volume curve between 3 and 5 minutes after venous distention at 30 cm H_2O; D. Calibration curve. Each step represents shortening or lengthening of the mercury-filled rubber tubing by one turn (0.6 mm) of the adjusting nut on the gauge. (From Simon G *et al.*, ref. 15. By permission.)

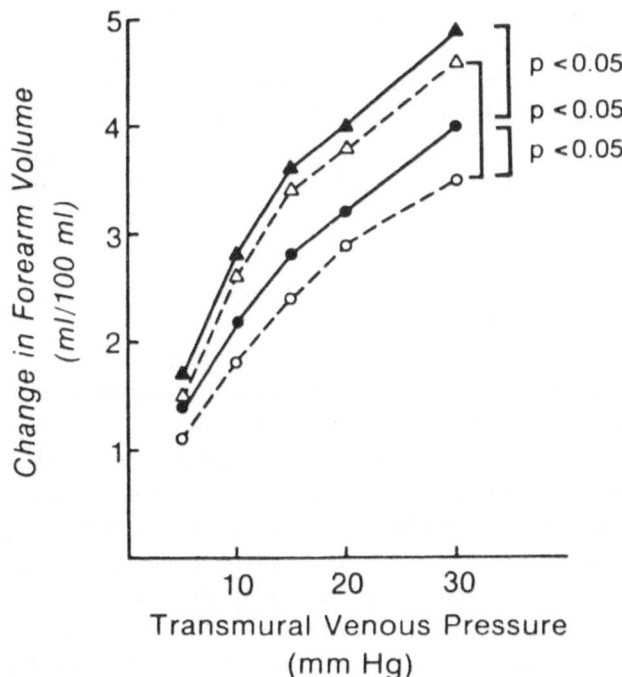

Figure 4. Forearm venous pressure-volume curves (inflation phase) in 5 subjects with borderline hypertension (circles) and 5 normotensive subjects (triangles) before (solid lines) and after (dashed lines) phentolamine 5 mg iv. (From Takeshita A *et al.*, ref. 16. By permission.)

70 mm Hg occluding pressure was 2.29 ml/100 ml. These numbers are low (see Fig. 4 for comparison). When the results are plotted on a pressure-volume curve, the rapidly rising portion of a typical distensibility curve is never reached. Thus, a difference in distensibility in the higher effective intravenous pressure ranges between hypertensives and normotensives could have been missed by the authors. Wood also used water plethysmography but was careful to set initial effective intravenous pressure in a large vein of the forearm to 1 mm Hg in each subject by inflating the congesting cuff slightly. Pressure-volume measurements were obtained during inflation of the congesting cuff. The lack of difference in forearm venous distensibility between hypertensive and normotensive subjects in Wood's study could have been due to the small number of subjects (10 hypertensive, 14 normotensive) and, perhaps, to the exclusion of the hand from the circulation by inflation of a wrist cuff to suprasystolic pressure, which results in sluggish and non-uniform filling of veins (see above).

The first report of decreased venous distensibility in human hypertension was by Caliva and coworkers [13]. They studied a highly specialized vascular bed, the finger tip, using a pneumoplethysmograph. The authors had to contend with a sizeable artifact in their measurements due to the close proximity of the congesting cuff to the plethysmograph. Following occlusion of venous outflow, the time course of volume increase in the fingertip was measured until outflow pressure exceeded the occlusion pressure. The pressure-volume curves of hypertensive subjects were steeper than those of normotensive subjects. In the systemic circulation about 70 percent of blood is contained in veins, therefore, a steeper pressure-volume curve can be interpreted to be due to reduced venous compliance. However, in the highly specialized vascular bed of the fingertip with its numerous AV shunts, a major contribution of small arteries to vascular capacitance cannot be excluded.

More convincing evidence for reduced venous distensibility in human hypertension resulted from the work of Walsh and coworkers [14]. The authors used an electrocapacitance plethysmograph to measure forearm venous pressure-volume relationships during deflation phase and with the hand included. These modifications resulted in smooth pressure-volume curves which were highly reproducible in the same sitting. The day-to-day reproducibility of measurements was much less. This has been the experience of the majority of plethysmographers indicating that the measurements are subject to day-to-day variations in the characteristics of the apparatus which are not easily controlled for. It has to be realized that at a venous occlusion pressure of 30 mm Hg the absolute increment in forearm circumference is about 6–7 mm, which one tries to measure accurately by translating changes in electrical conductance into changes in girth. This type of investigation would be aided by obtaining several measurements in the same subjects on different days and using average values from each subject for group comparisons. Walsh and coworkers did this in some of their subjects. They found a marked shift of forearm venous pressure-volume curves toward the pressure axis in hypertensive subjects in comparison to those in normotensive subjects. All but one of their hypertensive subjects were black in contrast to the normotensive group of subjects which was half black and half white or oriental. The mean arterial pressure of hypertensive subjects was 120 mm Hg (mean, range 103–158). The severity of hypertension had no significant bearing on venous forearm volume at 30 mm Hg distending pressure (VV 30). A small increase in VV 30 was detected in subjects who received antihypertensive therapy with guanethidine or reserpine for at least one month.

Our group has studied forearm venous distensibility in white men with mild-to-moderate essential hypertension and closely matched normotensive men [15]. We used the same mercury-in-rubber strain-gauge plethysmograph throughout the study. For more accurate measurement of venous occluding pressure, a water manometer was used. Minimal occluding pressure was determined at the beginning of the experiments and venous distending pressure was defined as the cuff pressure minus minimal occluding pressure. The inflation and deflation of the congesting cuff were timed, and venous pressure-volume curves were recorded during deflation. A wrist cuff was not used. Capillary filtration rate was also measured. VV 30 (cm of H_2O) was reduced and forearm venous pressure-volume curves were shifted toward the pressure axis in hypertensive subjects, but the differences between hypertensives and normotensives were smaller than in the study of Walsh *et al.* Capillary filtration rate was slightly higher in hypertensives than in normotensives, which reduced the differences in VV 30 between the two groups.

Takeshita and Mark studied forearm venous distensibility in white men with borderline hypertension, using a water plethysmograph [16]. Venous pressure was measured directly through an indwelling catheter, and the initial pressure in a large forearm vein was set at about 1.5 mm Hg by raising the water level in the plethysmograph to 23 cm above the upper aspect of the forearm. Changes in forearm volume were recorded during stepwise increases in transmural venous pressure. Transmural venous pressure was increased slowly to minimize non-uniform filling of veins and was held constant at each step until changes in forearm volume became stable. Compared to normotensive control subjects, forearm venous distensibility in young men with borderline hypertension was reduced (Fig. 4). Measurements were repeated after phentolamine 5 mg iv. Despite a small degree of venodilation, the differences in venous distensibility between hypertensives and normotensives persisted (Fig. 4).

Reports of reduced venous distensibility in essential hypertension are supported by experimental data. Shifts of pressure-volume curves toward the pressure axis in isolated veins and venous beds were demonstrated in dogs with one-kidney, one wrapped, rats with two- and one-kidney, one clip, and rats with spontaneous hypertension (Fig. 5) [17–20]. The isogravimetric method was used to demonstrate similar changes in the veins of dogs with deoxycorticosterone-salt and rats with spontaneous hypertension [21, 22].

Pathophysiology of reduced venous distensibility in hypertension

Characteristics of venous pressure-volume relationships in human hypertension and the way these measurements were obtained suggests that active venoconstriction did not significantly contribute to the findings. The methodology is such that 3–5 minutes are required after venous distention to complete the measurements. During this time stretch relaxation will occur, and active venoconstriction to a large extent will be overcome. The investigators who found a shift of venous pressure-volume curves toward the pressure-axis in human hypertension have either made these measurements during deflation of the venous congesting cuff or inflated the cuff slowly in stepwise fashion to minimize non-uniform filling of veins. The initial state of active venoconstriction has only a minor influence on pressure-volume curves observed during emptying or slow congestion of veins (see above and Fig. 2). The reported venous pressure-volume curves in human hypertension are curvilinear with convexity toward the volume axis. This type of curve is seen when active venoconstriction is eliminated by venodilator agents or by prolonged stretch and stretch relaxation (see above and Fig. 1). The shift of the venous pressure-volume curves persisted in the higher pressure ranges, where the resistance to stretch is provided by the connective tissue elements of veins. Using forearm venous plethysmography, it has been difficult to demonstrate either active venoconstriction by, for instance, tilting of subjects, or active venodilation by intravenous phentolamine (Fig. 4). The demonstrated changes have been minor and poorly reproducible, indicating that the method is more suitable for detecting passive (structural) than active compliance changes. Phentolamine resulted in a shift of forearm venous pressure-volume curves toward the volume axis in subjects with borderline hypertension but the differences in venous distensibility between hypertensives and normotensives persisted (Fig. 4), suggesting that there was a structural component to reduced venous distensibility in hypertension [16]. There was only a minor increase in VV 30 of hypertensive subjects after long-term guanethidine or reserpine treatment [14].

It was possible to examine the nature of venoconstriction in greater detail and under extreme circumstances in the experimental models of hypertension. The findings indicate that reduced venous compliance in experimental hypertension is predominantly structural in nature. Reduced compliance was demonstrated during both filling and emptying of veins (Fig. 5) and *in vivo* and *in vitro* [18–20]. Anti-adrenergic agents, venodilators and metabolic inhibitors did not reverse the shift of venous pressure-volume curves toward the pressure axis [17, 18]. Compliance changes persisted for several weeks after the reversal of hypertension in rats with one-kidney, one clip hypertension [23].

While there is evidence that reduced venous distensibility in human hypertension is predominantly structural in nature, the pathologic basis of this alteration is unclear. There is a paucity of pathologic examination of veins in human hypertension. We have examined the water, electrolyte, and glycosaminoglycan content of

796

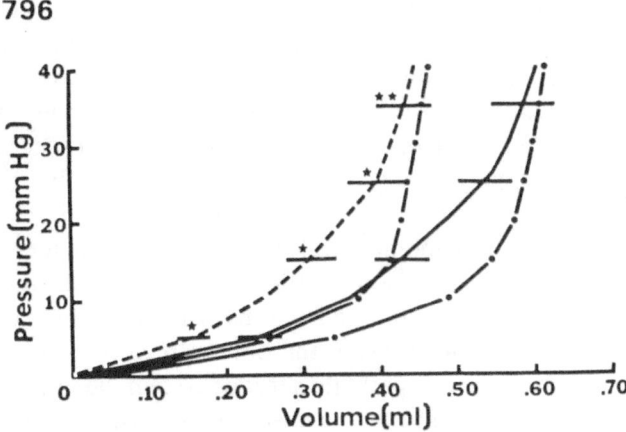

Figure 5. In vivo mesenteric vein pressure-volume curves (injection phase) in dogs with chronic one-kidney, one wrapped hypertension (dashed line, N = 15) and normotensive control dogs (solid line, N = 15). Dash-dot lines represent withdrawal phase. (From Simon G *et al.*, ref. 18. By permission.)

saphenous veins removed from hypertensive and normotensive patients undergoing coronary artery bypass surgery [24]. We found a small increase in the water and glycosaminoglycan content of veins from hypertensive subjects, but the electrolyte contents of their veins were unchanged. Our studies were hampered by the concomitant use of multiple medications, including diuretics, especially, by hypertensives, and the presence of complicating diseases. Extensive biochemical examination of veins has been carried out in the experimental models of hypertension. The principal finding has been the demonstration of waterlogging and increased sodium content of veins in experimental renal hypertension [19, 23, 25]. However, waterlogging and increased sodium content of veins do not fully explain reduced compliance because water and electrolyte changes may occur in the absence of demonstrable compliance changes and vice versa. In parabiotic rats, one unoperated and the other renal-hypertensive, we found increased water and sodium content of veins in both members of the pair, but venous pressure-volume changes were demonstrable only in the hypertensive rat [26]. Increased water and sodium content of veins in rats with one-kidney, one clip hypertension was reversed by reversing the hypertension but venous pressure-volume changes persisted for several weeks after the procedure [23]. Changes in the connective tissue elements of veins appear to play a more important role in the pathogenesis of reduced compliance than water and electrolyte changes. In rats with severe one-kidney, one clip hypertension, we found increased glycosaminoglycan content of veins [27]. The collagen content of veins, expressed per kg dry weight, was unchanged but changes in the physicochemical properties of collagen, making it less distensible, could not be ruled out [28, 29]. In spontaneously hypertensive rats, venous smooth muscle hypertrophy appears to be the cause of reduced venous distensibility [30].

The pathogenesis of human hypertension is not known; nor is the pathogenesis of reduced venous distensibility in hypertension. The structural changes in the wall of veins which maintain reduced compliance are not likely to be secondary to increased intraluminal pressure because venous pressure changes in human (and experimental) hypertension appear to be minor and transient. Rather, they must be the result of chronically acting neural or humoral stimuli. Because of the unpredictable and gradual onset of hypertension in human subjects, the investigation of the role of neural and humoral stimuli in the pathogenesis of reduced venous distensibility in this condition is difficult. In rats with chronic one-kidney, one clip hypertension, neonatal sympathectomy with guanethidine and bilateral adrenal medullectomy did not prevent the development of venous compliance changes, suggesting that the sympathetic nervous system did not play a predominant role in their pathogenesis [31]. We have provided several lines of evidence for the role of circulating humoral factors in the pathogenesis of increased water and sodium content of vascular tissue in the experimental models of renal hypertension, but these changes do not directly account for reduced venous compliance (see above) [26, 32, 33]. However, they may be markers for changes in the physicochemical properties of the connective tissue elements of the vessel wall, which may result in reduced compliance [29]. Based on parabiotic experiments with spontaneously hypertensive and Wistar-Kyoto normotensive rats, Greenberg also suggested that a circulatory humoral factor may be responsible for venous muscle hypertrophy and reduced compliance in hypertensive rats [34]. The identity and source of these putative humoral agents are not known.

Summary

Measured by plethysmography, forearm venous distensibility is reduced in chronic established and borderline essential hypertension. The reduction in venous distensibility is not reversed by either acute or chronic administration of anti-adrenergic agents. Characteristics of venous pressure-volume relationships in human hypertension suggest that active venoconstriction did not significantly contribute to reduced compliance. Venous compliance is also reduced in experimental animals with chronic renal, deoxycorticosterone-salt and spontaneous hypertension. Reduced venous compliance in the experimental models of hypertension has been shown to be predominantly structural in nature. The structural basis of reduced venous compliance in human and experimental hypertension appears to be the accumulation of ion-binding connective tissue polysaccharides in the wall of veins. An as yet unidentified circulating humoral agent may play a role in the pathogenesis of reduced venous distensibility in hypertension.

Supported by research grants from the Veterans Administration and by National Heart, Lung, and Blood Institute Research Grant HL-21673.

References

1. Alexander RS (1963): The peripheral venous system. In: Handbook of Physiology, Circulation, edited by Hamilton WE. Baltimore, Md: Williams and Wilkins Co., Vol. 2, pp 1075–1098.
2. Bader H (1963): The anatomy and physiology of the vascular wall. In: Handbook of Physiology, Circulation, edited by Hamilton WE. Baltimore, Md: Williams and Wilkins Co., Vol. 2, pp 865–888.
3. Wiederhielm CA (1965): Distensibility characteristics of small blood vessels. Fed Proc 24: 1075–1084.
4. Rothe CF (1983): Venous system: physiology of capacitance vessels. In: Handbook of Physiology, The Cardiovascular System, edited by Geiger SR. Bethesda, Md: Williams and Wilkins Co., Vol. 3, pp 397–452.
5. Shepherd JT, Vanhoutte PM (1975): Veins and Their Control. WB Saunders Co.
6. Anderson RM (1954): Intrinsic blood pressure. Circulation 9: 641–647.
7. Harrison LH, Frohlich ED (1970): Forearm venous reflex activity in normal and essential hypertensive subjects. Angiologica 7: 204–211.
8. Wood JE (1963): The Veins. Normal and Abnormal Function. Boston, Little, Brown and Co.
9. Whitney RJ (1953): The measurement of volume changes in human limbs. J Physiol 121: 1–27.
10. Bevegard SB, Shepherd JT (1965): Effect of local exercise of forearm muscles on forearm capacitance vessels. J Appl Physiol 20: 968–974.
11. Abramson DI, Fierst SM (1942): Resting blood flow and peripheral vascular responses in hypertensive subjects. Am Heart J 23: 84–96.
12. Wood EJ (1961): Peripheral venous and arteriolar responses to infusions of angiotensin in normal and hypertensive subjects. Circ Res 9: 768–772.
13. Caliva FS, Napodano RJ, Lyons RH (1963): Digital hemodynamics in the normotensive and hypertensive states. II. Venomotor tone. Circul 28: 421–426.
14. Walsh JA, Hyman C, Maronde RH (1969): Venous distensibility in essential hypertension. Cardiovasc Res 3: 338–349.
15. Simon G, Franciosa JA, Cohn JN (1979): Decreased venous distensibility in essential hypertension: lack of systemic hemodynamic correlates. Angiology 30: 147–159.
16. Takeshita A, Mark A (1979): Decreased venous distensibility in borderline hypertension. Hypert 1: 202–206.
17. Overbeck HW (1972): Hemodynamics of early experimental renal hypertension in dogs: normal limb blood flow, elevated limb vascular resistance and decreased venous compliance. Circ Res 31: 653–663.
18. Simon G, Pamnani MB, Dunkel JF, Overbeck HW (1975): Mesenteric hemodynamics in early experimental renal hypertension. Circ Res 36: 791–798.
19. Simon G, Pamnani MB, Overbeck HW (1976): Decreased venous compliance in dogs with chronic renal hypertension. Proc Soc Exp Biol Med 152: 122–125.
20. Simon G (1976): Altered venous function in hypertensive rats. Circ Res 38: 412–418.
21. Brock TA, Diana JN (1979): Effect of DOCA-NaCl hypertension on pre- and post-capillary resistance in isolated hindlimbs of dogs. Am J Physiol H586–H591.
22. Nilsson H, Folkow B (1980): Structurally reduced compliance of the venous capacitance vessels in spontaneously hypertensive rats. Acta Physiol Scand 110: 215–217.
23. Simon G (1980): Reversibility of arterial and venous changes in renal hypertensive rats. Hypert 2: 192–197.
24. Simon G, Conklin DJ, Altman S (1981): Abnormal saphenous vein composition in human hypertension. Clin Exp Hypert 3: 69–83.
25. Pamnani MB, Overbeck HW (1976): Abnormal ion and water composition of veins and normotensive arteries in coarctation hypertension in rats. Circ Res 38: 375–378.
26. Simon G (1978): Venous changes in renal hypertensive rats: role of humoral factors. Blood Vessels 15: 311–321.

27. Simon G, Altman S, Conklin DJ (1980): Venous wall electrolytes and hexosamines in hypertensive rats. Proc Soc Exp Biol Med 165: 13–16.
28. Simon G, Altman S (1978): Venous wall composition in hypertensive rats. Fed Proc 37: 349 (abstr).
29. Comper WD, Laurent TC (1978): Physiological function of connective tissue polysaccharides. Physiol Rev 58: 255–315.
30. Greenberg S, Palmer EC, Wilborn WM (1978): Pressure-independent hypertrophy of veins and pulmonary arteries of spontaneously hypertensive rats. Clin Sci Mol Med 55: suppl: 31–36.
31. Simon G (1981): Effect of sympathectomy on arterial and venous changes in renal hypertensive rats. Am J Physiol 241: H449–H454.
32. Simon G (1979): Angiopathic serum factor in perinephritic hypertensive dogs. Hypert 1: 197–201.
33. Simon G (1983): Passive transfer of pressor hyper-responsiveness from renal hypertensive to normotensive rats. Proc Soc Exp Biol Med 174: 356–362.
34. Greenberg S, Gaines K, Sweatt D (1981): Evidence for circulating factors as a cause of venous hypertrophy in spontaneously hypertensive rats. Am J Physiol 241: H421–H430.

Cardiac mechanoreceptors in hypertension

ALLYN L. MARK

Introduction

There is renewed awareness of the role of neurogenic mechanisms in the pathogenesis of hypertension. For many years, the interest in reflex mechanisms in
hypertension focused on arterial baroreceptors. However, with the recognition
that cardiac mechanoreceptors contribute physiologically to the regulation of
sympathetic nerve activity, renin release and vasopressin secretion, several investigators have evaluated the possibility that these receptors might be involved in
the pathophysiology of arterial hypertension.

In this chapter, I review briefly recent studies on cardiac mechanoreceptors in
spontaneously hypertensive rats; in the Dahl strain of salt-sensitive and resistant
rats; in renal hypertensive animals; and in humans with hypertension.

Several conclusions emerge from these studies. First, hypertension is frequently associated with an increase in the pressure threshold for cardiac mechanoreceptor discharge and a decrease in the discharge of these receptors over the
physiological range of cardiac filling pressures. Second, these alterations may be
offset by increases in the stimulus to cardiac mechanoreceptors so that the
inhibitory influence of these receptors may be normal or augmented rather than
decreased in hypertension. Third, cardiac mechanoreceptor function in hypertension is not static. Instead, it appears to vary with the severity or duration of
hypertension (presumably with the magnitude and duration of cardiac hypertrophy) and with sodium balance. Fourth, alterations in cardiac mechanoreceptor
function may contribute to abnormalities in sodium excretion, vascular resistance
and arterial pressure as well as renin and vasopressin in hypertension.

Spontaneously hypertensive rats (SHR)

The function of cardiac mechanoreceptors in SHR has been described in a series
of studies by Ricksten, Noresson and Thoren [1–6].

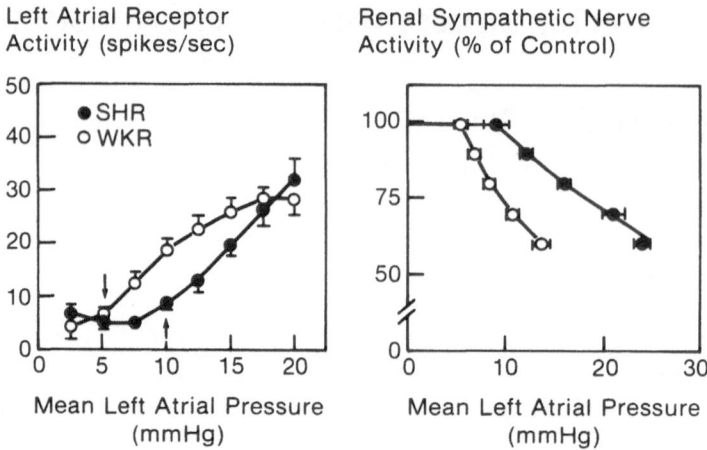

Figure 1. Abnormalities in cardiac sensory receptor function in spontaneously hypertensive rats compared with function in normotensive Wistar-Kyoto rats. The left panel shows resetting of the threshold for left atrial receptor activity to a higher pressure in spontaneously hypertensive rats than in Wistar-Kyoto rats (10.2 versus 4.6 mm Hg). The right panel shows the threshold and sensitivity for cardiac vagal afferent inhibition of renal sympathetic nerve activity during increases in left atrial pressure. The threshold was higher in spontaneously hypertensive rats than in Wistar-Kyoto rats (9.2 versus 5.4 mm Hg), and the slope of the curve relating atrial pressure to inhibition of sympathetic nerve activity tended to be flatter in spontaneously hypertensive rats. (From Ricksten, Noresson and Thoren [1, 2].)

The pressure threshold for high-frequency left atrial endings was elevated in SHR compared to normotensive Wistar-Kyoto rats (Fig. 1). As a result the pressure-discharge curve was shifted to the right in SHR although the maximal discharge of the left atrial endings did not differ in SHR and WKY (Fig. 1). The higher threshold of the atrial endings in SHR was accompanied by a corresponding alteration in the vagal afferent inhibition of renal sympathetic nerve activity. During volume expansion, a higher left atrial pressure was needed to inhibit renal sympathetic nerve activity in SHR than in WKY (Fig. 1). Furthermore, over a physiological range of left atrial pressures, e.g. 5 to 12 mm Hg, decreases in sympathetic nerve activity were less in SHR than WKY.

These alterations would be expected to decrease cardiac mechanoreceptor restraint on sympathetic activity in SHR. However, subsequent studies revealed that the higher pressure threshold of atrial endings in the SHR is offset (and perhaps even caused) by an elevation of left atrial pressure in the SHR [3]. The elevation of atrial pressure (10.3 mm Hg in SHR vs 4.6 mm Hg in WKY) results from a decrease in peripheral venous distensibility [4]. The decrease in venous distensibility also augments the increases in atrial pressure produced by volume expansion in SHR (Fig. 2).

As a result of the higher atrial pressures, the inhibition of sympathetic nerve activity during a 10% blood volume expansion is slightly greater in SHR than

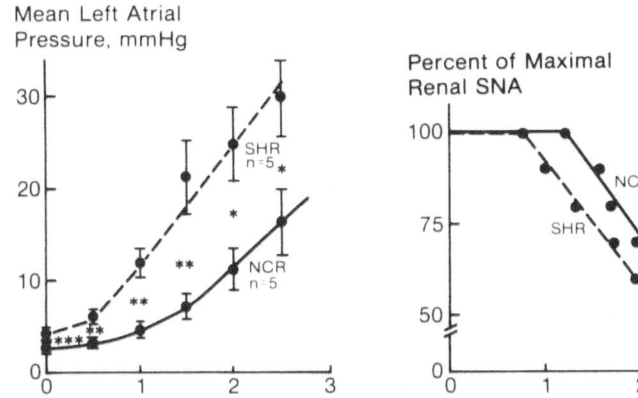

Figure 2. Increases in mean left atrial pressure and decreases in renal sympathetic nerve activity (SNA) during volume expansion in SHR and in Wistar-Kyoto normotensive control rats (NCR). Volume expansion caused greater increases in atrial pressure and a slightly greater inhibition of renal SNA in SHR. This indicates that the greater stimulus to cardiac mechanoreceptors in SHR (i.e. greater increases in atrial pressure) compensates for the higher pressure threshold of atrial endings in SHR. (From Ricksten, *et al.* [5].)

WKY (Fig. 2). In other words, the decreases in venous distensibility and the exaggerated increases in artrial pressure more than compensate for the higher pressure threshold of atrial endings in SHR so that the inhibitory influence of cardiac mechanoreceptors on renal sympathetic activity is augmented in SHR.

The augmented cardiac mechanoreceptor inhibition of renal sympathetic nerve activity in SHR appears to contribute to exaggerated natriuresis during volume expansion in SHR (Fig. 3) since the exaggerated natriuresis is attenuated by renal sympathetic denervation [6, 7].

The functional significance of the augmented cardiac receptor influence is also demonstrated by the work of Hoka *et al.* [8], who found that vagotomy produced greater increases in vascular resistance in young (12 weeks) SHR than in young WKY (Fig. 4). This demonstrates augmented cardiac vagal afferent modulation of vascular resistance in SHR with early established hypertension.

Thus, studies by investigators in Sweden and Japan indicate that the inhibitory influence of cardiac mechanoreceptors with vagal afferents is augmented in SHR with early established hypertension.

This augmented influence of cardiac vagal afferents disappears, however, in older SHR with chronic established hypertension [8]. Interrupting vagal afferents produced smaller increases in vascular resistance in old SHR compared with old WKY (35 weeks old). This decrease in cardiac vagal afferent influence in older SHR with chronic established hypertension occurred despite persistent elevation in atrial pressure. These observations indicate that with severe chronic hypertension, progressive impairment in cardiac sensory endings exceeds compensatory adjustments so that cardiac vagal afferent function decreases.

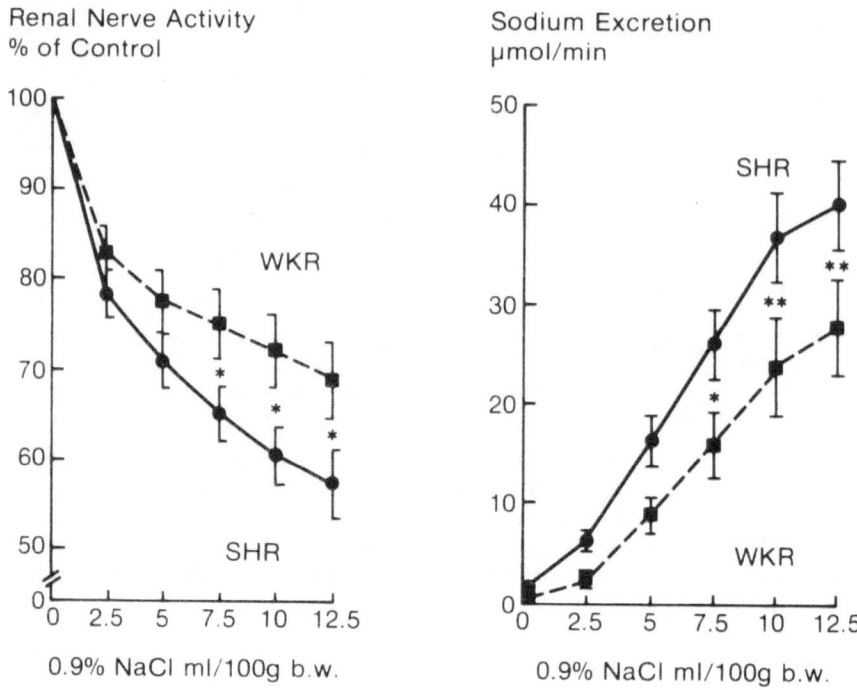

Figure 3. During volume expansion, there is an exaggerated inhibition of renal sympathetic nerve activity (SNA) in conscious SHR (solid lines) compared with normotensive Wistar-Kyoto rats (WKR) (broken lines). This is accompanied by exaggerated natriuresis in the SHR (from Ricksten, DiBona, *et al.* [6]). In a separate study [7], it was shown that the exaggerated natriuresis is attenuated by renal denervation.

Dahl salt-sensitive rats

Dahl genetically salt-sensitive (S) rats develop hypertension when fed a low sodium diet, but remain normotensive when fed a rigorously low sodium diet. Dahl S rats thus afford a valuable opportunity to study hypertension-prone animals in a prehypertensive phase and to examine mechanisms of salt-dependent hypertension. Dahl salt-resistant (R) rats remain normotensive with either low or high salt diet. Dahl R rats thus afford an opportunity to explore mechanisms of salt resistance.

Based on studies employing parabiosis and interstrain renal transplantation, Dahl and colleagues proposed that humoral and renal factors are paramount in the pathogenesis of the salt-induced hypertension in Dahl rats [9, 10]. Subsequent studies have implicated alterations in neurogenic control of vascular resistance in Dahl salt-dependent hypertension [11, 12]. These alterations in neurogenic control may relate partially to peripheral adrenergic [11] or central neural mecha-

Increase in hindlimb
resistance (%)

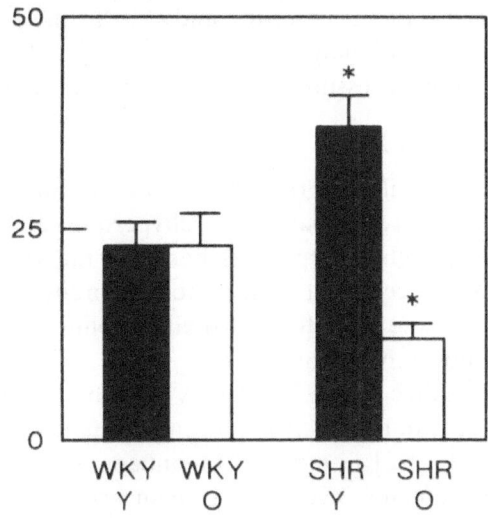

Figure 4. Effects of interrupting vagal afferents on hindlimb vascular resistance in young (12 weeks) and old (35 weeks) WKY and SHR. In young animals, vagotomy produced greater (* p<0.05) increases in resistance in SHR compared with WKY. In old animals, vagotomy produced smaller (* p<0.05) increases in resistance in SHR compared with WKY. This indicates that vagal afferent modulation of vascular resistance is augmented in young SHR and decreased in old SHR. (From Hoka, Takeshita *et al.* [8].)

nisms [13, 14], but recent studies in our laboratory have also identified abnormalities in afferent mechanisms [15–18], including cardiac mechanoreceptors with vagal afferents [18].

Ferrari *et al.* [18] compared cardiac mechanoreceptor function in prehypertensive Dahl S and R rats fed a low salt (0.4% NaCl) diet before increases in arterial or cardiac filling pressures and before the development of cardiac hypertrophy. Arterial baroreceptors were denervated and splanchnic sympathetic nerve activity was recorded during stimulation of cardiac baroreceptors by volume expansion with dextran. Volume expansion caused greater increases in cardiac filling pressures in Dahl S than in Dahl R rats [18]. Despite the greater stimulus to cardiac baroreceptors in S rats during volume expansion, there was less inhibition of sympathetic nerve activity in S compared with R rats so that cardiac baroreflex gain, calculated as percent inhibition of SNA divided by the increase in left ventricular end diastolic pressure was reduced in hypertension-prone S rats (-3.2 ± 0.2 in S vs -4.9 ± 0.6 in R; p<0.05).

This difference in cardiac baroreflex function appears to relate in large part to alterations in cardiac vagal afferents. Thoren *et al.* [19] found that atrial receptors with vagal unmyelinated afferents had a higher threshold in S rats (10 ± 1 mm Hg) than in R rats (6 ± 1 mm Hg).

Although the pressure threshold for atrial endings was reset to a higher level in the S rats, the maximal gain of the atrial endings was not different in S and R rats [19]. However, because of the resetting and shift to the right of the pressure-discharge curve, the increase in discharge of the atrial endings over a physiological range of cardiac filling pressures, e.g. 5 to 12 mm Hg, was less in S than R rats [19].

This resetting of the cardiac baroreceptors does not appear to relate to an alteration in the mechanical properties of the heart in S rats since Ferrari *et al.* [18] found no significant difference between prehypertensive S and R rats in atrial distensibility or heart weights. It appears, therefore, that the most likely explanation for the resetting of cardiac baroreceptors in prehypertensive DS rats is a genetic abnormality in the receptors, in their coupling to cardiac tissues, or in their humoral and ionic environment.

The resetting of cardiac baroreflexes may have hemodynamic consequences which could predispose to hypertension during sodium and volume loading. For example, Ferrari *et al.* [18] found that in sinoaortic denervated rats, volume expansion produced greater increases in mean arterial pressure in S ($+43 \pm 4$ mm Hg) than in R ($+28 \pm 5$ mm Hg) rats. This difference was abolished by interrupting vagal afferents ($+44 \pm 5$ in S vs $+41 \pm 4$ in R). This suggests that alterations in the cardiac mechanoreceptors with vagal afferents impair buffering of the pressor response to volume expansion in Dahl S rats.

Plasticity of mechanoreceptors in Dahl rats

There is recent evidence that the gain or sensitivity of cardiac baroreflexes is influenced by dietary sodium intake. Victor *et al.* [20] found that the gain of cardiac baroreflex inhibition of sympathetic nerve activity was augmented by a high salt diet in Dahl R rats, but was attenuated by high salt diet in S rats (Table 1). These changes parallel alterations in aortic baroreceptor afferent function in R

Table 1. Effects of dietary sodium on the gain of cardiac baroreflex in Dahl resistant and sensitive rats.

	Cardiopulmonary baroreflex gain		
	Low salt diet (0.1% NaCl)		High salt diet (8% NaCl)
Dahl resistant rats	-4.38 ± 0.37	$p < 0.05$	-6.24 ± 0.49
Dahl sensitive rats	-3.59 ± 0.44	$p = ns$	-2.49 ± 0.47

Cardiopulmonary baroreflex gain is expressed as the percentage decrease in sympathetic nerve activity per mm Hg increase in left ventricular end diastolic pressure produced by acute volume expansion in sinoaortic denervated rats. High salt diet augmented the gain in R rats, but tended to decrease gain in S rats. (Adapted from Victor *et al.* [20].)

and S rats during changes in dietary sodium [21]. High salt diet augments aortic baroreceptor discharge sensitivity in R but not in S rats. Thus, chronic increases in dietary salt sensitize both cardiac and arterial baroreceptor function in Dahl resistant rats. This plasticity in cardiac baroreceptor function, which might help protect against salt-induced hypertension, is lacking in Dahl sensitive rats, perhaps because of the development of hypertension and cardiac hypertrophy.

The mechanism of the salt-induced sensitization of cardiac mechanoreceptors in Dahl resistant rats is not clear. It does not appear to relate to salt-induced changes in cardiac distensibility [20]. It may involve ionic or humoral mechanisms. There is evidence for ionic sensitivity of cardiac [22] as well as arterial mechanoreceptors [23]. Thus, one possible explanation for salt-induced changes in cardiac baroreflexes might be salt-induced changes in the ionic environment of sensory endings in the heart. High salt diet does not alter concentrations of sodium and potassium in serum or arterial walls of Dahl rats [21, 24] which mitigates against these factors, but salt-induced changes in extracellular calcium remain a possible factor. Another possibility includes receptor sensitization by humoral factors released by high salt diet including the purported natriuretic hormone which inhibits Na-K ATPase [25]. Inhibition of Na-K ATPase with cardiac glycosides sensitizes both cardiac and arterial baroreceptors [26, 27].

Renal hypertension

Kezdi in 1976 reported the first studies of cardiac mechanoreceptor reflexes in hypertension [28]. He compared cardiac vagal afferent control of vascular resistance in normotensive and renal hypertensive dogs and observed that the cardiac pressure threshold for reflex vasodilation was higher in hypertensive dogs although the sensitivity of the cardiac vagal afferent reflex appeared to be preserved.

Thames and Johnson [29] recently studied vagal cardiopulmonary reflex control of renal sympathetic nerve activity in renal hypertensive and normotensive rabbits. In rabbits with arterial baroreflexes eliminated by sinoaortic denervation, stimulation of vagal afferents with volume expansion produced substantially smaller decreases in renal sympathetic nerve activity in renal hypertensive rabbits (Fig. 5).

These studies demonstrate that there is an increased pressure threshold and an impairment of the sensitivity of cardiac mechanoreceptors with vagal afferents in renal hypertensive animals. These observations indicate that alterations in cardiac mechanoreceptor function are found in acquired as well as spontaneous hypertension. The locus and mechanisms of these abnormalities are unclear.

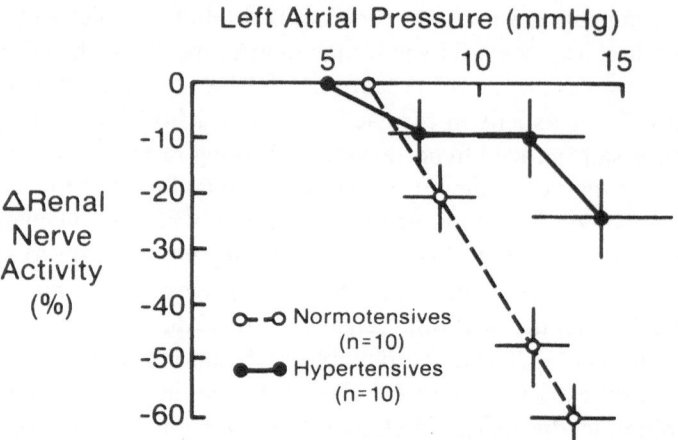

Figure 5. Relationship between changes in renal nerve activity and left atrial pressure during graded volume expansion in normotensive and renal hypertensive rabbits following sinoaortic baroreceptor denervation. Note the striking impairment of the inhibition of renal nerve traffic in the hypertensive group. Data are mean ± SE. (From Thames and Johnson [29].)

Hypertension in humans

Abnormalities in control of vascular resistance in human hypertensives have been attributed in part to abnormal neurogenic control. Bevegard *et al.* [30] and Kerber and I [31] studied reflex vasoconstrictor responses to inhibition of low pressure baroreflexes during decreases in cardiac filling pressure produced by lower body negative pressure (LBNP) in mild to moderately hypertensive men. Reflex forearm vasoconstrictor responses to LBNP were exaggerated in the hypertensive compared to normotensive subjects whereas reflex vasoconstrictor responses during inhibition of carotid baroreceptors with neck pressure were reduced in the hypertensive subjects (Fig. 6).

The augmented vasoconstrictor response could not be attributed to a non-specific influence of increased baseline resistance or to a generalized abnormality in reflex control since vasoconstrictor responses to another reflex stimulus, i.e. the cold pressor test, did not differ in the hypertensive and normotensive men [31].

The exaggerated reflex responses to LBNP in hypertensive subjects cannot be explained by an exaggerated influence of arterial baroreceptors since vasoconstrictor responses to neck pressure were less, not greater, in the hypertensive than in the normotensive subjects (Fig. 6).

The finding that the vasoconstrictor response to reducing the influence of cardiac mechanoreceptors is exaggerated in mild to moderately hypertensive humans suggests that the tonic inhibitory influence of cardiac mechanoreceptors

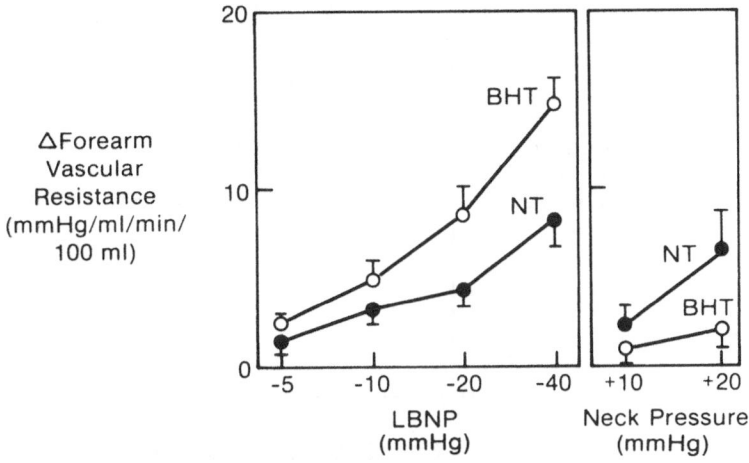

Figure 6. Forearm vascular responses to,lower body negative pressure (LBNP) and neck pressure in patients with borderline hypertension (BHT) and normotensive subjects (NT). Forearm vasoconstrictor responses to lower body negative pressure were augmented whereas forearm vasoconstrictor responses to neck pressure were impaired in the hypertensive subjects. This finding supports the view that cardiopulmonary baroreflexes are augmented and carotid baroreflexes are impaired in young men with borderline hypertension. (From Mark [31].)

is augmented in these subjects.

These observations have been extended by London *et al.* [32] who found a potentiated reflex forearm vasodilator response to stimulation of cardiac mechanoreceptors during head down tilting in patients with essential hypertension. This augmented reflex vasodilation was accompanied by greater increases in central venous pressure in the hypertensives, presumably secondary to decreased venous distensibility.

Several factors may contribute to the augmented inhibitory influence of cardiac mechanoreceptors. First, there is increasing evidence that cardiac filling pressures are elevated in human hypertensives, probably as a result of the decreased peripheral venous distensibility. Thus, the augmented influence of cardiac mechanoreceptors might reflect in large part a greater mechanical stimulus during diastole. Second, the higher left ventricular systolic pressure in hypertension may enhance the firing of left ventricular mechanoreceptors. Third, impaired arterial baroreflexes might contribute to the augmented inhibitory influence of cardiac mechanoreceptors. There is a central interaction of arterial and cardiac baroreceptors such that the inhibitory or buffering influence of cardiac baroreceptors is heightened when the inhibitory input from arterial baroreceptors is reduced as appears to be the case in chronic hypertension [33]. The possibility that this interaction may contribute to the augmented influence of cardiac mechanoreceptors in human hypertensives receives support from the observation that the slope of the relationship between central venous pressure and forearm vascular resis-

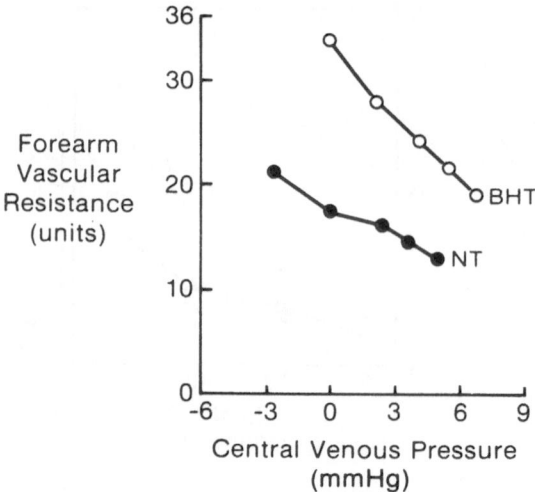

Figure 7. Relationship between central venous pressure and forearm vascular resistance in normotensive (NT) and borderline hypertensive (BHT) subjects. From right to left, the five values for each group were obtained in supine resting state and during lower body negative pressure (LBNP) at -5, -10, -20, and -40 mm Hg, respectively. The slope of the increases in forearm resistance divided by the decreases in central venous pressure during LBNP was significantly greater ($p<0.05$) in BHT (-1.92 ± 0.43) than in NT (-1.00 ± 0.28). (From Mark and Kerber [30].)

tance was steeper in hypertensive compared to normotensive subjects (Fig. 7).

We speculate that an augmented inhibitory influence of cardiac mechanorecep-tors might help explain several previous observations regarding humans with mild hypertension. During orthostatic stress, patients with borderline or mild hyper-tension have exaggerated increases in systemic vascular resistance [34–36] and plasma renin activity [37, 38]. These have been attributed at least partly to abnormalities in central neural or efferent mechanisms, but could relate partly to the finding of augmented cardiopulmonary baroreflex control. In mildly hyper-tensive subjects in the supine position, cardiopulmonary baroreceptors appear to exert an exaggerated inhibitory or buffering influence. Removal or reduction of this augmented inhibitory input during orthostatic stress (similar in effect to LBNP) might contribute to exaggerated reflex increases in vascular resistance and perhaps renin in BHT.

Conclusion

There is mounting evidence for alterations in cardiac mechanoreceptors in hyper-tension. These include an increase in the pressure threshold for mechanoreceptor discharge and a decrease in discharge of the receptors over a physiological range of cardiac filling pressures. These alterations in cardiac mechanoreceptor function are often offset by decreases in peripheral venous distensibility and increases in cardiac filling pressure, i.e. increases in the stimulus to the cardiac mechanoreceptors. As a result the inhibitory influence of cardiac mechanoreflexes may be normal or increased rather than decreased in hypertension. Cardiac mechanoreceptor function can differ in various models and stages of hypertension and with factors such as sodium balance so that the inhibitory influence of cardiac mechanoreceptors in hypertension is dynamic. There is increasing evidence that the alterations in cardiac mechanoreceptor function have implications for altered control of sodium excretion, vascular resistance and arterial pressure in hypertensive states.

Acknowledgments

I want to acknowledge the contribution of Drs. Alberto Ferrari, Ronald Victor, Peter Thoren and Frank Gordon and Mr. Donald Morgan who have participated in studies in the author's laboratory on cardiac receptors in hypertension. I also thank Ms. Sara Jedlicka and Ms. Nancy Davin for secretarial assistance.

The studies from the author's laboratory which are described in this review were supported by a program project grant HL14388 from the National Heart, Lung and Blood Institute and by research funds from the Veterans Administration.

References

1. Thoren P, Noresson E, Ricksten SE (1979): Resetting of cardiac C-fibers endings in the spontaneously hypertensive rat. Acta Physiol Scand 107: 13–18.
2. Ricksten SE, Noresson E, Thoren P (1979): Inhibition of renal sympathetic nerve traffic from cardiac receptors in normotensive and spontaneously hypertensive rats. Acta Physiol Scand 106: 17–22.
3. Noresson E, Ricksten SE, Thoren P (1979): Left atrial pressure in the spontaneous hypertensive rat. Acta Physiol Scand 107: 9–12.
4. Ricksten SE, Yao T, Thoren P (1981): Peripheral and central vascular compliance in conscious normotensive and spontaneously hypertensive rats. Acta Physiol Scand 112: 169–177.
5. Ricksten SE, Thoren P (1980): Reflex inhibition of sympathetic activity during volume load in awake normotensive and spontaneously hypertensive rats. Acta Physiol Scand 110: 77–82.
6. Ricksten SE, Yao T, DiBona GF, Thoren P (1981): Renal nerve activity and exaggerated natriuresis in conscious spontaneously hypertensive rats. Acta Physiol Scand 112: 161–167.
7. DiBona GF, Sawin LL (1986): Exaggerated natriuresis in experimental hypertension. Proc Soc Exp Biol Med 182: 43–51.
8. Hoka S, Takeshita A, Yamamoto K, Ito N, Ashihara T, Nakamura M (1984): Altered control of hindlimb vascular resistance by vagal afferents in spontaneously hypertensive rats. Circ Res 55: 763–772.
9. Dahl LK, Heine M (1975): Primary role of renal homografts in setting chronic blood pressure in rats. Circ Res 36: 692–696.

92

10. Knudsen KD, Iwai J, Heine M, Leitl G, Dahl LK (1969): Genetic influence on the development of renoprival hypertension in parabiotic rats. Evidence that a humoral hypertensinogenic factor is produced in kidney tissue of hypertension-prone rats. J Exp Med 130: 1353–1365.

11. Takeshita A, Mark AL (1978): Neurogenic contribution to hindquarters vasoconstriction during high sodium intake in Dahl strain of genetically hypertensive rats. Circ Res 43: I86–I91.

12. Takeshita A, Mark AL, Brody MJ (1979): Prevention of salt-induced hypertension in the Dahl strain by 6-hydroxydopamine. Am J Physiol 236: H48–H52.

13. Goto A, Ikeda T, Tobian L, Iwai J, Johnson MA (1981): Brain lesions in the paraventricular nuclei and catecholinergic neurons minimize salt-hypertension in Dahl salt-sensitive rats. Clin Sci 61: 53S–55S.

14. Brody MJ, Fink GD, Buggy J, Haywood JR, Gordon FJ, Knuepfer M, Mow M, Mahoney L, Johnson AK (1979): Critical role of the anteroventral third ventricle (AV3V) region in development and maintenance of experimental hypertension. Perspect Nephrol Hypertension 6: 76–84.

15. Gordon FJ, Matsuguchi H, Mark AL (1981): Abnormal baroreflex control of heart rate in prehypertensive and hypertensive Dahl genetically salt-sensitive rats. Hypertension 3: I135–I141.

16. Gordon FJ, Mark AL (1983): Impaired baroreflex control of vascular resistance in prehypertensive Dahl genetically salt-sensitive rats. Am J Physiol 245: H210–H217.

17. Gordon FJ, Mark AL (1984): Impaired baroreceptor function in prehypertensive Dahl salt-sensitive (DS) rats. Circ Res 54: 378–387.

18. Ferrari A, Gordon FJ, Mark AL (1984): Impairment of cardiopulmonary baroreflexes in Dahl salt-sensitive rats fed low salt. Am J Physiol 247: H119–H123.

19. Thoren P, Morgan DA, Mark AL (1985): Resetting of left atrial endings in Dahl sensitive rats on low salt diet. Circ 72: III248.

20. Victor RG, Morgan DA, Thoren P, Mark AL: Contrasting effects of high salt diet on cardiopulmonary baroreflexes in Dahl resistant and sensitive rats. Hypertension 8: II21–II27, 1986.

21. Ferrari A, Mark AL (1983): Adjustments of baroreceptor function to high salt intake in Dahl rats: a preliminary report. J Hypertension I(supp 2): 212–213.

22. Kunze DL, Orlea CJ (1980): The influence of calcium and potassium on atrial receptor discharge. Sleight P (ed) Arterial Baroreceptors and Hypertension, New York: Oxford Univ. Press, pp 88–90.

23. Kunze DL (1979):Calcium and magnesium sensitivity of the carotid baroreceptor reflex in cats. Circ Res 45: 815–821.

24. Abel PW, Trapani A, Matsuki N, Ingram MJ, Ingram FD, Hermsmeyer K (1981): Unaltered membrane properties of arterial muscle in Dahl strain genetic hypertension. Am J Physiol 241: H224–H227.

25. DeWardener HE (1977): Natriuretic hormone. Clin Sci Mol Med 53: 1–8.

26. Gillis RA, Quest JA (1978): Neural actions of digitalis. Ann Rev Med 29: 73–79.

27. Thames MD, Waickman LA, Abboud FM (1980): Sensitization of cardiac receptors (vagal afferents) by intracoronary acetyltrophanthidin. Am J Physiol 239: H628–H635.

28. Kezdi P (1976): Cardiac reflexes conducted by vagal afferents in normotensive and renal hypertensive dogs. Clin Sci Mol Med 51: 353S–355S.

29. Thames MD, Johnson LN (1985): Impaired cardiopulmonary baroreflex control of renal nerves in renal hypertension. Circ Res 57: 741–747.

30. Bevegard S, Castenfors J, Lindblad LE (1980): Effects of changes in blood volume distribution on circulatory regulation in young man with moderate hypertension. Sleight P, (ed) Arterial Baroreceptors and Hypertension, New York: Oxford Univ. Press, pp 492–498.

31. Mark AL, Kerber RE (1982): Augmentation of cardiopulmonary baroreflex control of forearm vascular resistance in borderline hypertension. Hypertension 4: 39–46.

32. London GM, Levenson JA, Safar ME, Simon AC, Guerin AP, Payen D (1983): Hemodynamic effects of head-down tilt in normal subjects and sustained hypertensive patients. Am J Physiol 245: H194–H202.

33. Abboud FM, Thames MD (1983): Interaction of cardiovascular reflexes in circulatory control. Shepherd JT and Abboud FM (eds) *Handbook of Physiology*, Am Physiol Soc, Bethesda, MD, pp,675–753.
34. Frohlich E, Tarazi R, Ulrych M, Dustan H, Page I (1967): Tilt test for investigating a neural component in hypertension. Circulation 36: 387–393.
35. Julius S, Esler M (1975): Autonomic nervous cardiovascular regulation in borderline hypertension. Am J Cardiol 36: 685–696.
36. Safar M, Weiss Y, Levenson J, London G, Milliez P (1973): Hemodynamic study of 85 patients with borderline hypertension. Am J Cardiol 31: 315–319.
37. Esler M, Nestel P (1973): Sympathetic responsiveness to head-up tilt in essential hypertension. Clin Sci 44: 213–226.
38. Kuchel O, Cuche J, Hamet P, Boucher R, Barbeau A, Genest J (1972): The relationship between adrenergic nervous system and renin in labile hyperkinetic hypertension. In: Genest J, Koiw E (eds) Hypertension. New York: Springer-Verga, pp 118–125.

Venous system, extracellular fluid volume and the kidney in essential hypertension

G.M. LONDON and M.E. SAFAR

The regulation of extracellular fluid (ECF) is a remarkable example of home-ostasis. Despite large and discontinuous variations in the salt and water intake, both ECF and plasma volume are held constant. The ECF regulation implicitly expresses the concept that volume is not regulated per se but is controlled relative to the holding capacity of the vascular and interstitial spaces. In fact, ECF control is nearly similar to the control of circulatory fullness, i.e. the control of mean circulatory pressure and filling pressure of the heart so as to ensure adequacy of the circulation, especially of the cardiac output. Changes in circulatory capaci-tance have a direct effect on circulatory filling pressure, with two consequences for ECF volume control. The first can be regarded as purely mechanical: the changes in circulatory filling pressure can influence the Starling forces regulating transcapillary fluid movements. The second is triggering of the response of various cardiac pulmonary mechanoreceptors affecting: (i) peripheral vascular resistances and the pre-to-postcapillary resistance ratio, and (ii) the renal mecha-nisms of excretion of sodium and water through changes in renal haemo-dynamics, plasma renin activity and other hormonal substances [1].

Venous compliance and the distribution of extracellular fluid volume

It has been reported that extracellular fluid volume is slightly, but significantly, increased in hypertension. However, in most of these studies, analyzed exten-sively in references [2], [3] and [4], an appreciable number of patients with renal parenchymal disease, cardiac impairment or malignant hypertension were in-cluded. Increased values of EFV and exchangeable sodium have also been observed in several (but not all) patients with primary aldosteronism [2–3]. But if the data presented in different reports are restricted to patients with uncompli-cated sustained essential hypertension, there is no increase in EFV and ex-changeable sodium [4].

The finding of reduced plasma volume (see Part II, p. 53ff.) and normal ECF in hypertension would suggest a disturbance in distribution between the intravascular and the interstitial compartments of ECF. Indeed, a decrease in the ratio between PV and interstitial fluid volume (IFV) has been shown in patients with sustained essential hypertension [2]. The decrease is found to be significant in severe [2–5], but not in mild hypertensives [6], reflecting a negative correlation between PV/IFV and blood pressure [5].

A normal EFV with reduced PV/IFV ratio suggests some disturbance in the mechanisms regulating EFV distribution. It has been established that any difference in resistance between the pre- and post-capillary vessels affects capillary hydrostatic pressure, and modifies capillary filtration [2]. Capillary filtration, which also depends on several factors such as arterial pressure, right atrial pressure and filtration coefficient, determines the distribution of body fluids between the intravascular and interstitial compartments. Thus, the decrease in the PV/IFV ratio could indicate an increase in filtration across the capillaries. Indeed, an increase in the transcapillary escape rate of albumin and Evans blue dye has been observed in essential hypertension [7–8]. The direct correlation of the transcapillary escape rate with the mean arterial pressure [7–8] was assumed to reflect an elevated capillary filtering pressure for which two explanations are possible: (i) inadequate protection by the precapillary sphincters and arterioles from the high systemic pressure, and (ii) changes in the post-capillary segment, mainly in venular distensibility and resistance. The findings of an inverse relationship between the intravascular volume and the PV/IFV ratio with blood pressure or total peripheral resistance could be taken to support the former possibility [2–5]. However, the correlation of arterial pressure with PV/IFV is weak, which excludes the precapillary factors from being the dominant mechanism of the decreased PV/IFV ratio [9]. It is more likely that the reduced PV/IFV ratio is related to decreased compliance of the venous bed. As well established [10], decreased venous compliance increases venous and cardiac filling pressures, thus directly influencing capillary hydrostatic pressure and fluid volume distribution. The strongly positive correlation observed between effective vascular compliance and the PV/IFV ratio (Fig. 1) in hypertensive supports this possibility and indicates the importance of venous factors in the mechanism of the decreased PV/IFV ratio [9].

Low pressure system, extracellular fluid volume and renal indices

In patients with sustained essential hypertension, glomerular filtration rate is normal and renal plasma and blood flow (RPF, RBF) are reduced. Thus the renal filtration fraction (FF) is increased [3]. In past years, the relationship between the kidneys and hypertension has been explored in man by studying the correlations between RFP or FF with blood pressure [2–11]. Although the kidney has a dominant role in the control of fluid volumes [12], no attempt was made to detect

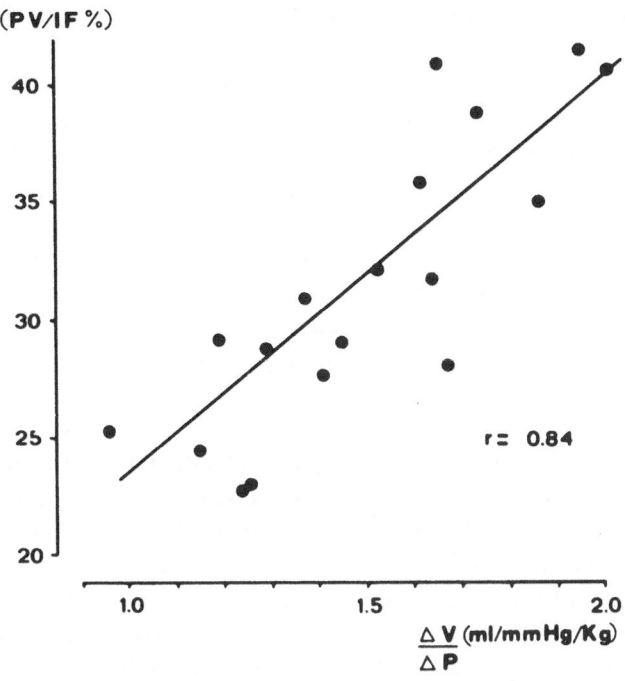

Figure 1. Sustained essential hypertension: relationship between the effective compliance of the vascular bed ($\triangle V/\triangle P$) and the ratio between plasma (PV) and interstitial (IF) fluid volumes (with courtesy of Circulation; see reference 9).

correlations between fluid volumes and renal indices. Such relationships are difficult to observe in normal subjects. However, they were found in hypertensives studied under steady-state conditions.

The first observation in hypertensives, taking fluid volume into consideration, concerned the finding of a pressure (or resistance) – volume disturbance. Indeed, several investigators have shown that, in essential hypertension, blood pressure and blood (or plasma) volume are inversely related [2]. A similar relationship has been observed between blood (or plasma) volume and the total peripheral resistance [2–3]. The latter correlation is more significant than the pressure–volume relationship and has been found in different types of hypertension, including borderline and sustained essential hypertension, renal artery disease, primary aldosteronism and pheochromocytoma. The pressure–volume and the resistance–volume relationships do no seem to depend on the methodology used for estimating blood volume. In addition, whatever reference to body size (weight, height, body surface area) is used to express blood volume, the relationships do not change [2, 5, 13, 14]. The negative pressure–volume relationship suggested an adaptive process between pressure and volume in man, i.e. when pressure is increased, volume is decreased, and thus contributes to maintain pressure within the normal range. Study of a large population of normotensive and hypertensive men of the same age facilitated the interpretation of the pressure (or resistance)–volume relationship [13–15]. When studied over a wide range of diastolic pressure (from 50 to 150 mm Hg), the pressure (or resistance)–volume curve was found to be curvilinear even using a semi-logarithmic scale [13–15]. Further, it can be clearly shown that the slope of the curve relating pressure (or resistance) and blood volume (dV/dP) was significantly steeper in normal and normotensive subjects than in hypertensive patients. The dV/dP value was shown to correlate well with RBF: the greater the inability to decrease the volume per unit rise in pressure, the greater the reduction in renal blood flow [13–15]. This suggested that, in essential hypertension, the blood volume was too high for the level of blood pressure, suggesting some modification in vascular compliance [16, 17].

Changes in vascular capacity could be partly responsible for the maintenance of sodium balance in hypertension. Lowenstein and coworkers [18] have found that renal venous pressure was higher in essential hypertensives than in normals and increased more during volume load [18]. Such modifications could account for the normal basic natriuresis and possibly explain the phenomenon of exaggerated natriuresis after sodium load in patients with essential hypertension [18]. Recent data of our laboratory [19] showed that the increase in hydrostatic forces in the low-pressure system could compensate for the increased peritubular oncotic forces in hypertensive kidneys. The renal filtration fraction is negatively related to vascular capacitance (Fig. 2) [17] and a negative correlation is observed between peritubular oncotic pressure and vascular compliance. Moreover, a positive correlation is observed between central venous pressure and postglomerular oncotic pressure [19]. Thus, the increase in 'low-pressure system' filling pressure due to decreased systemic capacitance may cause an abnormal fluid movement in the systemic capillaries with a fluid shift and a decreased PV/IF ratio and the same hydrostatic force, at the renal peritubular capillary level, may correct and cancel the higher oncotic pressure, equilibrating the Starling forces [3].

Cardiopulmonary receptors and the low pressure system

The reduced vascular compliance in hypertensives is associated with increased cardiac filling pressure and normal cardiopulmonary blood volume. This creates favorable conditions for cardiopulmonary mechanoreceptors stimulation and neurohumoral control of the ECF volume and systemic circulation. This is especially true in conditions of acute volume load, since CVP and cardiopulmonary blood volume increase more in hypertensive patients than in controls [9, 20], resulting in a higher stretch of cardiac mechanoreceptors. In the absence of cardiac hypertrophy, such an increased stretch could induce an exaggerated

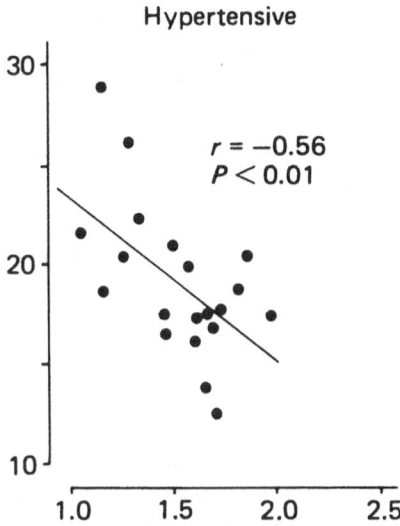

Figure 2. Sustained essential hypertension: relationship between effective compliance of the vascular bed (ordinate) and the renal filtration fraction (abcissa) in comparison with normotensive subjects (with courtesy of Kidney International; see reference 17).

reflex response while, in the presence of cardiac hypertrophy, such a modification could maintain normal reflex responses [21–23]. In patients with essential hypertension, information about the cardiopulmonary reflexes is scarce. Only the reflex regulation of forearm blood flow and plasma renin activity received particular attention [23–25].

Control of the forearm resistive vessels in man is under the influence of cardiopulmonary receptors [26–28]. Increase in central venous pressure and/or cardiopulmonary blood volume induces a reflex vasodilation of the forearm circulation and vice versa [23–25]. In borderline and established essential hypertension, an augmentation of forearm vascular reflexes has been observed [23–25]. In patients with established hypertension, this augmentation is due to an increased reflexogenic stimulus, i.e. a higher elevation in central venous pressure during central blood volume expansion [24]. The intensity of the reflex response is correlated with the basal degree of 'venous constriction', a fact which supports the role of the mechanical properties of capacitance system in the circulatory reflex control [24]. The nature of augmented forearm response in patients with borderline hypertension seems different since the changes in central venous pressure were similar in controls and in borderline hypertensive subjects [23]. However, the interpretation is difficult since, in patients with borderline hypertension, the changes in cardiopulmonary blood volume were not evaluated at the same time [23].

In normal man, the study of the response of plasma renin activity to changes in cardiopulmonary blood volume and/or presssure indicates that these changes are reciprocal, i.e. an increase in central volume and pressure induces a decrease in plasma renin activity and vice versa [29, 30]. In patients with sustained essential hypertension the relationship between plasma renin activity and cardiopulmonary blood volume (or pressure variations) is not well documented. It seems that hypertensive patients respond normally to changes in central venous pressure, i.e. plasma renin activity decreases when cardiopulmonary blood pressure increases, and, to the contrary, plasma renin activity increases when central venous pressure decreases [24]. The role of the capacitance system in the reflex control remains still unclear, but the decrease in compliance of veins seems to be responsible for a 'resetting' of the reflex both in animals and in men [22, 24].

The role of venous compliance in the maintenance of cardiopulmonary blood volume and pressure could, theoretically, have many consequences on the regulation of several hormonal systems, especially those responsible for the 'natriuretic' activity of the plasma. The maintenance of a diastolic stretch of the cardiopulmonary circulation in hypertensives could explain the finding of elevated circulating concentrations of natriuretic substances [31]. On the other hand, during acute sodium and volume load, the higher cardiopulmonary expansion which occurs in hypertensives could also produce a higher concentration of natriuretic factors and thus participate to the phenomenon of 'exaggerated natriuresis' observed in patients with essential hypertension [31, 32].

Acknowledgments

This study was performed with a grant from the Institut National de la Santé et de la Recherche Médicale (INSERM), the Association pour l'Utilisation du Rein Artificiel (AURA), the Ministère de la Recherche, Paris. We thank Miss Danièle Saquè for her excellent assistance.

References

1. Gauer OH, Henry JP, Behn C (1970): Regulation of extracellular fluid volume. Annu Rev Physiol 32: 547–595.
2. Tarazi RC: Hemodynamic role of extracellular fluid in hypertension. Circ Res Suppl 2: 38, 73–83.
3. Safar ME, London GM, Simon ACh, Chau NPh (1983): Volume factors, total exchangeable sodium and potassium in hypertensive disease, in hypertension: Physiopathology and treatment. Genest J Edit, 2nd ed. 42–54.
4. Schalekamp MADH, Birkenhager WH, Lever AF (1977): Volume factors, total exchangeable sodium and potassium in hypertensive disease. In: Hypertension Physiopathology and Treatment. Edited by Genest, E. Koiv, O. Kuchel, New York, pp 49–58.
5. Simon ACh, Safar ME, Levenson JA, Aboras NE, Alexandre JM, Pauleau NF (1979): Extracellular fluid volume and renal indices in essential hypertension. Clin Exp Hypertension 1 (5): 557–576.

6. Bauer JH, Brooks CS (1979): Volume studies in men with mild to moderate hypertension. Am J Cardiol 44: 1163–1169.

7. Parving HH, Gyntelberg F (1973): Transcapillary escape rate of albumin and plasma volume in essential hypertension. Circ Res 32: 643–651.

8. Ulrych M (1973): Plasma volume decrease and elevated Evans blue disappearance rate in essential hypertension. Clin Sci Mol Med 45: 173–181.

9. London GM, Safar ME, Simon ACh, Alexandre JM, Levenson JA, Weiss YA (1978): Total effective compliance, cardiac output and fluid volumes in essential hypertension. Circulation 57: 995–1000.

10. Echt M, Duweling J, Gauer OH, Lange L (1974): Effective compliance of the total vascular bed and the intrathoracic compartment derived from changes in central venous pressure induced by volume changes in man. Circ Res 20: 581–589.

11. Kaplan NM (1979): The Goldblatt Memorial lecture; Part II: The role of the kidney in hypertension. Hypertension 1: 456–461.

12. Guyton AC, Coleman TG, Cowley AW, Scheel KW, Manning RE, Norman RA (1974): Arterial pressure regulation. Overriding dominance of the kidneys in long-tem regulation and in hypertension. In: Hypertension Manual, Laragh JH (ed), New York, Dun-Donnelley, pp 111–134.

13. Safar ME, London GM, Weiss YA, Milliez PL (1975): Altered blood volume regulation in sustained essential hypertension: a hemodynamic study. Kidney International 8: 42–47.

14. London GM, Safar ME, Weiss YA, Corvol PL, Lehner JP, Menard JM, Simon AC, Milliez PL (1977): Volume-dependent parameters in essential hypertension. Kidney International 11: 204–208.

15. Safar ME, Chau NPh, Weiss YA, London GM, Simon ACh, Milliez PL: The pressure-volume relationship in normotensive and permanent essential hypertensive patients. Clin Sci Mol Med 50: 207–212.

16. Seely JF, Levy M (1981): Control of extracellular fluid volume. In: The Kidney, edit by Brenner BM and Rector FC. Philadelphia: Saunders, pp 371–407 and 733.

17. London GM, Safar ME, Levenson JA, Simon AC, Temmar MA (1981): Renal filtration fraction, effective vascular compliance, and partition of fluid volumes in sustained essential hypertension. Kidney International 20: 97–103.

18. Lowenstein J, Beranbaum ER, Chasis H, Baldwin DS (1970): Intra-renal pressure and exaggerated natriuresis in essential hypertension. Clin Sci 38: 359–374.

19. London GM, Levenson JA, London AM, Simon AC, Safar ME (1984): Systemic compliance, renal hemodynamics and sodium excretion in hypertension. Kidney Int 26: 342–350.

20. Safar ME, London GM, Levenson JA, Simon ACh, Chau NPh (1979): Rapid dextran infusion in essential hypertension. Hypertension 1: 615–623.

21. Ricksten SE, Yao T, Thoren P (1981): Peripheral and central vascular compliances in conscious normotensive and spontaneously hypertensive rats. Acta Physiol Scand 112: 169–175.

22. Hallback-Nordlander M, Noresson E, Thoren P (1979): Hemodynamic consequences of left ventricular hypertrophy in spontaneously hypertensive rats. Am J Cardiol 44: 986–991.

23. Mark AL, Kerber RE (1982): Augmentation of cardiopulmonary baroreflex control of forearm vascular resistance in borderline hypertension. Hypertension 4: 46–49.

24. London GM, Levenson JA, Safar ME, Simon AC, Guerin AP, Payen D (1983): Hemodynamic effects of head-down tilt in normal subjects and sustained hypertensive patients. Am J Physiol 245 (Hear Circ Physiol 14): H194–H198.

25. Bevegard BS, Castenfors J, Lindblad LE (1977): Effects of changes in blood volume distribution on circulatory variables and plasma renin activity in man. Acta Physiol Scand 99: 237–245.

26. Shepherd JT, Vanhoutte PM (1975): The veins and their control. Philadelphia, Saunders, vol 1, p 269.

27. Roddie IE, Shepherd JT (1963): Nervous control of the circulation in skeletal muscle. Brit Med Bull 19: 115–119.

102

28. Zoller RR, Mark AL, Abboud FM, Schmid PG, Heistad DD (1972): The role of low-pressure baroreceptors in reflex vasoconstriction response in man. J Clin Invest 51: 2967–2972.
29. Epstein M, Saruta T (1971): Effects of water immersion on renin-aldosterone and renal sodium handling in normal man. J Appl Physiol 31: 368–374.
30. Kiowski W, Julius S (1978): Renin response to stimulation of cardiopulmonary mechanoreceptors in man. J Clin Invest 62: 656–663.
31. DeWardener HE, McGregor GA (1982): The natriuretic hormone and essential hypertension. Lancet 1: 1450–1454.
32. Bates ER, Shenker Y, Grekin RJ (1986): The relationship between plasma level of immunoreactive atrial natriuretic hormone and hemodynamic function in man. Circulation 73, No 6, 1155–1161.

Part III

Large vessels and the concept of arterial compliance

Systolic hypertension in the elderly

EDWARD D. FROHLICH and FRANZ H. MESSERLI

The overall problem of hypertension in the aging patient has received increasing attention in recent years. Appreciation of this major concern has increased for several reasons: (1) the elderly segment of most Western industrialized populations (i.e., individuals older than 65 years of age) has more than doubled during this generation to upwards of 10 to 15 percent of the total population [1, 2] and this proportion is still increasing; (2) upwards of 50 percent of this elderly population have either diastolic or isolated systolic hypertension [3, 4]; (3) relatively recent reports demonstrate that the rise of arterial pressure with aging is neither a 'normal' nor an innocuous physiological phenomenon [5–10]; (4) reduction of arterial pressure in elderly individuals may be expected to be associated with an overall reduction in cardiovascular morbidity and mortality [11–14]; and (5) the recent emphasis on the feasibility of reducing isolated systolic arterial pressure elevation by pharmacological means [15] has led to a large multicenter study designed to demonstrate the safety and efficacy of its pharmacological treatment.

Although much emphasis has been put over the past three decades on the role of the pharmacological treatment of diastolic pressure elevation with its ensuing improvement of morbidity and mortality we must bear in mind the clear lessons from epidemiological data: systolic pressure elevation is most likely a better predictor of the cardiovascular complications of hypertension than diastolic pressure elevation [8]; and isolated systolic hypertension imparts a two- to five-fold excess risk of cardiovascular death [9], an incidence of stroke 2.5 times more than for those without isolated systolic hypertension [10], and a 51 percent excess mortality as compared with age-matched normotensive controls [16].

Epidemiological considerations

Classification

In the United States and elsewhere, severity of hypertension has been classified primarily by the height of diastolic pressure [17, 18]. However, the upper limit of normal has recently been defined in the United States as 89 mm Hg; and a level of 'high normal blood pressure' has also been defined as occurring in patients whose diastolic pressures fall between 85 and 89 mm Hg [17]. It was reasoned that these latter individuals were at a higher risk of developing hypertension and other cardiovascular problems later in life [19]. Another difference occurred with the definition of mild essential hypertension. In the recent Joint National Committee's third report this was defined as diastolic pressure falling between 90 through 104 mm Hg [17], whereas the World Health Organization has defined this range of diastolic pressures as between 95 through 104 mm Hg [18]. It is important to recognize these definitions with respect to diastolic pressure in order to identify patients classified with respect to systolic pressures (Table 1).

According to the Joint National Committee's third report, systolic pressure elevation has been said to occur in those individuals whose systolic pressure is in excess of 139 mm Hg. Patients whose diastolic pressures are less than 90 mm Hg but whose systolic pressures fall between 140 through 159 mm Hg are said to have borderline systolic hypertension; and if the systolic pressure is 160 mm Hg and greater (with diastolic pressure <90 mm Hg), they have *isolated systolic hypertension*. It is this latter group of patients whose problem falls under the purview of this discussion.

Prevalence of Isolated Systolic Hypertension (ISH)

There have been two major reports that have focused on the prevalence of patients with ISH, one from the Evans County Study [20] and the other from the Hypertension Detection and Follow-Up Program (HDFP) [21]. Earlier, the National Center for Health Statistics reported an 8.5 percent prevalence of ISH in

Table 1. Classification of blood pressures [17].

Pressure range (mm Hg)	Classification
Systolic (when diastolic <90):	
<140	Normal blood pressure
140–159	Borderline isolated systolic hypertension
≥160	Isolated systolic hypertension
Diastolic:	
<85	Normal blood pressure
85–89	High normal blood pressure
90–104	Mild hypertension
105–114	Moderate hypertension
≥115	Severe hypertension

elderly individuals 65 through 74 years of age (the 1971–74 census) [22]. This finding compares favorably to the 8.4 percent prevalence of ISH for individuals whose ages fell between 40 and 90 years of age in Evans County [20] and a 6.8 percent prevalence in the HDFP study [21]. These prevalence data, however, are at variance with the present definitions outlined above since ISH was defined as occurring when diastolic pressures were less than *95 mm Hg* (not 90 mm Hg). Further differences related to the means of obtaining the pressure measurements: the Evans County study pressure measurements were obtained in the study clinics whereas in the HDFP study pressures were also obtained in the individuals' home settings. From these data, the HDFP reported an all-cause mortality rate (adjusted for age, race, and sex) of 17.6 percent in people with ISH as compared with a 7.7 percent in those whose systolic pressures were less than 160 mm Hg [21].

Implications

The implications of these epidemiological findings are clear. ISH in the elderly is a frequent finding that imparts a definite excess risk of 'all-cause' as well as cardiovascular mortality (and morbidity). As indicated from the prospectively conducted Framingham Study this abnormality confers an increased predisposition for later development of coronary heart disease, sudden death, congestive heart failure, and stroke. Since these data are clear-cut two natural questions follow: (1) will control of the elevated isolated systolic pressure result in a reduced morbidity and mortality; and (2) what is the best means of achieving this pressure

Table 2. Hemodynamic differences in younger and older men with isolatd systolic hypertension data represent the mean ($\pm$ ISEM) [24].

	Younger men (<35 years)		Older men (>35 years)	
	Normal	ISH	Normal	ISH
Number of men	11	13	7	13
Age (years)	23 (1.5)	27 (1.0)	45 (3.1)	49 (1.6)
Arterial pressures (mm Hg):				
Systolic	120 (3.3)	155 (1.5)*	132 (5.8)	159 (1.9)*
Diastolic	74 (1.6)	87 (1.4)*	76 (1.8)	87 (1.3)*
Mean	91 (2.0)	110 (1.1)*	95 (3.1)	112 (1.1)*
Heart rate (bpm)	65 (1.6)	74 (3.9)*	70 (5.2)	67 (2.2)
Cardiac index (L/min/m²)	2.9 (0.1)	3.3 (0.1)	3.2 (0.16)	2.5 (0.1)*
Left ventricular ejection rate				
index (ml/sec/m²)	145 (7.8)	171 (8.1)*	152 (4.5)	127 (7.5)*
Total peripheral resistance				
index (μ/m²)	33 (2)	35 (2)	29 (1)	45 (2)*

* Denotes statistical significance with a p-value of at least <0.05.

control? A recent small multicenter feasibility study conducted by the National Heart, Lung, and Blood Institute [15] suggested that a larger study be initiated and that the use of a thiazide congener diuretic might provide the best form of therapy [23]. These studies are, at best, preliminary and the overall results will not be forthcoming for several years. Nevertheless, a better insight into the disease and its treatment should be achieved from an understanding of the fundamental pathophysiological alterations associated with ISH. This will be the substance of most of this discussion.

Pathophysiological considerations

Despite the high prevalence of the problem, as indicated from the foregoing discussion of its epidemiological considerations, there has been a paucity of reports detailing the pathophysiological changes associated with an isolated arterial pressure rise. Most of our physiological information concerning these changes has been inferred from information obtained from patients with systolic hypertension coexisting with diastolic pressure elevation. The following discussion will be concerned primarily with isolated systolic hypertension. Where information is available related to patients with both systolic and diastolic pressure elevation this will be so delineated.

Systemic hemodynamics

Several years ago, in the first systematic study of this problem, we compared systemic hemodynamic changes in younger (under 35 years of age) and older (over 35 years) individuals with systolic arterial pressure elevation who were matched with normotensive individuals of the same age, race, and sex [24]. Several important findings became apparent. First, even though systolic pressures were elevated by design of the study and patients with diastolic pressure elevation were likewise excluded, the patients with the 'isolated systolic hypertension' had significantly higher diastolic pressures than age- and sex-matched normotensive control subjects – whether older or younger than 35 years. Secondly, the elevated systolic pressure elevation in the younger individuals was associated with a hyperdynamic circulation manifested by an increased heart rate, elevated cardiac output and a greater index of left ventricular contractility. In contrast, the systolic pressure elevation of the 'older' patients was associated with a significantly reduced cardiac output and left ventricular ejection rate and an increased total peripheral resistance. Thirdly, the intravascular (plasma) volume was normal in the younger patients but was *contracted* significantly in the older patients. Our succeeding studies, performed in different patients and with different associates, continued to demonstrate that the elevated arterial pressure of aging subjects was associated with (1) a normal or reduced cardiac output heart rate, and myocardial contractility; (2) an increased total peripheral resistance; and (3) a contracted plasma volume (18.2 ± 0.8 vs. 16.4 ± 0.4 ml/cm) [24]. In one recent study, however, we found that the systolic pressure was significantly higher and diastolic pressure lower in elderly hypertensive patients (average age 73 years) whose mean arterial pressure was matched with young subjects [25] (Fig. 1). In another study from our laboratory with a different group of patients whose age averaged 50 years [26], we confirmed the systemic hemodynamic characteristics of older patients with ISH that we had reported earlier [24].

In a study conducted similarly to those reported from our laboratory, but designed primarily to evaluate the compliance of the larger arteries, Simon and his associates demonstrated that the ISH of their older group of patients (age 51 years) was associated with a significant reduction in arterial compliance (as estimated from the monoexponential blood pressure-time curve during diastole [27]. These data, from several different laboratories, strongly demonstrate that vastly different hemodynamic mechanisms underlie the pathophysiological changes in younger and older patients with ISH. Thus, in the younger patients the systolic pressure elevation is associated with a hyperdynamic circulation that may be driven by adrenergically mediated factors. In contrast, the elevated systolic pressure of the older patients was maintained by factors subserving an increased total peripheral resistance and reduced compliance of the larger arteries.

Notwithstanding this implication of potentially different mechanisms underlying the ISH (i.e., adrenergic participation in the younger and loss of arterial elasticity and distensibility in the older patients) two important additional concepts are apparent. First, in these studies the initial thought – that atherosclerosis may underlie the alterations that make the arteries less compliant in the older individual – may not be the sole explanation. These older patients were, on the average, 51 and 49 years in the Simon et al. studies, and ours, respectively. Clinically significant large arterial atherosclerotic vascular disease was not present and the physiological alteration was not fixed since pharmacological agents that dilated the arteries reversed the compliance changes [27]. Secondly, there was a contraction in plasma volume in the older patients. Volume contraction would not be possible with only a precapillary pressure rise, and therefore a certain degree of postcapillary constriction must have taken place to permit the transcapillary exchange of plasma from the intravascular compartment. And, in this regard, it is of interest that large arterial constriction may not be the sole explanation for the increased total peripheral resistance; arteriolar constriction may also participate since, in our early study, patients with systolic hypertension also had significantly higher diastolic pressures than the matched normotensive subjects.

110

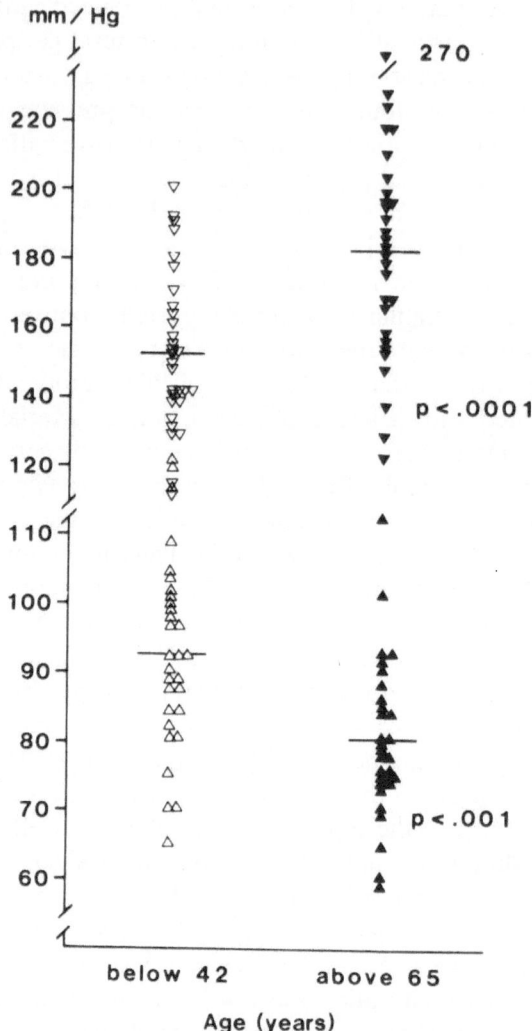

Figure 1. Systolic and diastolic pressures of elderly patients with hypertension (right column) who were matched with younger patients (left column) according to mean arterial pressure. ▼ = systolic pressure; ▲ = diastolic pressure.

Reduced large arterial compliance

An important hemodynamic consideration, particularly when one must consider the possibility of therapeutic options, is the role of the larger arterial vessels as well as the smaller arterioles that account for the increased total peripheral resistance. The large arterial vessels contribute a certain degree of active constriction mediated by an increased state of contractility of the vascular smooth muscle in the wall of these vessels. But, in addition, other factors compound this increased resistance to the forward flow of blood by reducing arterial distensibility. This latter factor may be explained on the basis of an altered viscoelastic state of these larger arteries [28–31]. These changes are observed in hypertension even in the absence of advancing age or clinically significant atherosclerosis [26, 27, 31–36] and have been explained, in part, on the basis of structural changes that have been associated with hypertensive vascular disease [26–28, 33–38]. It is possible however, that these changes may be related to still other complicating factors including aging and atherosclerosis, processes that are most difficult to dissociate from the hypertensive disease [39–43]. Moreover, in a few elderly subjects the arterial stiffening may become so excessive as to interfere with the measurement of arterial pressure by cuff (pseudohypertension). This entity may be suspected clinically by a palpable radial artery even after the ipsilateral occlusion of blood flow by cuff pressures exceeding systolic values (Osler's maneuver) [44].

That these changes of reduced arterial compliance and distensibility are, most likely, at least in part related to the problem of hypertensive vascular disease may be inferred by its presence in patients with borderline or mild essential hypertension who are in their late 30s or early 40s [34–36, 43–48]. Moreover, were these alterations exclusively related to fixed structural changes brought about by aging and atherosclerotic changes they would not likely be reversed, at least to some extent, immediately by pharmacological interventions [27] or with a variety of forms of prolonged antihypertensive therapy including diuretics [23, 48–51].

That these patients with ISH may not be volume-dependent [24] and may demonstrate a spectrum of plasma renin activity by 'renin-profiling' and responsiveness to antihypertensive therapy with diuretic therapy as well as angiotensin converting enzyme or beta-adrenergic receptor inhibiting therapy [52] suggests that there may be no one pathophysiological factor that will explain ISH. Once again, then, the mosaic of factors underlying the control of arterial pressure is suggested [53, 54]. It therefore seems reasonable to conclude that the large (and small) arterial changes that account for the elevated total peripheral resistance and reduced compliance and distensibility in patients with ISH are not solely explained by fixed structural changes associated with aging or atherosclerosis.

Conclusion

Earlier reports seemed to relate the changes of isolated systolic hypertension to increased stroke volume, and increased rate of systolic ejection; however these findings are not supported by recent and more controlled studies. Increased arterial stiffness, explained on the bases of aging and atherosclerosis, was the explanation for the changes; but, as suggested by Koch-Weser, were this the case diastolic pressures should be reduced and this is not the usual finding [55]. In fact, as suggested by our earlier report [24], diastolic pressures may be even higher than in an age-, sex-, and racially matched group of normotensive subjects. Thus, more information is needed to explain more clearly the physiological mechanisms that subserve these functional derangements of increased arteriolar resistance and reduced arterial compliance in ISH. As suggested above, these mechanisms most likely are interdependent with one another and in some patients one or more may participate more than others. To conclude prematurely that one form of therapy is more likely than others to be effective may exclude those therapeutic options such as the possibility of monotherapy and reducing the chances of drug interactions and side effects. In an older population who may be using other drugs for coexistent diseases or who may be more predisposed to side effects because of those drugs, this may be an unwise and precipitous therapeutic decision. Thus, it seems entirely appropriate to draw from our clinical and investigative experiences over the years in patients with essential hypertension to view ISH as another expression of multifactorial essential hypertension.

References

1. Health and Nutritional Examination Study (HANES), 1971–1974 Vital and Health Statistics Series II, No. 203 (1977): Blood pressure levels of persons 60–74. U.S. National Center for Health Statistics, Department of Health, Education, and Welfare.
2. Office of Population Consensus and Surveys (1971): Population projections, 1970–2010. London, H.M.S.O.
3. Ostfeld AM, Shekelle RB, Klawans H, Tufo HM (1974): Epidemiology of stroke in an elderly welfare population. Am J Pub Healh 64: 450–458.
4. Drizd T, Dannenberg A, Engel A: Blood presssure levels in persons 18–74 years of age in 1976–80, and trends in blood pressure from 1960–80 in the United States. *Vital Health Stat* 1986; 11, DHHS Publication No. (PHS) 86–1684.
5. Page LB (1980): Hypertension and atherosclerosis in primitive and acculturating societies. In: Hypertension Update: Mechanisms, Epidemiology, Evaluation, and Management, Hunt JC (ed), Bloomfield, NJ, Health Learning Systems, pp 1–12.
6. Genest J, Larochelle P, Kuchel O, Hamet P, Cantin M (1983): Hypertension in the elderly: athero-arteriosclerotic hypertension, Chapter 56. In: Hypertension: Physiopathology and Treatment, 2nd ed, Genest J, Kuchel O, Hamet P, Cantin M (eds), New York, McGraw-Hill Book Company, pp 913–921.
7. Atherosclerosis Study Group: Kannel WB, Doyle JT, Ostfeld AM, Jenkins CD, Kuller L, Podell RN, Stamler J (1984): Optimal resources fom primary prevention of atherosclerotic diseases. Circulation 70: 157A–205A.
8. Kannel WB (1976): Some lessons in cardiovasular epidemiology from Framingham. Am J Cardiol 37: 269–282.
9. Kannel WB (1981): Implications of Framingham study data for treatment of hypertension: Impact of other risk factors. In: Frontiers in Hypertension Research, Laragh JH, Bühler FR, Seldin DW (eds), New York, Springer-Verlag, pp 17–21.
10. Shekelle RB, Ostfeld AM, Klawans HL Jr (1974): Hypertension and risk of stroke in an elderly population. Stroke 5: 71–75.
11. Hypertension Detection and Follow-Up Program Cooperative Group (1979): Five-year findings of the Hypertension Detection and Follow-Up Program. II. Mortality by race, sex and age. JAMA 242: 2572–2577.

12. Hypertension Detection and Follow-Up Program Cooperative Group (1982): Five-year findings of the Hypertension Detection and Follow-Up Program. III. Reduction in stroke incidence among persons with high blood pressure. JAMA 247: 633–638.

13. National Heart Foundation of Australia (1981): Treatment of mild hypertension in the elderly: Report by the Management Committee. Med J Aust 2: 398–402.

14. Amery A, Birkenhäger W, Brixko P, Bulpitt C, Clement D, Deruyttere M, De Schaepdryver A, Dollery C, Fagard R, Forette F, Forte J, Hamdy R, Henry JF, Joossens JV, Leonetti G, Lund-Johansen P, O'Malley K, Petrie J, Strasser T, Tuomilehto J, Williams B (1985): Mortality and morbidity results from the European Working Party on High Blood Pressure in the Elderly Trial. Lancet 1(8442): 1349–1354.

15. Hughes G, Schnaper HW (1982): The isolated systolic hypertension in the elderly program. International Journal of Mental Health 2: 76–97.

16. Blood Pressure Study 1979. Chicago: Society of Actuaries and Association of Life Insurance Medical Directors of America, 1980.

17. The Joint National Committee on the Detection, Evaluation and Treatment of High Blood Pressure (1984): The 1984 report of the Joint National Committee on Detection, Evaluation, and Treatment of High Blood Pressure. Arch Intern Med 144: 1045–1057.

18. Report of WHO Expert Committee (1978): Arterial Hypertension, World Health Organization Technical Report Series, No. 628. Geneva, Switzerland, World Health Organization.

19. Final Report of the Subcommittee on Definition and Prevalence of the 1984 Joint National Committee (1985): Hypertension prevalance and the status of awareness, treatment, and control in the United States. Hypertension 7: 457–468.

20. Wing S, Aubert RE, Hansen JP, Hames CG, Slome C, Tyroler HA (1982): Isolated systolic hypertension in Evans County. I. Prevalence and screening considerations. J Chronic Dis 35: 735–742.

21. Curb JD, Borhani NO, Entwisle G, Tung B, Kass E, Schnaper H, Williams W, Berman R (1985): Isolated systolic hypertension in 14 communities. Am J Epidemiol 121: 362–370.

22. National Center for Health Statistics, Blood Pressure Levels of Persons 6–74 years. United States, 1971–1974,, Series 11, No. 203. Rockville, MD: National Center for Health Statistics, 1977. (DHEW publication no. [HRA] 78–1648).

23. Hulley SB, Furberg CD, Gurland B, McDonald R, Perry HM, Schnaper HW, Schoenberger JA, Smith WMcF, Vogt TM (1985): Systolic hypertension in the elderly program (SHEP): Antihypertensive efficacy of chlorthalidone. Am J Cardiol 56: 913–920.

24. Adamopoulos PN, Chrysanthakopoulis SG, Frohlich ED (1975): Systolic hypertension: Non-homogeneous diseases. Am J Cardiol 36: 697–701.

25. Messerli FH, Sundgaard-Riise K, Ventura HO, Dunn FG, Glade LB, Frohlich ED (1983): Essential hypertension in the elderly: Haemodynamics, intravascular volume, plasma renin activity, and circulating catecholamines. Lancet 2: 983–986.

26. Messerli FH, Ventura H, Aristimuño GG, Suarez DH, Dreslinski GR, Frohlich ED (1982): Arterial compliance in systolic hypertension. Clin Exper Hyper A4: 1037–1044.

27. Simon AC, Safar MA, Levenson JA, Kheder AM, Levy BI (1979): Systolic hypertension: Hemodynamic mechanisms and choice of antihypertensive treatment. Am J Cardiol 44: 505–511.

28. Hallock P, Benson IC (1937): Studies on the elastic properties of human isolated aorta. J Clin Invest 16: 595–602.

29. Peterson LH, Jensen RE, Parnell J (1960): Mechanical properties of arteries in vivo. Circ Res 8: 622–639.

30. Gow BS, Taylor MG (1968): Measurement of viscoelastic properties of arteries in the living dog. Circ Res 23: 111–122.

31. O'Rourke MF (1970): Arterial hemodynamics in hypertension. Circ Res 27 (II): 123–133.

32. Finberg MH (1927): Systolic hypertension: its relationship to atherosclerosis of the aorta and larger arteries. Am J Med Sci 173: 835–842.

33. Wolinski H (1972): Response of the rat aortic media to hypertension. Circ Res 30: 301–309.
34. Tarazi RC, Magrini F, Dustan HP (1975): The role of aortic distensibility in hypertension. In: International Symposium On Recent Advances in Hypertension, Miller P, Safar ME (eds), Monte Carlo, Boehringer Ingelheim, pp 133–142.
35. Randall OS, Esler MD, Calfee RV, Bullock GF, Maisel AS, Culp B (1976): Arterial compliance in hypertension. Aust NZ J Med 6 (II): 49–59.
36. Alicandri CL, Agabiti-Rosei E, Fariello R, Beschi M, Boni E, Castellano M, Montini E, Romanelli G, Zaninelli A, Muiesan G (1982): Aortic rigidity and plasma catecholamines in essential hypertensive patients. Clin Exper Hyper A4: 1073–1083.
37. Hallbäck M, Lundgren Y, Weiss L (1974): The distensibility of the resistance vessels in spontaneously hypertensive rats (SHR) as compared with normotensive control rats (NCR). Acta Physiol Scand 90: 57–68.
38. Mulvany MJ, Halpern W (1977): Contractile properties of small arterial resistance vessels in spontaneously hypertensive and normotensive rats. Circ Res 41: 19–26.
39. Landowne M (1958): The relation between intraarterial pressure and impact pulse wave velocity with regard to age and atherosclerosis. J Gerontol 13: 153–162.
40. Abboud FM, Huston JH (1961): The effects of aging and degenerative vascular disease on the measurement of arterial rigidity in man. J Clin Invest 40: 933–939.
41. Abboud FM, Huston JH (1961): Measurement of arterial aging in hypertensive patients. J Clin Invest 40: 1915–1921.
42. Folkow B (1978): Cardiovascular structural adaptation; its role in the initiation and maintenance of primary hypertension. Clin Sci Mol Med 55: 3s–22s.
43. Gribbin B, Pickering TJ, Sleight P (1979): Arterial wall distensibility in normal and hypertensive men. Clin Sci 56: 413–417.
44. Messerli FH, Ventura HO, Amodeo C (1985): Osler's maneuver and pseudohypertension. N Eng J Med 312: 1548–1551.
45. Simon AC, Safar ME, Levenson JA, London GM, Levy BI, Chau NP (1979): An evaluation of large arteries compliance in man. Am J Physiol 237: H550–H554.
46. Safar ME, Simon AC, Levinson JA (1984): Structural changes of large arteries in sustained essential hypertension. Hypertension 6 (Suppl. 3): 117–121.
47. Ventura HO, Messerli FH, Oigman W, Suarez DH, Dreslinski GR, Dunn FG, Reisin E, Frohlich ED (1984): Impaired systemic arterial compliance in borderline hypertension. Am Heart J 108: 132–136.
48. Smulyan H, Vardau S, Griffiths A, Gribbin B (1984): Forearm arterial distensibility in systolic hypertension. J Am Coll Cardiol 2: 387–393.
49. European Working Party on High Blood Pressure in the Elderly. Antihypertensive therapy in patients above age 60 with systolic hypertension. Clin Exper Hypertension 4: 1151–1176.
50. Seligmon AW, Alderman MH, Davis TK (1979): Systolic hypertension: occurrence and treatment in a defined community. J Am Geriat Soc 27: 135–138.
51. Niarchos AP, Weinstein DL, Laragh JH (1984): Comparison of the effects of diuretic therapy and low sodium intake in isolated systolic hypertension. Am J Med 77: 1061–1068.
52. Niarchos AP, Laragh JH (1984): Renin dependency of blood pressure in isolated systolic hypertension. Am J Med 77: 407–414.
53. Page IH (1967): The mosaic theory of arterial hypertension – its interpretation. Perspect Biol Med 10: 325–333.
54. Frohlich ED (1983): Mechanisms contributing to high blood pressure. Ann Intern Med 98: 709–714.
55. Koch-Weser J (1973): Correlation of pathophysiology and pharmacotherapy in primary hypertension. Am J Cardiol 32: 499–510.

Large arteries in borderline and sustained essential hypertension

ALAIN SIMON and JAIME LEVENSON

The large arteries are important to consider in hypertension, because they serve two important functions: a) to conduct the blood from the heart to the capillary beds; and b) to store a fraction of ventricular outflow in their distensible walls in order to buffer the pulsatile hemodynamics generated by the heart [1]. Another reason of interest is that large arteries represent the specific site of the circulation where the degenerative vascular damage occurs [2]. However, until recently, the large arteries have received little attention in clinical investigation, because of the serious difficulties in measuring non-invasively and quantitatively their state and function in man. Recent innovations in vascular technology have reversed this situation and led to important gains in knowledge of human large arteries especially in hypertension, which is the most common pathological model which affects early the arterial system in man. Because the large arteries include multiple branches from the proximal aorta to the peripheral arteries, only some of them have focused attention to date: the aorta, which is the main distensible chamber of the arterial tree and the brachial artery which represents the clinical site of pressure measurements [2].

I. The aorta

Two kinds of techniques are available for the quantification of human aorta properties: (i) the aortic imput impedance, which relates simultaneously re-corded aortic pressure and flow waveforms under specific mathematical condi-tions and operations and (ii) the systemic arterial compliance which is defined from the quantitative analysis of the morphology of the aortic pressure curve.

1. The imput impedance of the aorta

Aortic imput impedance represents one measure of the opposition to pulsatile ventricular outflow presented by the physical properties of the systemic arteries and of the blood. It is calculated as the instantaneous ratio of pressure and flow waves in the ascending aorta [3]; practical calculation of this pressure-flow ratio requires to transform pressure and flow pulses into a sum of sinusoidal waves, or harmonics, superimposed on the mean pressure and flow, according to the Fourrier theorem, by using an analog-to-digital converter and a computer. Each harmonic of pressure and flow is a complex number, described by its modulus (amplitude), phase angle (timing in relation to other harmonics) and frequency (multiple of the fundamental frequency equal to heart rate). Harmonics of impedance are calculated as the ratio of pressure and flow modulus and as the difference between pressure and flow phases at the same frequency and are represented (impedance spectrum) as a plot of moduli and phases of the impedance against the frequency of its harmonic [3].

In human hypertension, the general form of aortic impedance spectrum exhibits several differences with normal state [4, 6] (Table 1). The elevation of peripheral resistance reflects the reduction in the caliber of arterioles which is classically admitted as the hall-mark of sustained essential hypertension. The increase in impedance moduli at low frequencies (especially in the first harmonic) has not got a clear physiological signification, but it implies that more ventricular energy than in normal state is lost in vascular pulsations [7]. The shift to the right of modulus minimum and phase cross-over reflects a functional reflection site nearer from the heart than in normal because the frequency of modulus minimum and phase cross-over represents the frequency at which reflecting sites are one quarter wave length away [3]; this nearer reflecting site can be explained by enhanced constriction of the peripheral arterioles and also by increased pulse wave velocity, as observed in the hypertensive human aorta [5], so contributing to earlier return of wave reflection. The increased characteristic impedance is the more specific feature of hypertensive aorta which is not dependent on age since it persists when hypertensive patients are compared to age-matched normal subjects [10]; characteristic impedance which represents the impedance of the aorta, considered as an open tube in the absence of reflections [3], is directly related to the elastic properties of the aortic walls but inversely related to its cross-sectional area [3]; since the aorta radius was reported to be increased in hypertension [5],

Table 1. Effects of hypertension on the general form of aortic impedance spectrum comparatively with the normotensive state.

Impedance Patterns	Effects of Hypertension
Peripheral resistance	Increase
Impedance moduli at low frequencies	Increase
Minimum of impedance moduli	Shift to the right
Characteristic impedance	Increase

the enhanced characteristic impedance implies a loss of aortic distensibility even in the presence of compensatory effect of its larger cross-sectional area.

Thus, the alterations of the impedance spectrum at the entrance of hypertensive aorta imply profound changes in the distensible properties of the aorta. The question is raised if the hypertensive changes in impedance reflect only the effect of elevated distending pressure itself on the stretch of the aortic walls [8]; indeed arteries become stiffer as they are distended, presumably because more and more of the wall stress is borne by collagen as the diameter increases [8]. This fact can be observed for the elevation of pressure that follows intravenous infusion of norepinephrine [9], or angiotensin [5] in normotensive subjects; the impedance spectrum of the aorta then exhibits modifications comparable to those observed in chronic hypertension; inversely the decrease in arterial pressure that follows intravenous infusion of sodium nitroprussid [5] in hypertensive subjects is accompanied by a decrease in the impedance moduli at low frequencies, a shift to the left of the frequency of the modulus minimum and a decrease of the characteristic impedance. These observations suggest that abnormality of the aortic impedance spectrum in hypertension could depend mainly on the elevated transmural pressure; however, the modifications observed with vasoactive substance impair the interpretation of the role of pressure 'per se' because their pharmacological action may also alter the active tension of smooth muscles of the arterial wall [10]. Thus to date, it cannot be concluded if increased aortic impedance in hypertension depends only on elevated transmural pressure or rather on structural adaptive changes of the arterial walls consecutive to chronic state of hypertension as suggested by experimental studies [11].

2. The systemic arterial compliance

Systemic arterial compliance, or absolute volume distensibility of the aorta and peripheral elastic arteries is the ratio of arterial volume rise to the accompanying rise in pressure (dV/dP) [11]; its evaluation is based on the analysis of the morphology of the arterial pressure wave via a reasonably simple model of the arterial circulation [12, 13]. The analysis of the pressure wave as function in time, is facilitated when it is restricted to the diastolic segment of the pressure curve because, during the diastole, the aortic valves are closed [13]; thus the diastolic waveform can be considered as the transient response of the arterial system to the pressure change occurring in systole [14]; the general shape of diastolic pressure assumes a simple mono-exponential form [14] with some oscillations superimposed, principally in the first part of diastole [12]. The fact that the oscillations of the pressure curve are practically absent in the last part of diastole, is related to the fact that the last part of diastole contains mainly the low frequencies of the impedance spectrum [15]; the lack of pressure fluctuations in telediastole permits with some exceptions to use the mono-exponential decline in pressure to calculate arterial compliance on the basis of a simple 'Windkessel' model [13]. The fundamental property of this model is that the product between the compliance and the resistance equals the reciprocal of the semilogarithmic linear slope of the exponential decline in pressure – i.e. the time constant of the system – (Fig. 1). Thus the compliance of large arteries, or systemic arterial compliance, can be simply calculated as the ratio between the time constant of the mono-exponential pressure decay in the last two-thirds of diastole (Fig. 1), and the resistance of the arterial tree assumed to be the total peripheral resistance; this latter assumption is justified by the existence of a close linear relation through zero between the time constant of the diastolic pressure and the total peripheral resistance calculated as the mean arterial pressure divided by cardiac output [13]. In practice, arterial pressure was directly recorded from a punction into the brachial artery rather than from aortic catheterisation because the diastolic portion of the pressure wave, has few significant distortions during its travel from the aorta to the brachial artery [16].

In human hypertension, the reduction in systemic arterial compliance is a constant pathological feature which was observed at different stages of the disease, such as juvenile borderline hypertension [12], sustained systolodiastolic hypertension [13] and systolic hypertension in elderly patients [19]. The observation that systemic arterial compliance is reduced in young borderline hypertensive patients comparatively to normal subjects of similar age is of interest. It shows that the decrease in compliance of the large arteries begins early in the development of hypertensive disease; one might argue that this decreased arterial compliance could be caused by the elevated pressure [8] 'per se' because of the non-uniform elastic composition of human large arteries; however, the 30% decrease in arterial compliance observed in these patients was associated with an only 9% increase in mean arterial pressure compared with that of the normal subjects, so that arterial compliance was clearly inappropriately more reduced than would be expected from the slight increase in arterial pressure alone. Thereby it seems likely that other factors involving the activation of the sympathetic nervous system contribute to reduce arterial compliance in borderline hypertensive patients. Further morphological and biochemical studies are, however, necessary to document and delineate such factors in humans with borderline hypertension. In chronic systolo-diastolic hypertension, systemic arterial compliance is strongly decreased comparatively with normotensive state [12, 13] at similar age (Fig. 2); then the reduction in arterial compliance could reflect the decrease in arterial distensibility which occurs with pressure increase, because of the non-linear elastic properties of human arteries [8] or the adaptative change of arterial walls to chronic hypertension [11, 17]. The first possibility is supported by the fact that intravenous angiotensin infusion in normotensive subjects decreased sytemic arterial compliance concomitantly to pressure elevation toward values observed in chronic hypertension [18]. However, this observation did not demonstrate the exclusive role in pressure for decreasing arterial compliance; pressure

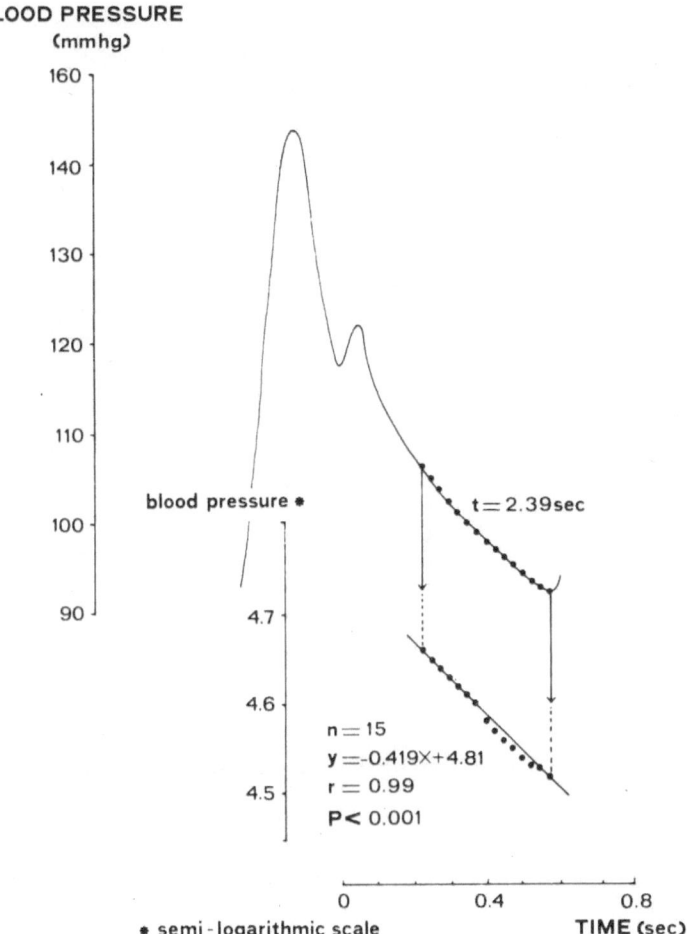

Figure 1. Method for calculation of the time constant of the diastolic pressure decay. From Simon *et al.* [13] with permission.

changes are induced in acute and not in long-term situation, and vasoactive agents may modify the active tension of the arterial wall [10]. In isolated systolic hypertension (systolic level above 160 mm Hg and diastolic level less than 95 mm Hg) of patients over 50 years of age systemic arterial compliance was found to be strongly decreased comparatively to age-matched normotensive controls (Fig. 2); and inversely related to the value of systolic arterial pressure [19]. Moreover, intravenous infusions of sodium nitroprusside or nitroglycerine increased systemic arterial compliance and decreased concomitantly systolic pressure toward normotensive values [19]. These observations suggest that isolated systolic hypertensive of patients over 50 years of age is directly related to a reduction of compliance of the aorta and large arteries. The mechanism of this arterial

120

ARTERIAL COMPLIANCE IN HYPERTENSION

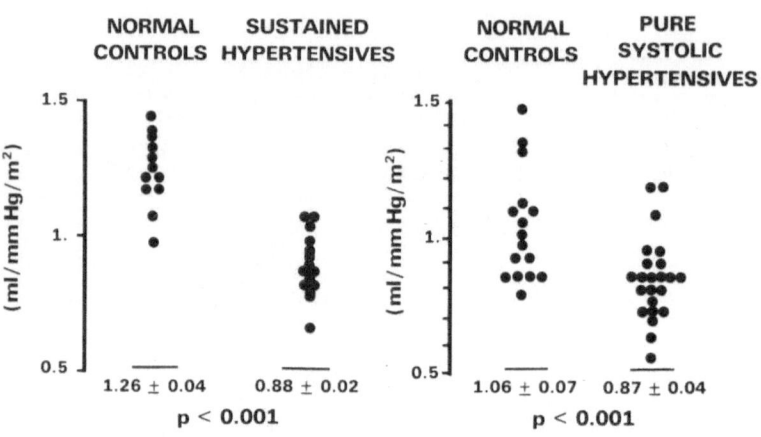

SYSTEMIC ARTERIAL COMPLIANCE

FOREARM ARTERIAL COMPLIANCE

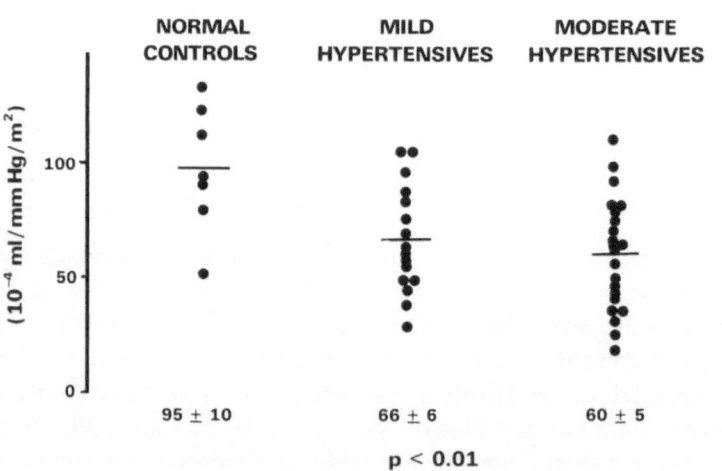

Figure 2. Systemic and forearm arterial compliance in normotensive subjects and in hypertensive patients. Values are mean ± 1 SEM. Pure systolic hypertensives denote isolated systolic hypertension in the elderly, while hypertensives (mild, moderate, sustained) denote hypertension in the middle aged.

compliance reduction cannot be related to a distending pressure effect since diastolic and mean level of blood pressure are not different in patients and in controls [19]. Thus it remains that the reduced arterial compliance reflects a chronic increased rigidity of the walls of the large arteries, which is consistent with the frequency of arterial calcifications or atherosclerotic lesions in older patients with systolic hypertension [20].

II. The brachial artery

Although it supplies the forearm circulation which is not a site particularly affected by vascular complications, the brachial artery is of primary importance in human hypertension because it represents the site of pressure measurements in clinical and epidemiological studies. Its investigation is based upon two types of methodology: (i) estimation of pulse wave velocity and (ii) pulsed Doppler arterial measurements.

1. Pulse wave velocity

The velocity with which a pulse wave (pressure or flow) travels along an artery is accepted as a good measure of arterial distensibility and commonly used in clinical studies to express the relative volume distensibility according to the equation of Bramwell and Hill [21].

$$C^2 = 1/\varrho D$$

D is the relative volume distensibility which represents the ratio between the percent change in arterial volume dV/V and the unit rise in pressure dP; p is the blood density. Transforming the equation of Bramwell and Hill for a circumferential tube whose radius is R and length L, the absolute volume distensibility per unit length of artery, or arterial compliance (dV/dP), can be expressed as follows [22, 23]:

$$dV/dP = \pi R^2/\varrho C^2$$

From this equation it appears that a simple measurement of pulse wave velocity along an artery permits to estimate arterial compliance, providing that the arterial radius is concomitantly evaluated [23]. The most common method of determining the pulse wave velocity along the brachial artery is to apply, non-invasively, two strain-gauge tranducers to the skin, over the course of the vessel, and to measure the ratio of the distance between the two transducers to the time-delay between the two pulses curves recorded. The time delay can be measured from the foot of the curves – i.e. the point at which the curves begin to rise at the end of diastole (foot-to-foot velocity) because this point has been found little affected by reflections, and closely related to the apparent or 'true phase velocity' [23, 24].

In human hypertension pulse wave velocity was reported increased in the brachial artery which indicates that distensibility is reduced in hypertensive patients comparatively to normotensive subjects [23]. However, the precise mechanism of these arterial changes is questioned. Age is the first variable to be taken into consideration since pulse wave velocity was found to increase with age probably because of loss of arterial distensibility due to the process of aging [25, 26]. Another factor to discuss is the distending arterial pressure which can 'per se' increase pulse wave velocity because the elastic modulus of the artery becomes greater as it is stretched by increase in pressure. To elucidate the role of these two factors in the increased pulse wave velocity of hypertensive patients, the patients were compared in terms of the continuous gradation that occurs in normal subjects between pulse wave velocity, and the product of age and arterial pressure [23] (Fig. 3). Such relations are supposed to express the effect of the natural aging process on arterial properties, and the product of age and pressure represents a quantitative expression of the accelerating effect of pressure on this aging phenomenon [26]. In some hypertensive patients pulse wave velocity was observed to be higher than the value corresponding to the normal aging and pressure effect. This observation permitted the classification of hypertensive patients according to whether their pulse wave velocity was inside (Group 1) or outside (Group 2) the 95% confidence bands of normal regression of pulse velocity with the product of age and pressure. These two groups of patients had similar values of age and pressure but showed marked differences with respect to the state and function of large arteries (Fig. 4). In Group 1, the observation that pulse wave velocity increased within the limits of the normal regression with the product of age and pressure indicates that 1) the aging factor is related to these arterial modifications by the same relationship as in normal subjects and 2) pressure elevation acts in concurrence with the normal evolution of aging as an accelerating factor of this aging process. In addition to exhibiting the same aging process as that seen in Group 1, patients of Group 2 exhibited marked arterial changes. Their pulse wave velocity was more elevated than expected from their level of age and pressure. Their brachial artery diameter failed to increase significantly above the normal value, in contrast to Group 1 and despite having the same pressure and age levels as the latter (Fig. 4). This finding gives an additional indication of abnormal stiffness of their arterial walls. Moreover, this lesser arterial dilatation could not compensate for the marked elevation of pulse wave velocity, which would explain the decrease in arterial compliance and abnormal elevation in characteristic impedance of these patients (Fig. 4). One consequence of the alteration of their arterial function was an increased amplitude of pulse pressure inversely related to the level of arterial compliance. The mechanisms responsible for the arterial modifications of patients of Group 2 are unclear. In addition to the

123

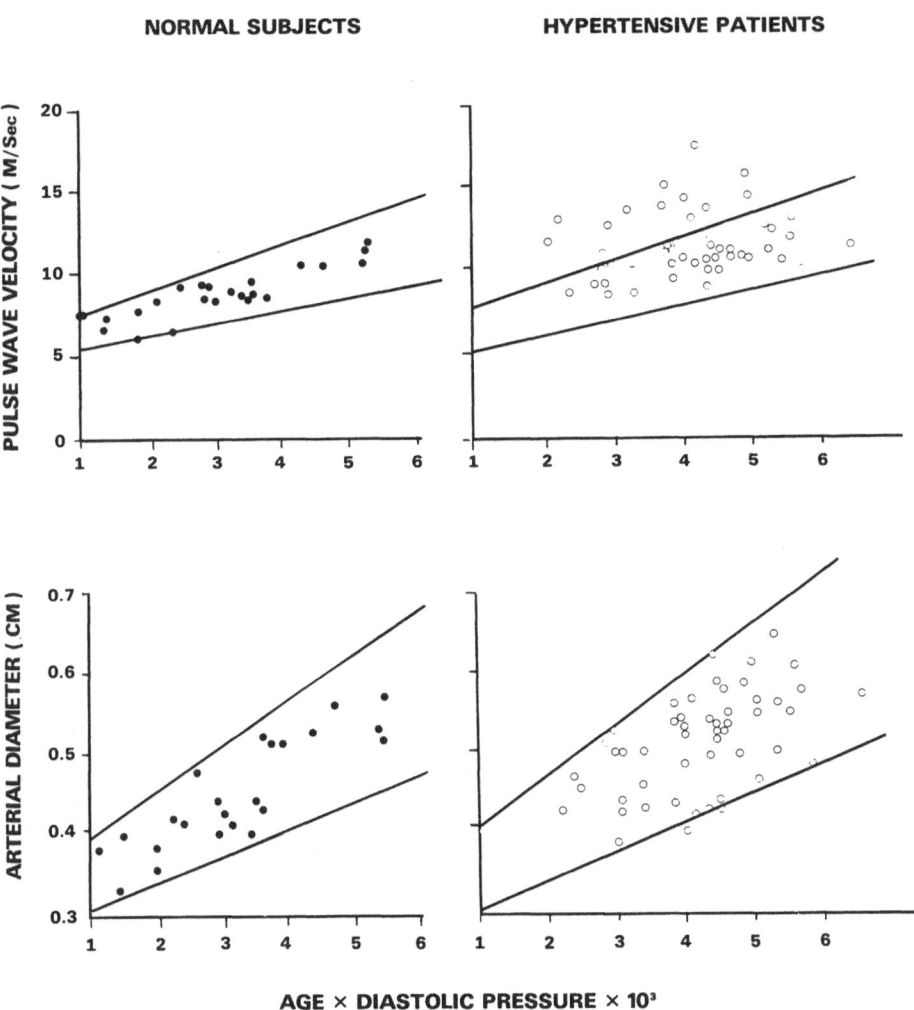

Figure 3. Nomograms of pulse wave velocity and arterial diameter according to the product of age and diastolic pressure in normal subjects and hypertensive patients. The dotted lines indicate the actual regression line, and the continuous lines designate the 95% confidence limits for normal date. From Simon *et al.* [23] with permission.

aging and pressure, they include other unidentified factors possibly related in part to subclinical atherosclerosis, as suggested by pulse wave velocity studies in animals [27]. Results from investigations of pulse wave velocity suggest that early modifications of large arteries of the forearm occur in essential hypertension. These changes, however, may be attributed to different mechanisms. The first change, which affected most of the hypertensive patients in this study, could be considered to be an accelerated aging process. The second form of arterial disease

124

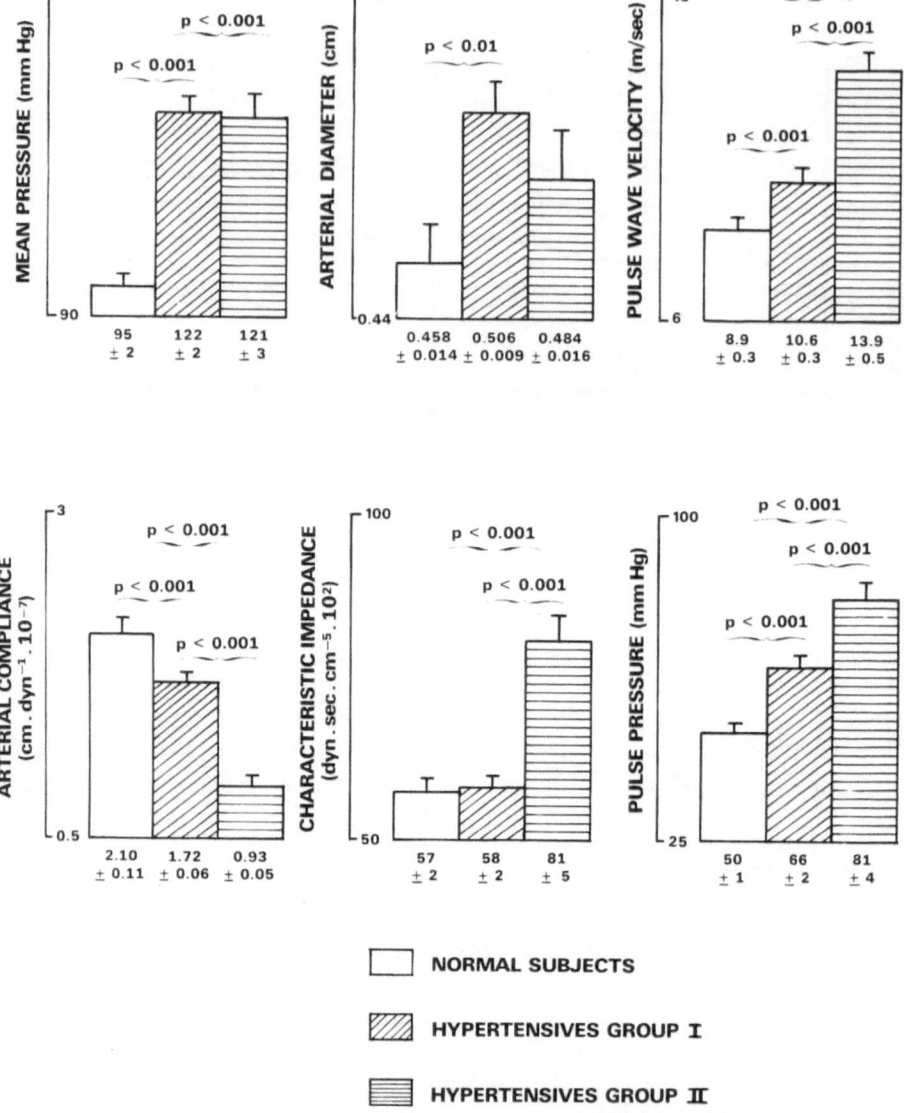

Figure 4. Comparison of mean pressure, arterial diameter, pulse wave velocity, arterial compliance, characteristic impedance, and pulse pressure between normal subjects, hypertensive patients of Group 1, and hypertensive patients of Group 2. Data are expressed as means ± SEM. From Simon *et al.* [23] with permission.

concerned a minority of patients and was associated with the natural aging process and the effects of other factors, perhaps atherosclerotic in nature.

2. Pulsed Doppler arterial measurements

Diameter, blood velocity and flow

The arterial diameter and the blood velocity of the brachial artery can be non-invasively measured by means of a pulsed Doppler velocimeter which operates at a frequency of 8 Mhz and has a double transducer probe and a range-gated time system of reception [28]. The two transducers are located in the tip of the Doppler probe and form between them an angle of 120° so that the velocity signals recorded by each transducer represent the two components of the blood column velocity vector projected on the axis of the ultrasonic beams emitted by each transducer; when the absolute values of these two velocity components are equal, simple geometry shows that the two ultrasonic beams are each at an angle of 60° to the blood column axis. The adjustable time system of reception permits to deduce the distance of the moving red cells from the transducer by means of a simple time-distance echographic relation and to calculate the width of the measurement volume giving the Doppler signals from the duration of the reception. When the measurement volume is focused to its smallest value and its distance from the transducer is increased step by step, the arterial lumen is crossed over by the measurement volume; which permits to record a peak-to-peak velocity profile where the first and the last peak velocity indicates the entering and the coming out of the vessel, thus enabling to deduce simply the internal diameter (D) of the artery. The cross-sectional velocity of the blood volume is determined by adjusting the width of the measurement volume to the value of the arterial diameter and its distance from the transducer to the value of the depth of the proximal arterial wall. The mean arterial blood flow Q is calculated with the following formula:

$$Q = \pi D/4 . \bar{V}$$

D is the internal arterial diameter and $\bar{V}$ the mean arterial blood velocity obtained from integration of the instantaneous blood velocity curve [28].

In human hypertension the mean brachial artery blood flow was found normal [27–29] but the Doppler measurements enabled us to observe that the internal diameter of the brachial artery was somewhat higher and the blood velocity inside the artery lower in hypertensive than in normotensives subjects. The elevation of arterial caliber was not found dependent of age, but directly related to the level of blood pressure suggesting, that, as the arterial pressure increases, the large arteries dilate in proportion; however, the question remains whether this arterial dilatation is a direct mechanical consequence of the distending pressure elevation, by increased stretch of the arterial walls, or whether it represents adaptative functional and/or structural change of the artery, related to a chronic state of hypertension; findings in chronic experimental hypertension suggest that dilatation of large arteries might rather reflect structural arterial modifications [17]. Whatever its precise mechanism, the dilated brachial artery caliber may appear as

126

a mechanism to maintain a normal arterial blood flow despite of the reduction in blood velocity in the forearm circulation of hypertensive patients.

Forearm arterial compliance
The elastic properties of the large arteries of the forearm can be adequately represented by the forearm arterial compliance which expresses the capacity of increase arterial volume of the forearm by unit rise in arterial pressure [30]. One estimation of forearm arterial compliance was deduced from the analysis of the diastolic pressure-flow curves in the brachial artery using a first-order model of the forearm arterial circulation [30]; in this procedure, intra-arterial pressure is recorded directly into the brachial artery, and flow is transcutaneously obtained by bidimensional pulsed Doppler velocimeter. The model of the forearm circulation consists of a capacitance, representing the large arteries, branched in series on a resistance representing the arterioles. During the last part of diastole, the outflow of the system (Qout) is approximately Poisseuillean (Qout = P/R, P being the pressure at any time in diastole, and R the forearm resistance) and the inflow of the system is approximately constant and represents the diastolic brachial artery blood flow (Q) which assumes during the last part of diastole a relatively stable plateau (Fig. 5). From these hypotheses the equation of the model during the diastole is:

$$Q_D = C \, dp/dt + P/R$$

and the pressure (P) solution of this equation is

$$P = RQ_D - (RQ_D - Po)\text{expo}(-t/RC)$$

Where Po is the value of pressure corresponding to the zero time of the model, and RQ the value of pressure extrapolated to infinite time (Rα). The pressure (P) predicted by the model has a mono-exponential form just as the actual recorded intra-arterial blood pressure; the exponential slope of pressure of the model (1/RC) and that of the actual recorded pressure during diastole (α) are equal and their equality permits to calculate the forearm arterial compliance (C) as follows:

$$C = 1/\alpha R$$

R the forearm resistance is calculated as the ratio between the mean arterial pressure and the mean brachial artery blood flow. The slope (α) of the exponential decay of brachial artery blood pressure during diastole is calculated by correlating semilogarithmically with time the difference between the brachial pressure P at any time in diastole and the pressure of the model extrapolated to infinite time, (Fig. 5) [30].

In human hypertension the forearm arterial compliance was found decreased

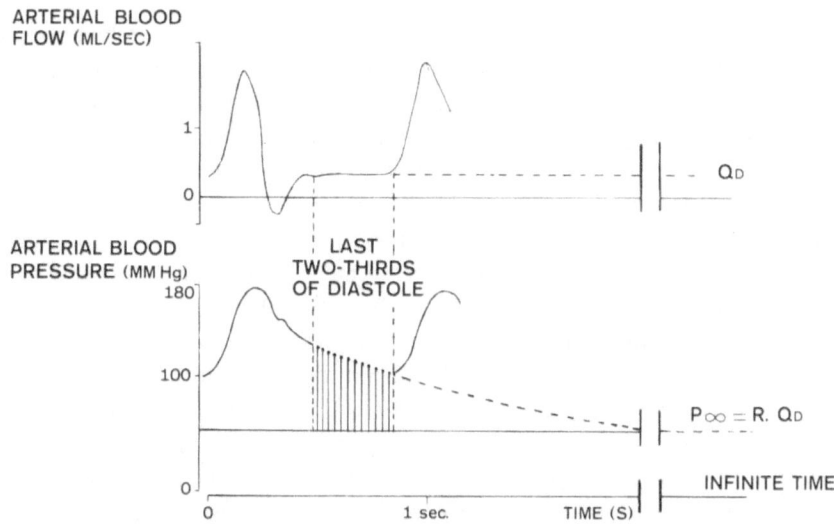

Figure 5. Simultaneous recording of flow and pressure waves in the brachial artery. The upper part shows a typical phasic flow contour with a stable plateau (Q) during diastole. The lower part shows the exponential pressure decay diastole. P is the value of pressure predicted by the model of the forearm circulation at infinite time and is equal to the product RQ, R, being the forearm resistance. The vertical lines represent the differences between pressure and P used in the exponential pressure-time correlation. Modified from Simon *et al.* [30].

comparatively with normal subjects [30] even at the stage of borderline hypertension; indeed, a recent study showed that a subgroup of young patients with borderline hypertension and normal cardiac output had forearm arterial compliance significantly lower than in normal controls of similar age [31]. Reduced arterial compliance of the forearm was also observed in middle-aged, systolo-diastolic hypertensive patients (Fig. 2); the role of pressure could explain these reductions in arterial compliance, because of the nonlinear elasticity of the human arteries. However, a predominant role of pressure 'per se' appears unlikely for several reasons. (i) in patients with borderline hypertension forearm arterial compliance is reduced despite the fact that blood pressure is not markedly elevated [31]; (ii) in sustained hypertension, patients with a normal resting intra-arterial pressure had the same degree of reduction of forearm arterial compliance as patients with more marked pressure elevation [30]; lastly (iii) patients with moderate hypertension whose arterial pressure was normalized with intravenous dihydralazine kept a reduced forearm arterial compliance [30]. Thus, the reduction of forearm arterial compliance observed at different phases of hypertension cannot be predominantly related to the magnitude of elevation in pressure 'per se'; and probably expresses functional and/or structural adaptive changes of the arterial walls consecutive to the chronic state of hypertension [17].

Imput impedance of the brachial artery
Another methodology for estimating the physical properties of the large arteries of the forearm is to calculate the imput impedance of the brachial artery, from the instantaneous ratio of pressure and flow waves in this vessel. Pressure and flow curves are obtained by punction of the brachial artery and transcutaneous pulsed Doppler velocimetry [32]. The pressure-flow ratio calculations were made on the harmonic waves of pressure and flow obtained by Fourier analysis of the recorded curves by means of an analog-to-digital converter and a computer. Imput impedance modulus at each harmonic frequency was calculated by dividing flow modulus into pressure modulus, and impedance phase by substracting the phase angle of flow from that a pressure. Impedance spectrum obtained in hypertensive subjects exhibits a classical form [32]: amplitude of modulus shows a sharp decrease during the six first harmonics, a minimum about the 6 harmonic, and a climb until the 10 harmonic. By decreasing systolic blood pressure with intravenous nitroglycerin, the impedance moduli curve becomes flatter with significant reduction in the low frequencies moduli and shifts to the right of the minimum of moduli [32]; this suggests an improvement of the viscoelastic properties of the forearm arteries with reduction in pressure of hypertensive subjects.

IV. Conclusion

The arterial hemodynamic findings reported in this review provide evidence that human essential hypertension at its different stages of evolution appears associated with marked changes in the physical properties of large arteries consisting in an increased arterial caliber, a decreased arterial compliance, an increased characteristic impedance and an increased pulse wave velocity. Among the responsible mechanisms of these large arteries abnormalities of hypertension, the distending arterial pressure is a critical variable because it governs the diameter and the distensibility of the arteries; indeed, an elevation in distending pressure by more stretching the arterial walls induces an increase in arterial diameter and, because of the non-linear elasticity of human arteries, a decrease in arterial distensibility. This net effect of distending pressure is difficult to analyse 'per se' because it is impossible to compare hypertensive patients and normotensive subjects at the same level of distending pressure without inducing pharmacological pressure changes which are also associated to modification of the smooth muscle lone of the arterial walls. However, several arguments obtained from the observation of arterial abnormalities in borderline hypertension [12, 31] or in mild sustained hypertension [30] tend to indicate that the direct role of elevation of distending pressure is not exclusive for explaining the alterations of the large arteries properties and that adaptive modifications of the arterial wall are surely implicated, as well demonstrated in hypertensive experimental animals [11, 17].

A second important point resulting from these arterial studies is that the functions of large arteries are modified in hypertension as a consequence to the alterations of their physical properties. The buffering function which results from the fact that the arterial distensibility acts as an elastic chamber for damping the pulsatile nature of pressure and flow, is altered in hypertension because of the decreased compliance of the large arteries. Modifications of pulsatile arterial hemodynamics ensue, consisting principally of an increase in the amplitude of the pulse pressure and an increase in the amplitude of the low frequencies moduli of the aortic impedance spectrum. The increase in the pulse pressure amplitude leads to an elevation of systolic arterial pressure disproportionate with the diastolic level; its more striking expression is achieved in isolated systolic hypertension of elderly subjects [19]. The elevation of systolic pressure reacts adversely against the cardiac function by increasing the internal ventricular work and the pulsatile external work of the ventricule [33]. The effects of increased pulsatile arterial dynamics appear also adverse against the large arteries themselves and could contribute to accelerate the process of degenerative change of their physical properties by increasing the pulsatile stress of their walls [33]. The conducting function of large arteries, which consists in delivering an adequate supply of blood to peripheral organs through the different branchs of the arterial tree, seems less altered than the buffering function in uncomplicated hypertension. Indeed, arterial blood flow remains unchanged although arterial caliber and blood velocity undergo profound variations. The hypertensive brachial artery is a typical example of this observation [23, 29]; its flow is normal whereas its caliber is abnormally elevated and its blood velocity reduced; thus, the reduction in arterial blood velocity which expresses the downstream opposition to flow induced by the increased arterioloresistence of the forearm, is compensated by the brachial artery dilatation which permits to maintain a normal flow. It is suggested that the increase in diameter of large arteries acts as a mechanism enabling to maintain the homeostasis of flow delivered to tissues.

References

1. O'Rourke MF (1982): Introduction. In: Arterial function in health and disese, Churchill, Livingstone, p. 3–10.
2. Pickering GW (1968): High blood pressure. Churchill London.
3. Mc Donald DA (1974): Arterial impedance. In: blood flow in arteries, 2nd edition. Williams and Wilkins, Baltimore, p. 309–388.
4. Nichols WW, Conti CR, Walker WV, Milnor WR (1977): Imput impedance of the systemic circulation in man. Circul Res 40: 451–458.
5. Merillon JP, Fontenier G, Chastre J, Lerallut JF, Jaffrin MY, Gourgon R (1980): Etude du spectre d'impédance chez l'homme normal et hypertendu. Effects de l'accroissement de fréquence cardiaque et des drogues vasomotrices. Archives des maladies du Coeur 73: 83–90.
6. Pepine CJ, Nichols WW (1982): Aortic imput impedance in cardiovascular disease. Progress in Cardiovasc Diseases XXIV: 307–318.
7. Milnor WR, Bergel DH, Bargainer JD (1966) Hydraulic power associated with pulmonary blood

130

flow and its relation to heart rate. Circ Res 19: 467–480.
8. Hallock P, Benson IC (1937): Studies on the elastic properties of human isolated aorta. J Clin Invest 16: 595–602.
9. Gabe IT, Karnell J, Porje IG, Rudewald B (1964): The measurement of imput impedance and apparent phase velocity in the human aorta. Acta Physiol Scand 61: 73–84.
10. Gow BS (1972): Influence of vascular smooth muscle on the viscoelastic properties of blood vessel. In: Bergel DH (Ed) cardiovascular fluid dynamics. Academic Press New York, p. 65–110.
11. Wolinsky H (1972): Long term effects of hypertension on rat aortic wall and their relation to concurrent ageing changes. Morphological and clinical studies. Circul Res 30: 301–309.
12. Ventura HO, Messerli FH, Oigman W et al. (1984): Impaired arterial compliance in borderline hypertension. Am Heart J 108: 132–136.
13. Simon ACh, Safar ME, Levenson JA, London GM, Levy BI, Chau NPh (1979): An evaluation of large arteries compliance in man. Amer J Physiol 237 (5): H550–H554.
14. Goldwyn RM, Watt TB (1967): Arterial pressure pulse contour analysis via a mathematical model for the clinical qualification of human vascular properties I.E.E.E. Trans Bio Med Eng BME 14: 11–17.
15. Noordergraaf A (1978): Circulatory System dynamics. New York Academic, p. 137–139.
16. Remington JW (1983): The physiology of the aorta and major arteries. In: Hamilton WF, Dow P (ed) Handbook of physiology, section 2. Circulation, Vol. II. (Hamilton WF, Dow P (Ed). Washington, DC, American Physiological Society, p. 799–838.
17. Wolinsky H (1972): Long-term effects of hypertension on the rat aortic wall and their relation to concurrent aging changes. Morphological and chemical studies. Circ Res 30: 301.
18. Levenson JA, Safar ME, Simon ACh, Kheder AI, Daou JN, Levy BI (1981): Systemic arterial compliance and diastolic runoff in essential hypertension. Angiology 32: 402–413.
19. Simon ACh, Safar ME, Levenson JA, Kheder AI, Levy BI (1979): Systolic hypertension: hemodynamic mechanism and choice of antihypertensive treatment. Am J Cardiol 44: 505–511.
20. Adamopoulos PN, Chrysanthakopoulis SG, Frohlich ED (1975): Systolic hypertension non homogenous diseases. Am J Cardio 36: 697–701.
21. Bramwell JC, Hill AV (1922): The velocity of the pulse wave in man. Proc Roy Soc B 93: 298–306.
22. Levenson JA, Simon ACh, Bouthier JA, Safar ME (1983): Post synaptic alpha blockade and the brachial arterial compliance in essential hypertension. J Hypertension 2: 37–41.
23. Simon ACh, Levenson JA, Bouthier J, Safar ME, Avolio AP (1985): Evidence of early degenerative changes in large arteries in human essential hypertension. Hypertension 7: 675–680.
24. Mc Donald DA (1974): Wave velocity and attenuation. In: Blood flow in arteries, second edition. Williams and Walkins, Baltimore, p. 389–419.
25. Avolio AP, Shang-Gong Chen, Ruo-Ping Wang, Chun-Lai Zhang, Mei-Feng LI, O'Rourke MK (1983): Effects of aging on changing arterial compliance and left ventricular load in a northern Chinese urban community. Circulation 68: 50–58.
26. Learoyd BM, Taylor MG (1966): Alterations with age in the viscoelastic properties of human walls. Circul Res 18: 347–349.
27. Farrar DJ, Green HD, Bond C, Wagner WD, Gobbee RA (1978): Aortic pulse wave velocity, elasticity, and composition in a nonhuman primate model of atherosclerosis. Cir Res 43: 52–62.
28. Levenson JA, Peronneau PP, Simon ACh, Safar ME (1981): Pulsed Doppler: determination of diameter, blood flow velocity and volumic flow of brachial artery in man. Cardiovascular Res 15: 164–170.
29. Safar ME, Peronneau PP, Levenson JA, Simon ACh (1981): Pulsed Doppler: diameter, velocity and flow of the brachial artery in sustained essential hypertension. Circulation 63: 393–400.
30. Simon ACh, Laurent S, Levenson JA, Bouthier JA, Safar ME (1983): Estimation of forearm arterial compliance in normal and hypertensive men from simultaneous pressure and flow measurements in the brachial artery, using a pulsed doppler device and a first-order arterial model during diastole. Cardiovasc Res 17: 331–338.

31. Simon ACh, Levenson JA, Maarek BC, Bouthier J, Safar ME (1986):Evidence of early arterial changes in borderline hypertension. J Cardiovasc Pharmacol 8 (Suppl. 5): S36–S38.
32. Simon ACh, Levenson JA, Levy BI, Bouthier JA, Peronneau PP, Safar ME (1982): Effect of nitroglycerin on peripheral large arteries in hypertension. Br J Clin Pharm 14: 241–246.
33. O'Rourke MF (1982): Vascular impedance and cardiac function. In: Arterial function in Health and disease, Churchill Livingstone, p. 153–169.

Pulse wave velocity and hypertension

A.P. AVOLIO

1. Introduction

Of the many factors implicated in the genesis and maintenance of elevated arterial pressure, the pulsatile function of the arterial system has received little attention in comparison to other cardiovascular related phenomena such as increase in peripheral resistance, regulation of cardiac output, the role of the autonomic nervous system, glomerular filtration and the renin-angiotensin axis. This, despite the fact that ventricular ejection is by necessity intermittent, generating a pulsatile aortic pressure wave which is propagated throughout the arterial vasculature at a finite speed.

The early descriptions of high arterial pressure as 'essential hypertension' equated the sustained state of high arterial pressure with chronic elevation of peripheral resistance [1]. However, other interpretations suggested that increase in peripheral resistance is only an adaptive mechanism secondary to overall regulation of cardiac output [2]. Although Guyton suggested that, in the quest for aetiology of hypertension, investigators need to consciously alter their perspective in relation to causes and effects of high blood pressure, there has been little integration of pulsatile mechanisms in the complex array of parameters involved in the relationship between arterial pressure and hypertension [2]. Since the early simple association of essential hypertension with peripheral resistance, the problem has become one of multifactorial dimensions resulting in descriptions of many forms of essential or 'primary hypertension' [3], with an uncertain delineation between causes and effects [4]. High arterial pressure is now known to exist in the presence of normal peripheral resistance [5] and in cases where increases in cardiac output are not necessary related to increases in blood volume [6].

Many of the apparent discrepancies or anomalies which exist in the current understanding of haemodynamics in hypertension could be resolved by considering the pulsatile function of large arteries as an important and integral factor in the genesis of high blood pressure. In the search for more efficacious antihypertensive treatment, recent investigations have focused on the structure and func-

function of large central and peripheral arteries [7, 8] where haemodynamics are determined by the relationship between oscillatory pressure and flow and by wave propagation characteristics of the arterial system. Although this has been a result of a series of progression of ideas, it is essentially a return to early concepts proposed by physicians such as Young [9] and Mahomed [10] in the 18th and 19th century, when understanding of the function of arteries and the arterial pulse was not confounded by the seemingly exaggerated importance of sphygmomano-metric measurement of diastolic pressure in the brachial artery [11]. Early inter-pretations of maximum (systolic) and minimum (diastolic) pressure in the brachial artery lead to such simplified and erroneous concepts as associating systolic pressure with the contractile force of the heart and diastolic pressure with peripheral resistance [11].

Fundamental investigations into dynamic relationships between blood pres-sure and flow [12] have emphasised the concept of arterial pressure being con-sidered as a steady pressure over which is superimposed an oscillatory pressure wave [13]. The steady component, determined by cardiac output and total pe-ripheral resistance, is essentially constant throughout the arterial system. The oscillatory component, however, varies in amplitude between central and pe-ripheral locations and is determined by geometric and elastic properties of the conduit arteries, timing and intensity of wave reflection and propagation proper-ties of the arterial system [12–14].

Pulse wave velocity is determined primarily by the distensibility of the arterial wall, and varies throughout the arterial system due to non-uniform elasticity. This elastic 'taper' [15], in addition to peripheral wave reflection, is responsible for the amplification of the travelling pressure pulse resulting in marked differences between systolic pressure in the central aorta and in the brachial artery [16].

Because the elastic modulus of the artery wall increases with circumferential tension [17], pulse wave velocity depends on arterial pressure: the higher the pressure, the faster the speed of wave travel. In hypertension this mechanism causes a state of positive feedback where increase in pressure causes increase in pulse wave velocity resulting in earlier return of reflected waves further augment-ing systolic pressure (Fig. 1). The positive feedback mechanism described by Folkow [3] in relation to structural adaptation of arterioles, where increase in pressure produces further increases in peripheral resistance, applies to the *steady* component of arterial pressure. Similarly, a positive feedback mechanism in the function of large elastic arteries is associated with increase in the *pulsatile* compo-nent of arterial pressure. This concept of positive feedback effect has been re-enforced recently by Korner [4] to include the functional role of the hyper-trophied heart and blood vessels as cardiac and vascular 'amplifiers' in the maintenance of elevated arterial pressure. The amplification effect, due to in-crease in stroke volume in the initial phase, becomes progressively attenuated by the amplification effect of the peripheral vasculature due to increase in peripheral resistance and to reduced 'cushioning' function of the large elastic conduit arteries [4, 13].

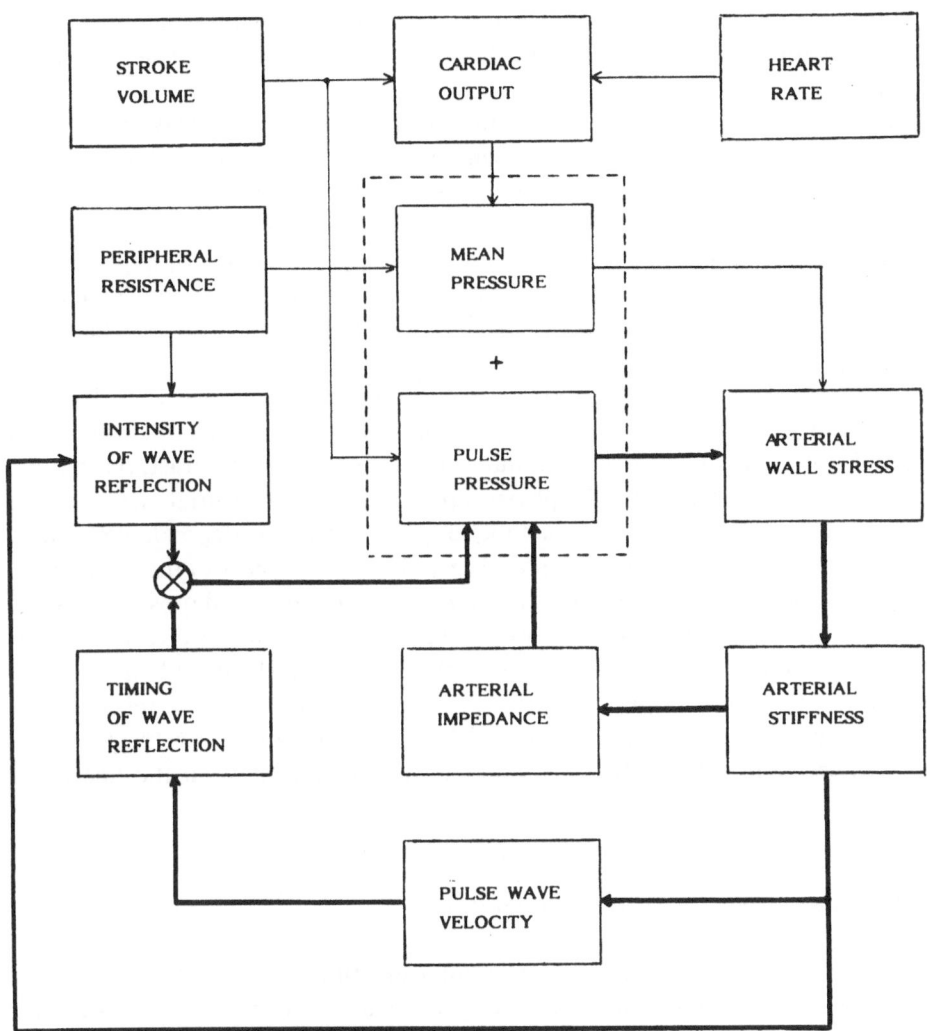

Figure 1. Schematic diagram of major determinants of arterial pressure considered in terms of steady (mean pressure) and oscillatory (pulse pressure) component. Pathways designated by heavy arrows indicate positive feedback loops affecting pulse pressure. The state of elevated arterial pressure (whether acute or chronic, as in essential hypertension) increases the 'gain' of parameters in the positive feedback loop resulting in further increase in the pulsatile component of arterial pressure.

Increase in peripheral resistance results in a concomitant increase in intensity of peripheral wave reflection. When this occurs together with increase in pulse wave velocity, the early return of reflected energy augments systolic pressure at the aortic root while the ventricle is still ejecting [13]. This results in increased systolic wall stress increasing myocardial oxygen consumption [18]. Reduction of pulse wave velocity such that reflected waves return after aortic valve closure has a beneficial effect on vascular-ventricular coupling by augmenting pressure at the aortic root during diastole increasing perfusion pressure in the coronary circulation [19].

The most important factor contributing to increase in pulse wave velocity in human populations is age [20–24]. This is due to increased arterial stiffness because of medial calcification and loss of elasticity with age [25]. Although this produces an increase in the pulsatile component of arterial pressure, this is not manifest in all human populations as an increasing prevalence of hypertension with age [26]. The increased arterial stiffness may be partly offset by decrease in stroke volume which occurs with age [27], resulting in little or no change in arterial pressure.

Arterial pressure is determined by ventricular ejection and the impedance of the arterial vasculature to both steady and pulsatile flow. It is a quantity which depends simultaneously on cardiac and arterial function. In contrast, pulse wave velocity depends entirely on the physical properties of the arterial system and is completely independent of cardiac function. It is, however, dependent on intra-arterial pressure which affects wall tension and so distensibility of the artery wall. Thus, measurement of pulse wave velocity, in addition to blood pressure, gives a more complete description of the 'cushioning' function of large arteries [13] and is an important parameter determining both cardiac afterload and the relation between central and peripheral pulsatile pressure. In hypertension, this property becomes more pronounced since it is a major component of the positive feedback loop where both arterial function and the interaction between the heart and arterial vasculature become compromised.

2. Pulse wave velocity and the arterial wall

The pressure pulse generated by ventricular ejection is propagated throughout the arterial tree at a speed determined by the elastic and geometric properties of the arterial wall and the density of blood. Since fluid is contained in a system of elastic conduits, energy propagation occurs predominantly along the wall of the distensible boundary (artery wall) and not through the incompressible medium (blood). The material properties of the artery wall, its thickness and the lumen calibre thus become the major determinants of the speed of propagation. These physical concepts have been formalised in many mathematical forms where the arterial segment is considered as a thin- [28] or thick-walled tube [29]. For large arteries, pulse wave velocity (c) is given by (i) the Moens-Korteweg equation:

$$c = \sqrt{Eh/2\varrho R}$$

(assuming a thin perfectly elastic wall and non-viscous fluid) or (ii) the Bramwell-Hill equation:

$$c = \sqrt{\Delta P \cdot V / \Delta V \cdot \varrho}$$

where

E = Young's Modulus of the wall

h = wall thickness

R = vessel radius

ϱ = blood density

$\Delta V, \Delta P$ = change in pressure and volume respectively

$\Delta P \cdot V / \Delta V$ = relative volume elasticity of the vessel segment

Volume distensibility (VD) may be calculated from pulse wave velocity using a modification of the Bramwell-Hill [20] equation:

$$VD = (3.5/c)^2$$

The main load-bearing components of the arterial wall are located in the media and consist of fibrous structures (elastin and collagen) and, in muscular arteries, smooth muscle cells. Elastin is arranged to form concentric lamellae [30] supported by a collagenous and cellular matrix. Throughout many mammalian species, the tension per lamellar unit in the aorta has been shown to be remarkably constant despite a 20-fold variation in vessel diameter. The increase in wall tension due to higher pressure or larger diameter is compensated by increase in wall thickness [30]. In man, this is complicated by the degenerative effects of age [31] where increase in size of arteries is accompanied by degradation of elastic properties of the arterial wall resulting in progressive deterioration of the 'cushioning' function of the whole arterial system. While there is abundant information (essentially qualitative) on pathological processes which occur in the arterial wall, to date there is little quantitative information on the precise mechanisms responsible for the progressive loss of function of the load-bearing components in ageing human arteries.

Alteration of structural and geometrical components of the arterial media leads to functional changes such as modification of vascular impedance and associated change in pulse wave velocity. Disintegration of elastic fibres caused by increased circumferential tension with high arterial pressure and fatiguing effects of cyclic mechanical stress [13], cross-linking of collagen, hypertrophy of smooth muscle cells and accumulation of calcium deposits within the media, all lead to increased stiffness of the artery wall resulting in decreased arterial compliance and increased pulse wave velocity.

An additional factor which influences functional properties of the artery wall is the accumulation of intracellular and extracellular water [32]. This becomes significant when increased arterial pressure is directly or indirectly related to fluid balance within the body. The direct effect on pulse wave velocity is not known, but this mechanism may be related to the increase in volume distensibility with diuretics observed in the brachial artery of hypertensive subjects [33] and the decrease in brachial artery compliance following saline infusion [34].

3. Measurement of pulse wave velocity

Arterial pulse wave velocity (c) is a parameter derived from measurements of pulse transit time (t) and the distance (d) travelled by the pulse between two recording sites: $c = d/t$. Transit time is determined from the time delay between two corresponding points on the proximal and distal pulse waves. Because of the effects of wave reflection, damping and dispersion [12], the foot of the wave is the time event which is least affected by these phenomena. Hence, accurate estimation of the 'foot' of the wave becomes extremely important in measurement of pulse wave velocity. In high fidelity intra-arterial recordings of pressure, the foot is identifiable as the beginning of the initial upstroke. When this is not readily obtained, the foot is estimated as the point of intersection of tangents drawn along the upstroke in early systole and through the latter part of diastole of the preceding wave [23].

Accurate measurements of the distance travelled by the pulse is obtained only with invasive procedures such as catheterisation or angiography. Non-invasive procedures allow only an estimate from superficial measurements of distance with possible corrections based on anatomical dimensions of the body [35]. Since arteries become tortuous with age [31], the path lengths determined from linear superficial measurements are generally underestimated and so the real pulse wave velocity in the elderly is actually higher than that calculated from surface measurements. Pulse wave velocity in the aorta is usually determined between the pulse detected in the region of the base of the neck and in the femoral artery, in the arm between the brachial and radial artery and in the leg between the femoral artery and post-tibial or dorsalis pedis artery. When aortic pulse wave velocity is obtained using the carotid pulse instead of the pulse in the aortic arch, the distance from the suprasternal notch to the carotid location is subtracted from the total distance to account for the pulse travelling in the opposite direction [23].

The arterial pulse may be detected and displayed as a time varying signal of pressure, flow velocity or vessel diameter, and the time delay obtained from any of these is identical. For invasive measurements, the method of choice is intra-arterial pressure using high fidelity transducers. If pressure-sensitive transducers are used for non-invasive procedures, measurement is restricted to superficial arteries where the pulse may be externally palpated. Ultrasound techniques, however, do not have this limitation, and transcutaneous Doppler transducers are often used to detect the flow velocity pulse in the aorta and other arteries [23, 24]. In severely hypertensive subjects, a major difficulty is often encountered in detecting the aortic pulse at the base of the neck: pulsations due to high systolic pressure cause large displacement of both arterial and muscular structures resulting in unreliable Doppler velocity waveforms (unpublished observations). In these situations the carotid pulse is detected more reliably and the appropriate corrections are applied for determination of pulse wave velocity.

4. Change of pulse wave velocity with blood pressure and age

Because of the non-linear stress-strain relationship of the arterial wall and its dependence on wall tension, the elastic modulus is a function of intra-arterial pressure [17]. Since pulse wave velocity is related to wall elasticity, it becomes directly related to distending pressure. For foot-to-foot velocity, it would seem logical that the corresponding pressure which determines wall tension would be diastolic pressure. However, varying correlation coefficients have been reported between pulse wave velocity and systolic, diastolic, and mean pressure [36]. This variation is probably attributable to the inherent variability in both pulse wave velocity and blood pressure within and across individual subjects. While some studies use changes in pulse transit time (measured non-invasively) to reflect direct changes in arterial pressure following psychological manoeuvers (e.g. conditioned response) in the same subject [37], other studies report variable relationships between blood pressure and pulse wave velocity. Eliakim *et al.* [38] found higher values in hypertensive subjects only after age 60. Population studies by Schimmler in German subjects [22] found definite increase of pulse wave velocity with mean arterial pressure at all ages (Fig. 2), whereas a less definite relationship was found by Avolio *et al.* [23, 24] in Chinese subjects, where age was the main determinant. This difference may be due to the relatively smaller numbers of subjects in the respective subgroups of age and blood pressure in the Chinese study compared with the much larger numbers in similar subgroups in the German study.

Measurement of local diameter, arterial compliance and pulse wave velocity in the brachial artery in normotensive and hypertensive subjects aged 17–63 years suggested that in many subjects the increase in pulse wave velocity could be related to the concomitant increase in blood pressure with age [39]. However, a subgroup of hypertensive subjects was identified which showed abnormally high pulse wave velocity, when normalised for age and blood pressure, indicating the presence of early degenerative changes in the arterial wall associated with acceleration of hypertension [39].

Other studies in the brachial artery, where the arm was placed in a pressurised box, have shown that increase in pulse wave velocity with increased intra-arterial pressure could be abolished if comparisons are made at similar transmural pressure [40]. Further studies based on these findings suggested that if age-related changes in blood pressure are taken into account, volume distensibility of the brachial artery actually increases with age [41]. Although there was considerable scatter in the data relating calculated volume distensibility in the brachial artery and transmural pressure, it was nonetheless concluded that increased arterial stiffness with age is a consequence rather than the cause of elevated arterial pressure [33]. While these findings may be a combination of many factors including measurements made from relatively short transit times (20–30 milliseconds) and individual variations of ageing effects on calculated volume disten-

140

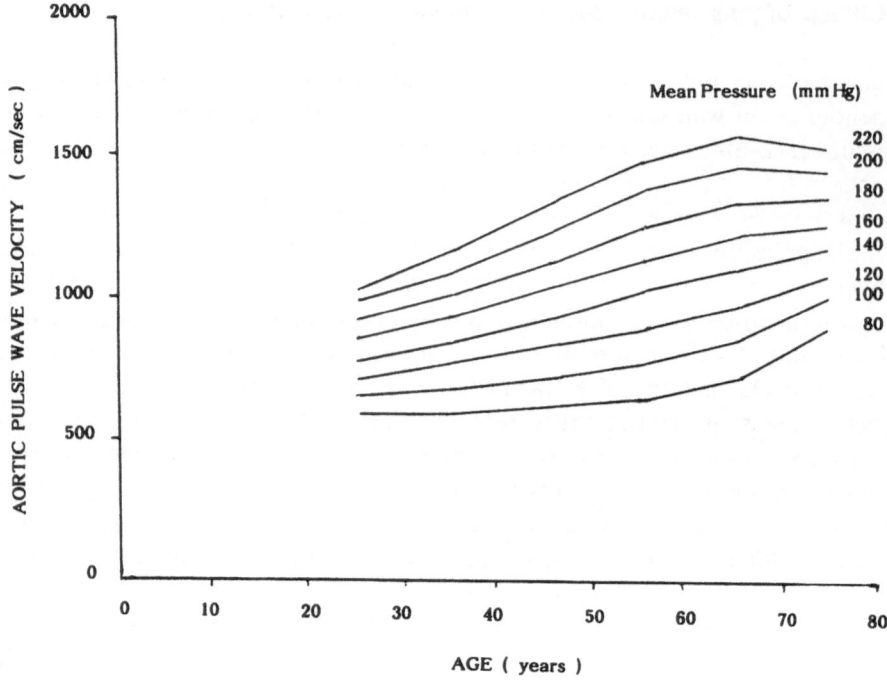

Figure 2. Aortic pulse wave velocity and age as a function of mean arterial pressure determined from external recordings of carotid and femoral pulses. Data obtained from Schimmler's study in 2500 German subjects [22].

sibility of the brachial artery, it is unclear how this relates to the aorta and other central large arteries which are known to exhibit definite age-related changes in structural components of the artery wall [25, 31].

The early findings of increased arterial pulse wave velocity with age described by Bramwell and Hill in 1922 [19] have been confirmed by subsequent studies in humans both in health and disease [13, 21–24, 38, 39]. While this is a well established property of the ageing cardiovascular system, the mechanisms responsible are as yet unclear. There are conflicting reports regarding the effects of age-related development of atherosclerosis on arterial distensibility. Some studies suggest that increase in pulse wave velocity could be an early indicator of development of atherosclerosis with diabetes mellitus [42]. Other studies showed no significant difference (compared to normals matched for age and blood pressure) in changes in pulse wave velocity (or volume distensibility) with age in subjects predisposed to high risk for atherosclerosis such as familial hypercholesterolaemia [43] nor in populations with different prevalence of atherosclerosis [22, 23, 44]. Similar findings were obtained in much earlier studies of pulse wave velocity by Haynes *et al.* in 1936 [45]. They found that aortic pulse wave velocity in patients with clinical and X-ray evidence of marked thickening and calcification of arteries, but with normal blood pressure, was not higher than that for age-matched controls.

Results from the same study also showed a significant relationship between aortic pulse wave velocity and pulse pressure when all data were pooled, with the exception of data from patients with aortic regurgitation (Fig. 3). The effect of increased pulse pressure is additive to the effect of age per se, since the mean age of each group was essentially similar, with the exception of the arterosclerosis group which was older, but having similar values of pulse wave velocity to the control group.

Although there has long been a qualitative association between the process of atherosclerosis with 'hardening of the arteries', pulse wave velocity studies indicate that hypertension contributes more than atherosclerosis to increased arterial stiffening with age [23, 24, 45].

5. Pulse wave velocity and the relation between aortic and brachial artery pulse pressure

The contour of the aortic pressure pulse alters as it travels toward the periphery. Pulse amplitude generally increases and the sharp incisura caused by aortic valve closure becomes progressively damped [13, 14, 16]. In the brachial artery, pulse pressure can exceed that in the aorta by more than 50% [14]. The relationship between proximal (aortic) and distal pressure is complex and depends on physical properties of the arterial segment between the two sites and on the vascular bed beyond the distal site [12]. Transmission (or transfer function) is frequency-dependent where different harmonic components of the wave are amplified (or attenuated) and delayed to different degrees [12, 13, 16]. Factors responsible for these characteristics are non-uniform arterial elasticity and peripheral wave reflection [12–16]. The difference in distensibility of the aorta and peripheral arteries is manifest as different values of pulse wave velocity found in the aorta and limbs. Aortic pulse wave velocity is generally lower but increases to greater degree with age.

Using a simple transmission line model, values of pulse wave velocity in the aorta and brachial artery can be used to estimate the amplification of the pulse due to non-uniform arterial elasticity. From the 'water hammer' formula [12], pulse wave velocity (c) is related to characteristic impedance (Zo, impedance in the absence of wave reflection) of an artery and blood density (ϱ) as

$$c = Zo \cdot \varrho$$

For a lossless transmission line which alters its characteristic impedance along its length, the ratio of proximal (Pp) to distal (Pd) pressure amplitude is proportional to the square root of the characteristic impedance [15]:

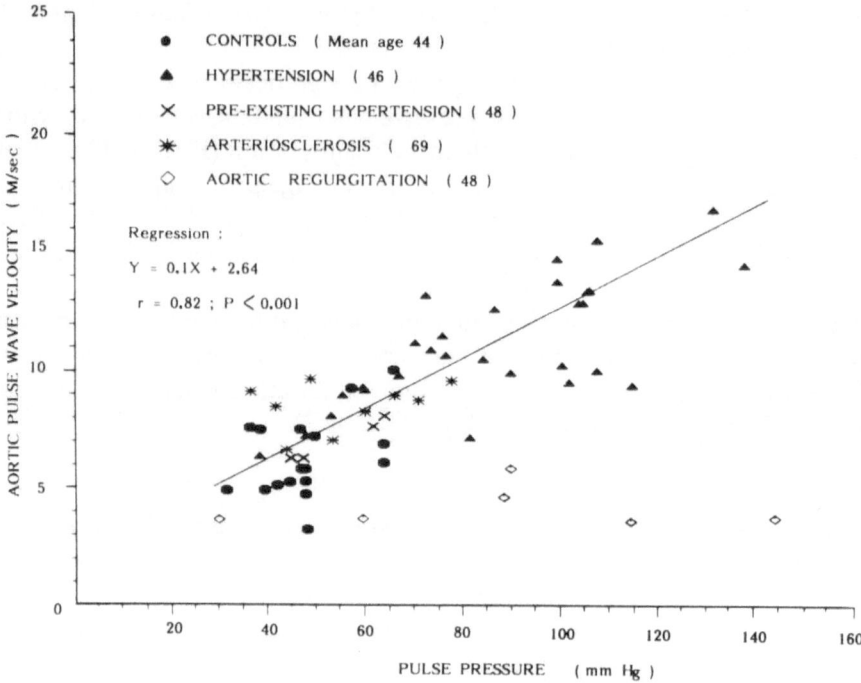

Figure 3. Aortic pulse wave velocity as a function of pulse pressure in control subjects (age range 18–79; mean 44) and in patients with arterosclerosis (age 50–76; mean 69), hypertension (age 16–77; mean 46), pre-existing hypertension (age 38–62; mean 48) and aortic regurgitation (age 22–58; mean 48). Note that patients with clinical evidence of arterosclerosis (thickening and calcification of the arterial wall) have pulse wave velocities within the normal range. In patients with aortic regurgitation, pulse wave velocity is independent of pulse pressure. This is because a high pulse pressure (eg. 160/15 mm Hg) corresponds to a relatively low mean pressure (61 mm Hg), hence the low values of pulse wave velocity. Regression equation for aortic pulse wave velocity (y, m/sec) and pulse pressure (x, mm Hg) was calculated for all data (n = 60) with the exception of data from patients with aortic regurgitation: y = 0.1x + 2.64; r = 0.82; p<0.001. Data from Haynes *et al.* [45].

$$Pp/Pd = \sqrt{Zo(prox)/Zo(dist)}$$

Hence, in terms of pulse wave velocity (c):

$$P(brachial)/P(aorta) = \sqrt{c(brachial)/c(aorta)}$$

This ratio was calculated for different ages (Fig.4) where it reaches a maximum of 24% below age 20 and drops to almost zero above age 70. This corresponded to a maximal difference of 10 mm Hg between brachial artery and aortic pulse pressure.

Because peripheral wave reflection is also responsible for pulse wave amplification, this calculated difference is an underestimation of the true value since it

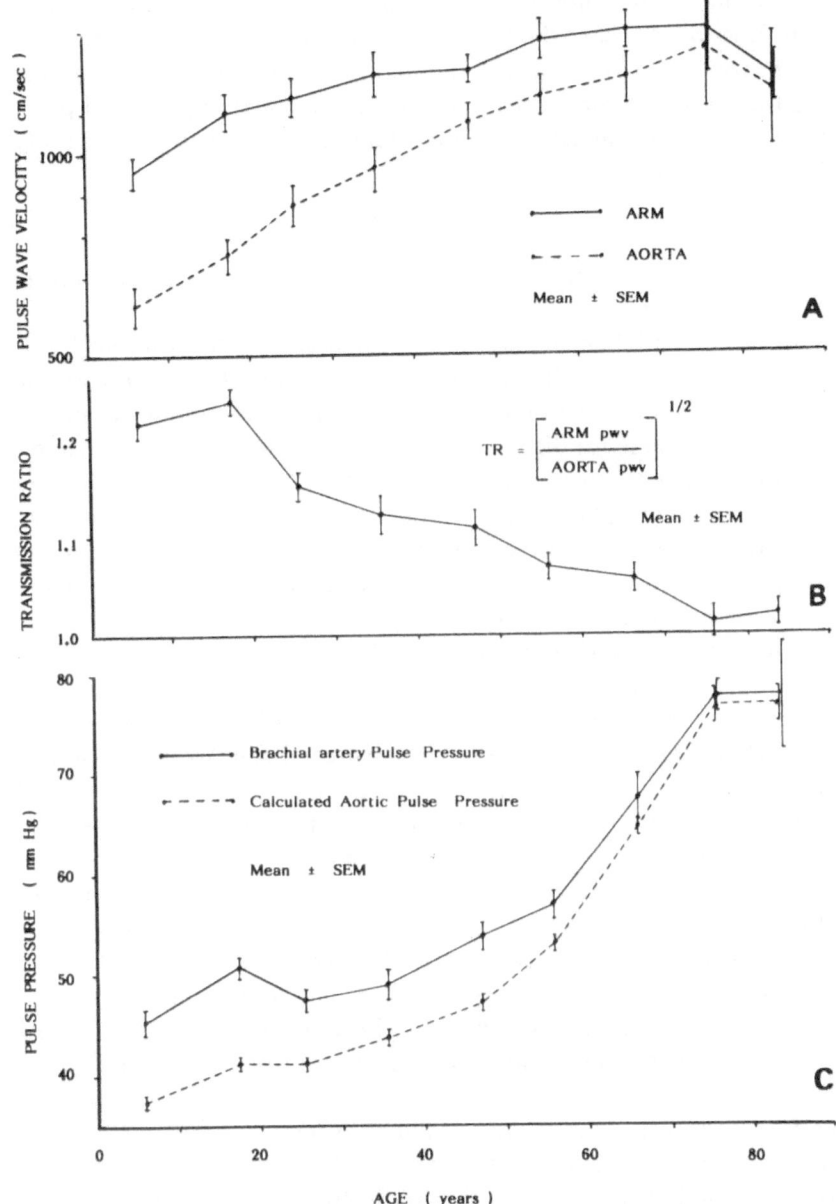

Figure 4. (A). Aortic and arm pulse wave velocity (PWV) in urban Beijing subjects as a function of age. (B). Transmission ratio (TR) calculated as TR = √arm PWV/aorta PWV. (C). Measured brachial artery pulse pressure (BPP) in the same subjects and calculated aortic pulse pressure (APP): APP = BPP/TR. Since total amplification is a combination of elastic non-uniformity and peripheral wave reflection, calculated difference between BPP and APP represents the minimum difference that might be expected. See text for explanation. Data from Avolio *et al.* [23].

is based only on the one mechanism of non-uniform elasticity and does not consider the possible effect of duration of ejection which has been shown to be a significant factor [14]. However, this method does provide a means of at least estimating the minimum difference in aortic and brachial artery pulse pressure which in itself is substantial, and is an important factor in measurement of blood pressure in the young.

6. Pulse wave velocity in populations with different prevalence of hypertension

Findings from epidemiological surveys in populations with different levels of acculturation have shown that increase in blood pressure with age is not a uniform occurrence in all human communities [46, 47], that dietary patterns and living standards are responsible for different prevalences of hypertension [47] and that westernisation leads to increase in prevalence of many forms of cardiovascular disease [48]. To minimise the age-related effects of atherosclerosis on cardiovascular function, as occurs in Western populations, studies were conducted in two Chinese populations with known low prevalence of atherosclerosis, but markedly different prevalence of hypertension.

The first study was conducted in 480 normal subjects, age 3 to 89 years, in urban Beijing during October-November, 1981 [23], and the second in 524 normal subjects, age 2 months to 94 years, in the rural districts of Guangzhou in October, 1983 [24]. Our findings of change in blood pressure with age were consistent with those of a recent nationwide study in a sample of over 4 million subjects [49] which showed distinct regional differences in prevalence of hypertension throughout China. Markedly different prevalence of hypertension was found between the two groups; overall prevalence of hypertension was: Guangzhou, 4.9%; Beijing, 15.6%, using the WHO criteria of supine systolic pressure >160 mm Hg or supine diastolic pressure >95 mm Hg. Pulse wave velocity measured in the aorta, arm and leg increased with age in both groups, but to a much greater degree in urban Beijing subjects. The following regression equations were obtained for pulse wave velocity (y, cm/sec) and age (x, years):

Urban Beijing (Overall prevalence of hypertension: 15.6%)
    Aorta: $y = 9.2x + 615$; $r = 0.673$; $p < 0.001$
    Arm: $y = 4.8x + 998$; $r = 0.453$; $p < 0.001$
    Leg: $y = 5.6x + 791$; $r = 0.630$; $p < 0.001$
Rural Guangzhou (Overall prevalence of hypertension: 4.9%)
    Aorta: $y = 5.1x + 533$; $r = 0.552$; $p < 0.05$
    Arm: $y = 0.61x + 817$; $r = 0.121$; $p < 0.05$
    Leg: $y = 4.4x + 718$; $r = 0.512$; $p < 0.005$

Although many studies have shown that the increase in pulse wave velocity with age is associated with a concomitant increase in blood pressure [22, 36, 38, 39], this comparative study was the first to show that the profile of aortic pulse wave velocity with age is similar to the profile of the increase in prevalence of hypertension with age (Fig. 5). In these two particular populations, a delay of some 25–30 years is found between similar levels of mean pressure, aortic pulse wave velocity and prevalence of hypertension.

Besides the known low prevalence of atherosclerosis in these communities, serum cholesterol was similar in both populations: Urban Beijing, 4.49 SE 0.11 mmol/L; Rural Guangzhou, 4.34 Se 0.10 mmol/L. Furthermore, notwithstanding the lower cholesterol levels in Chinese subjects compared to normal levels for Western populations, aortic pulse wave velocity in urban Beijing subjects was found to be markedly higher than in subjects from Germany, U.S.A., Canada, Israel, England, France [23] and Australia [50]. This provides further support for observations from other studies [43] that serum cholesterol does not contribute substantially to increasing arterial stiffness with age.

Results from the comparative studies in China strongly suggest that the accelerated increase in blood pressure and arterial stiffness with age in the Beijing community is due to the higher dietary salt intake which is common throughout northern China [24, 49].

7. Pulse wave velocity and salt intake

Findings from the comparative studies in China [23, 24] showed that while increase in pulse wave velocity with age was greater in the Beijing community with the higher prevalence of hypertension and higher salt intake, it was also higher in these subjects when compared at the same age and blood pressure with subjects from rural Guangzhou (Fig. 6). This suggested that the higher rate of increase of arterial stiffness with age in the Beijing group was largely independent of the difference in level of blood pressure but related to the marked difference in dietary salt. Salt intake, measured as mean 24 hour urinary sodium excretion was: Beijing, 230 SE 7 mmol; Guangzhou, 126 SE 6 mmol.

Although sodium is considered to play a direct role in hypertension, there is increasing evidence for the independent role of sodium in cardiovascular pathophysiology. It has been found that in salt-loaded hypertensive rats, vascular lesions precede the development of hypertension and may be partly responsible for the acceleration of increased arterial pressure [51]. In renal hypertensive rats, levels of dietary sodium restriction which did not reverse hypertension produced marked reduction in heart weight (31%), suggesting an independent role for sodium in cardiac hypertrophy [52].

Our own studies in normotensive Australian subjects on a voluntary low-salt diet confirm the possible independent role of sodium with respect to arterial distensibility [53]. Pulse wave velocity in low salt subjects (mean intake 44 mmol

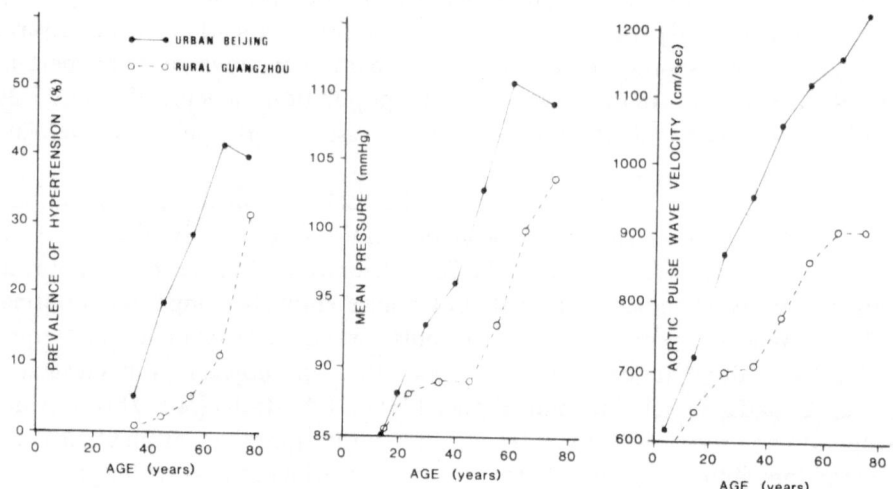

Figure 5. Change of prevalence of hypertension (WHO criteria. systolic/diastolic >160/95 mm Hg), arterial mean pressure and aortic pulse wave velocity with age in normal subjects in urban Beijing and rural Guangzhou. These profiles indicate that similar levels of prevalence of hypertension. mean pressure and aortic pulse wave velocity (and hence arterial stiffness) occur some 25–30 years later in the rural Guangzhou community compared with those in the urban Beijing community. From Avolio *et al.* [23] with permission.

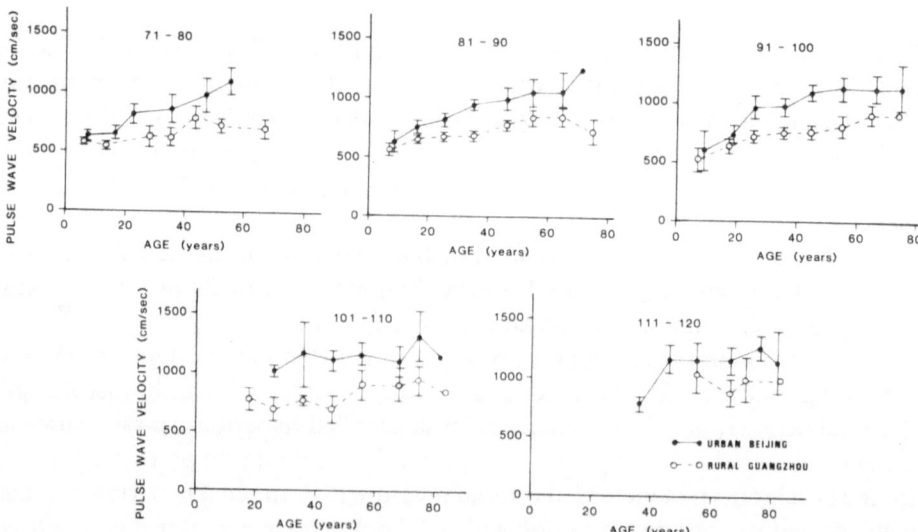

Figure 6. Comparison of aortic pulse wave velocity between normal subjects in urban Beijing and rural Guangzhou at five levels of mean arterial pressure. Values are Mean ± 2 SEM and arterial pressure is indicated at the top of each graph (mm Hg). For all pressure levels after the first decade, pulse wave velocity in the rural Guangzhou community is consistently lower than that in the urban Beijing community. From Avolio *et al.* [24] with permission.

Na/day) was compared with measurements in control subjects on a regular diet (mean intake 130–200 mmol/day) and matched for age and blood pressure. Subjects were divided into three age groups: Group I, 2–19 years; Group II, 29–44 years; Group III, 45–66 years. There was no significant difference in aortic pulse wave velocity in Group I (the youngest subjects with the poorest compliance with diet), but low-salt subjects in Groups II and III had significantly lower values (21.8%, $p<0.001$ and 22.7%, $p<0.05$ respectively) (Fig. 7).

The mechanism that might be responsible for the pressure-independent reduction of pulse wave velocity with reduced salt intake is unknown. However, these results are consistent with other findings of increased volume distensibility of the brachial artery of hypertensive subjects with diuretics [33] and of decreased arterial compliance with sodium infusion [34]. Similar results of increased compliance of large arteries observed with vasodilating agents such as nitroglycerine, calcium antagonists and converting enzyme inhibitors suggest that salt intake may have a direct effect on vascular smooth muscle affecting elasticity of the arterial wall.

In addition to providing further support for the observations made in the Chinese study, findings in Australian subjects on a low-salt diet suggest that arterial pulse wave velocity may be reduced when salt restriction is in effect for a relatively short period of time. Subjects in this study avoided salt from between 8 months to 5 years (average 24.8 months) whereas Chinese subjects differed in salt intake throughout life. Similar findings from a longitudinal study would provide definite confirmation of the role of sodium in improving arterial distensibility independently of its established anti-hypertensive action.

8. Pulse wave velocity, ascending aortic impedance and ventricular-vascular coupling

The development of ventricular hypertrophy in hypertension is due to compensatory increase in wall thickness secondary to increased systolic pressure leading to depressed contractility [54]. The elevated distending pressure within the arterial system increases vascular impedance by reducing arterial distensibility and also increases arterial pulse wave velocity. The combined effect of increased peripheral resistance and increased pulse wave velocity is to augment the early return of reflected energy such that it adds to the incident ejection wave throughout systole (Fig. 1) increasing peak pressure. This has adverse effects on the matching between the ejecting ventricle and the arterial hydraulic load.

In experimental animals, a near optimal ventricular-vascular coupling has been observed which is achieved by a combination of factors, including patterns of arterial branching, non-uniform elasticity, peripheral wave reflection, the eccentric anatomical location of the heart in relation to the upper and lower body, and an inverse relationship between heart rate and body length [13]. In man, this

148

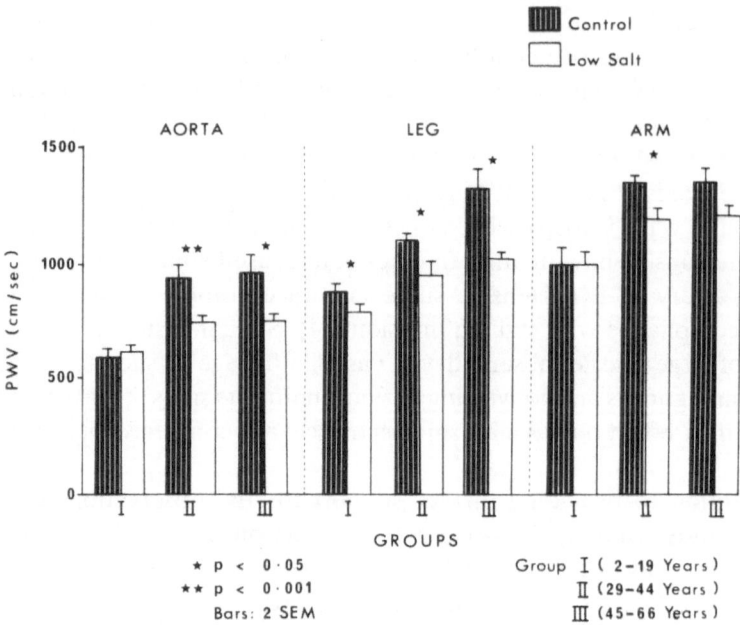

Figure 7. Pulse wave velocity (PWV) in the aorta, leg and arm in normotensive Australian subjects on a low-salt diet (average 44 mmol sodium/day) and in control subjects (average 130–200 mmol sodium/ day) matched for age and mean arterial pressure. Group I: 2–19 years; Group II: 29–44 years; Group III: 45–66 years. From Avolio *et al.* [53] with permission.

favourable relationship is disturbed as a result of progressive arterial degeneration and increase in pulse wave velocity and with elevation of arterial pressure.

Thus aortic pulse wave velocity per se is an important determinant of systolic pressure. Since it is directly related to characteristic impedance (according to the 'water hammer' formula) aortic pulse wave velocity provides a useful non-invasive measurement of left ventricular load [23]. The effects of increased arterial pulse wave velocity are manifest as an increase in low frequency aortic impedance modulus resulting in an increase in the pulsatile component of external left ventricular work [13].

Reduction of pulse wave velocity improves ventricular-vascular coupling by delaying wave reflection, reducing systolic pressure and myocardial oxygen consumption. Since stroke volume has been shown to depend on end-systolic pressure [55] for a given preload, reduction of systolic pressure, caused by delay of wave reflection into diastole, could improve ventricular ejection. Furthermore, delaying of wave reflection to augment pressure during diastole increases coronary perfusion pressure further improving the interaction between the ejecting ventricle and the arterial vasculature.

The interplay between reduction of intensity of reflected energy from peripheral arteries and arterial pulse wave velocity has been implicated to explain the beneficial effects of sublingual nitroglycerine on reduction of ventricular afterload in patients without cardiac failure [56]. In this study, the marked reduction in aortic systolic pressure (34%) could not be fully explained by the effects of nitroglycerine commonly attributed to reduction in preload. A small drop in mean pressure was associated with a concomitant reduction in stroke volume resulting in no significant change in total peripheral resistance. However, changes in aortic imput impedance spectra, including marked reduction in impedance modulus of the first harmonic, suggested a decrease in wave reflection. The dilation of large arteries known to occur with nitrates [8] was suggested to have caused negative wave reflection at branch points in the peripheral vasculature resulting in reduced intensity of reflected energy being propagated back to the aortic root [56]. While some reduction may have been achieved through a slight decrease in preload, most of the reduction of systolic pressure was attributed to the effect of decreased peripheral wave reflection resulting in the improvement of the already disturbed ventricular-vascular coupling.

Summary

Arterial distensibility is a major determinant of the pulsatile component of arterial pressure. Factors which alter the pulsatile function of the arterial system amplify the effect of elevated arterial pressure tending towards further increase in pressure via a series of positive feedback mechanisms. Quantitative changes in arterial distensibility due to age and increased arterial pressure are determined indirectly by non-invasive measurement of pulse wave velocity. Aortic pulse wave velocity is directly related to aortic characteristic impedance, and, together with arterial pressure, gives a measure of the arterial load on the ejecting ventricle; it is a major factor determining ventricular-vascular interaction. Increased pulse wave velocity and concomitant early return of peripheral wave reflection are precursors to elevated systolic pressure.

Pulse wave velocity studies in populations with different prevalences of hypertension and atherosclerosis have shown that hypertension, and not atherosclerosis, contributes predominantly to accelerated arterial stiffness with age. In communities with different prevalence of hypertension, the rate of increase in pulse wave velocity with age is similar to the age-related increase in prevalence of hypertension. Lower values of pulse wave velocity in normotensive subjects on a low-salt diet compared to controls matched for age mean arterial pressure suggest a direct influence of sodium on arterial distensibility, independent of its antihypertensive action.

150

References

1. Freis ED (1960): Hemodynamics of hypertension. Physiol Rev 40: 27–54.
2. Guyton AC (1980): Arterial pressure and hypertension. W.B. Saunders, Philadelphia.
3. Folkow B (1982): Physiological aspects of primary hypertension. Physiol Rev 62: 347–504.
4. Korner PI (1982): Causal and homoeostatic factors in hypertension. Clin Sci 63: 5s–26s.
5. Lund-Johansen P (1980): Haemodynamics in essential hypertension. Clin Sci 59: 343s–354s.
6. Dustan HP, Tarazi RC, Bravo EL (1975): Physiological characteristics of hypertension. In: Laragh JH (ed) 'Hypertension Mechanisms' Yorke Medical Books, NY, pp. 121–146.
7. Safar ME (1985): Focus on the large arteries in hypertension. J Cardiovasc Pharmacol 7: S1–S4.
8. Safar ME, Bouthier JA, Levenson JA, Simon AC (1983): Peripheral large arteries and the response to anti-hypertensive treatment. Hypertension 5 (Supp III): 63–68.
9. Young T (1809): On the function of the heart and arteries. The Croonian Lecture. Phil Trans Roy Soc 99: 1–31.
10. Mahomed F (1874): The aetiology of Bright's disease and the prealbumenuric stage. Med Chir Trans 57: 197–228.
11. O'Rourke MF (1983): Hypertension is a myth. Aust NZ J Med 13: 84–90.
12. McDonald DA (1974): Blood flow in arteries. Edward Arnold, London.
13. O'Rourke MF (1982): Arterial function in health and disease. Churchill Livingstone, Edinburgh.
14. O'Rourke MF (1970): Influence of ventricular ejection on the relationship between central aortic and brachial pressure pulse in man. Cardiovasc Res 4 (3): 291–300.
15. Taylor MG (1964): Wave travel and the design of the cardiovascular system. In: Attinger EO (ed): 'Pulsatile blood flow'. McGraw Hill, NY, pp. 343–367.
16. O'Rourke MF, Blazek JV, Morreels CL, Krovetz LJ (1968): Pressure wave transmission along the human aorta. Circ Res 23: 567–579.
17. Bader H (1967): Dependence of wall stress in the human thoracic aorta on age and pressure. Circ Res 20: 354–361.
18. Sarnoff SJ, Braunwald E, Welch GH, Stainsby WN, Macruz R (1958): Hemodynamic determinants of oxygen consumption of the heart with special reference to the tension-time index. Am J Physiol 192: 148–156.
19. Greg DE, Khouri EM, Rayford CR (1965): Systemic and coronary energetics in the resting dog. Circ Res 16: 102–113.
20. Bramwell JC, Hill AV (1922): The velocity of the pulse wave in man. Proc Roy Soc Lond (Biol) 93: 298–306.
21. Hallock P (1934): Arterial elasticity in man: relationship to age as evaluated by the pulse wave velocity method. Arch Intern Med 54: 770–798.
22. Schimmler W (1965): Untersuchungen zu Elastizitatsproblemen der Aorta. Arch Kreislaufforschung 47: 189–233.
23. Avolio AP, Chen SG, Wang RP, Zhang CL, Li MF, O'Rourke MF (1983): Effects of aging on changing arterial compliance and left ventricular load in a northern Chinese urban community. Circulation 68 (1): 50–58.
24. Avolio AP, Deng FQ, Li WQ, Luo YF, Huang ZD, Xing LF, O'Rourke MF (1985): Effects of aging on arterial distensibility in populations with high and low prevalence of hypertension: comparison between urban and rural communities in China. Circulation 71 (2): 202–210.
25. Milch RA (1965): Matrix properties of the aging arterial wall. Monographs Surg Sci 2 (4): 261–341.
26. Prior IAM, Stanhope JM (1980): Blood pressure patterns, salt use and migration in the Pacific. In: Kesteloot H, Joossens JV (eds), 'Epidemiology of arterial blood pressure' Martinus Nijhoff, The Hague, pp. 243–262.
27. Altman PL, Dittmer DS (eds) (1971): Respiration and Circulation. Biological Handbooks. Fed Amer Soc Exp Biol, pp. 319–320.
28. Womersley JR (1957): Oscillatory flow in arteries: the constrained elastic tube as a model of

arterial flow and pulse transmission. Phys Med Biol 2: 178–187.

29. Cox RH (1968): Wave propagation through a Newtonian fluid contained within a thick walled, viscoelstic tube. Biophys J 8: 691–709.

30. Wolinsky H, Glagov (1967): A lamellar unit of aortic medial structure and function in mammals. Circ Res 20: 99–111.

31. Mitchell JRA, Schwartz CJ (1965): Arterial disease. Blackwell, Oxford.

32. Tobian L (1975): A viewpoint concerning the enigma of hypertension. In: Laragh JH (ed) 'Hypertension Mechanisms' Yorke Medical Books. NY, pp. 25–52.

33. Smulyan H, Vardan S, Griffiths A, Gribbin B (1984): Forearm arterial distensibility in systolic hypertension. J Amer Col Cardiol 3 (2): 387–393.

34. Levenson JA, Simon AC, Maapek BE, Gitelman RJ, Fiessinger JN, Safar ME (1985): Regional compliance of brachial artery and saline infusion in patients with arteriosclerosis obliterans. Arteriosclerosis 5: 80–87.

35. Dellacorte M, Locchi F, Spinelli E, Scarpelli PT (1979): Effect of the anatomical structure of the arterial tree on the measurement of pulse wave velocity in man. Phys Med Biol 24 (3): 593–599.

36. Lyager-Nielson B, Straede-Nielsen J, Fabricus J (1968): Pressure wave velocity in the human aorta. J Amer Geriatrics Soc 16 (16): 647–657.

37. Dutch J, Redman S (1983): Psychological stress and arterial pulse transit time. NZ Med J 96: 607–609.

38. Eliakim M, Sapoznikow D, Weinman J (1971): Pulse wave velocity in healthy subjects and in patients with various disease states. Amer Heart J 82 (4): 448–457.

39. Simon AC, Levenson J, Bouthier J, Safar ME, Avolio AP (1985): Evidence of early degenerative changes in large arteries in human essential hypertension. Hypertension 7: 675–680.

40. Gribbin B, Pickering TG, Sleight P (1979): Arterial distensibility in normal and hypertensive man. Clin Sci 56: 413–417.

41. Smulyan H, Csermely TJ, Mookherjee S, Warner RA (1983): Effect of age on arterial distensibility in asymptomanic humans. Arteriosclerosis 3: 199–205.

42. Woolam GL, Schnur PL, Valibona C, Hoff HE (1962): The pulse wave velocity as an early indicator of atherosclerosis in diabetic subjects. Circulation 25: 533–537.

43. Avolio A, O'Rourke M, Clyde K, Simmons L (1985): Change of arterial distensibility with age in subjects with familial hypercholesterolaemia. Aust NZ J Med 15 (Suppl II): 516.

44. Nakashima T, Tanikawa J (1971): A study of human aortic distensibility with relation to atherosclerosis and aging. Angiology 22: 477–490.

45. Haynes FW, Ellis LB, Weiss S (1936): Pulse wave velocity and arterial elasticity in arterial hypertension, arteriosclerosis and related conditions. Am Heart J 11 (4): 385–401.

46. Maddocks I (1961): Possible absence of essential hypertension in two complete Pacific Island populations. Lancet 2: 396–399.

47. Sinnet PF, Whyte HM (1973): Epidemiological studies in a total highland population, Tukisenta, New Guinea. J Chron Dis 26: 265–290.

48. Marmot MG, Kagan A, Kato H (1980): Hypertension and heart disease in the Ni-Hon-San study. In: Kesteloot H, Joossens JV (eds), 'Epidemiology of arterial pressure', Martinus Nijhoff, The Hague, pp. 437–452.

49. Wu YK, Lu CQ, Gao RC, Yu JS, Liu GC (1982): Nationwide hypertension screening in China during 1979–1980. Chinese Med J 95: 101–108.

50. Ho KL, Avolio AP, O'Rourke MF (1983): Aortic pulse wave velocity, a non-invasive index of left ventricular afterload and aortic stiffening in an Australian community. Fed Proc 42: 1128.

51. Limas C, Westrum B, Limas CJ, Cohn JN (1980): Effect of salt on the vascular lesions of spontaneously hypertensive rats. Hypertension 2: 477–489.

52. Lindpainter K, Sen S (1985): Role of sodium in hypertensive cardiac hypertrophy. Circ Res 57: 610–617.

53. Avolio AP, Clyde KM, Beard TC, Cooke HM, Ho KL, O'Rourke MF (1986): Improved arterial

152

distensibility in normotensive subjects on a low salt diet. Arteriosclerosis 6: 166–169.
54. Takahashi M, Sasayama S, Kawai S, Kotoura H (1980): Contractile performance of the hypertophied ventricle in patients with systemic hypertension. Circulation 62 (1): 116–126.
55. Suga H, Kitabatke A, Sagawa K (1979): End-systolic pressure determines stroke volume from fixed end-diastolic volume in the isolated canine left ventricle under a constant contractile state. Circ Res 44: 238–249.
56. Yaginuma T, Avolio A, O'Rourke M, Nichols W, Morgan J, Roy P, Baron D, Branson J, Feneley M (1986): Effect of glycerol trinitrate on peripheral arteries alters left ventricular hydraulic load in man. Cardiovasc Res 20: 153–160.

Renin-angiotensin system and arterial wall in hypertension

VICTOR J. DZAU

Introduction

The renin-angiotensin system is a blood-borne biochemical cascade whose final product, angiotensin II, is a potent vasoconstrictor and a primary stimulus for aldosterone secretion. Numerous studies have demonstrated an important role for this circulating system in blood pressure, and electrolyte and fluid homeostasis. Our understanding of the contribution of the circulating renin-angiotensin system to cardiovascular and renal physiology has been made possible through the development of radioimmunoassay, and availability of synthetic peptides and pharmacologic inhibitors. More recently, using biochemical and molecular biologic techniques, a number of investigators also demonstrated the expression of renin and angiotensinogen genes in a variety of tissues, thus allowing for the possibility of local angiotensin production. As a result of these observations, the concept of the renin-angiotensin system as a hormonal system alone is now in question. Locally expressed renin-angiotensin systems may be involved in the regulation of individual tissue function, independent of the circulating counterpart. This emerging concept may be important in providing additional understanding of the renin-angiotensin system's role in physiology and the responses to pharmacologic inhibitors.

This paper will focus on the documentation and characterization of a local renin-angiotensin system in the blood vessel wall. The localization and cellular distribution of the components of this local system in the arterial tree, the possible function and role of vascular angiotensin in pathophysiology will also be examined.

Influence of angiotensin on blood vessels

Angiotensin II receptors are widely distributed throughout the vascular tree [1]. Specific angiotensin II binding sites have been identified in the intact rabbit aorta

[2], the subcellular fractions of rabbit and guinea pig aortas [3] and the rat mesenteric artery [4]. In addition, specific binding of angiotensins have been demonstrated in cultured aortic and mesenteric arterial smooth muscle cells [5, 6]. The binding of angiotensin to these receptors is stereospecific and saturable. Angiotensin can be displaced from receptors by structurally related agonists and antagonists. The dissociation constant K_d is approximately 10^{-10} M. Using in vitro autoradiographic techniques, several investigators have also localized angiotensin II binding sites in large, medium and small arteries, and in the vasa recta the kidney [1].

It is well known that systemic administration of angiotensin can result in blood pressure elevation due to increased systemic vascular resistance. Angiotensin also produces contractile response in the aortic strip or ring as well as in isolated femoral, carotid and coronary arteries. Indeed, infusion of angiotensin into various vascular beds has been shown to cause vasoconstriction in these vascular beds. On the other hand, heterogeneity of vascular responses to angiotensin also appears to exist. Toda and co-workers observed that the isolated canine renal arteries exhibited a relaxant response to angiotensin in contrast to the contractile responses of the femoral or the carotid arteries [7]. These investigators demonstrated that this vasorelaxant effect was due to angiotensin's stimulation of endothelial production of prostacyclin. Similarly, Nishimura observed that [Sar 1-Val 5] angiotensin II produced a vasorelaxant response in isolated chicken aorta [8]. This vasorelaxant effect may be mediated by endothelial-derived relaxant factor uniquely released by the chicken aorta in response to angiotensin. Arterioles also exhibit heterogeneous responses to angiotensin. The best example is the well-documented differential sensitivity of the renal efferent and afferent arterioles to angiotensin. Angiotensin II produces preferential efferent arteriolar constriction resulting in increased filtration fraction in the kidney [9]. This effect is particularly important in the maintenance of glomerular filtration rate during reduced renal perfusion pressure. The physiologic relevance of the heterogeneity of vascular response to angiotensin is supported by studies in intact animal or man, which demonstrate differential regional blood flow distribution in response to converting enzyme inhibitor administration. Angiotensin-converting enzyme inhibition results in selective increase in blood flow to the kidney and the heart in the sodium-depleted animal and in man with congestive heart failure [10–12]. Inhibition of the renin-angiotensin system also reduces filtration fraction in the kidney, such that in conditions associated with low perfusion pressure its inhibition may result in acute renal insufficiency [13, 14].

Vascular angiotensin receptors are regulated by sodium intake. In vivo studies have shown that the sensitivity of blood vessels to angiotensin II increases during sodium loading [15, 16]. The converse occurs during sodium depletion. The effects of a low-sodium diet on vascular receptors can be reproduced by infusion of angiotensin II and blocked by captopril, indicating that changes in circulating angiotensin II are responsible for the regulation of angiotensin II receptors [17].

Recent studies indicate that changes in glomerular angiotensin II receptors resemble those of vascular smooth muscle receptors with respect to sodium intake. The changes in number of glomerular angiotensin II receptors parallel the changes in glomerular contractility and dynamics and thus may be important in the regulation of glomerular filtration [18].

As mentioned earlier, the affinity of angiotensin II to bind its receptors has been reported in the nanomolar range, corresponding to the physiologically effective concentration [1]. However, the plasma concentration of angiotensin II is in the picomolar range. Recently, angiotensins have been detected in various tissues. Hence, it has been proposed that angiotensin II production occurred at tissue sites outside the circulation, and that local angiotensin II may be higher than plasma AII concentration and approximate that of receptor Kd [20].

Evidence for existence of a vascular renin-angiotensin system

In the last few years, renin-like enzymes have been described in a variety of tissues, including the blood vessels [9]. Several investigators have demonstrated that the renin-like activity in the aorta persisted for many hours in nephrectomized rats after plasma renin activity was no longer detectable [10, 11]. Aguirela et al. [15] were able to measure immunoreactive angiotensin II in the plasma of rats 24 hours after bilateral nephrectomy, at which time plasma renin activity was undetectable. These data suggest that angiotensin II production may occur at sites outside the plasma and that the peptide was released from the tissue of production into the circulation. The concept of local synthesis of angiotensin II in vascular wall was suggested by the data of Swales and Thurston [19], who reported that the amount of angiotensin antiserum required to inhibit exogenous angiotensin effect in sodium-loaded rats was in marked excess of that predicted. These investigators believed that the data could not be explained solely by alterations of angiotensin receptor or sensitivity, and they interpreted the findings to suggest local synthesis of angiotensin II in the vascular wall, which influenced the response to antiserum.

The renin-like activity in the blood vessel wall has been shown to be primarily derived from immunoreactive renin based on the ability of antirenin antibody to neutralize its activity and the presence of positive immunostaining by antirenin [20]. Angiotensin-converting enzyme and immunoreactive angiotensins have also been demonstrated in the vasculature [20]. Thus, the blood vessel wall contains the essential components of the renin-angiotensin system which persist after binephrectomy, suggesting the existence of a local system independent of the circulating system [21, 22]. Indeed, aortic renin-angiotensin activities are elevated in animal models of hypertension with normal plasma renin and converting enzyme activities, e.g. the spontaneously hypertensive rat (SHR) and the chronic 2 kidney-1 clip (2K–1C) hypertensive rat. In the spontaneously hypertensive rat,

156

blood pressure correlated closely with aortic renin concentration [23]. Similarly, in the chronic 2 kidney-1 clip rat, chronic hypertension was associated with the increase in aortic-converting enzyme activity [24]. Converting enzyme inhibitor administration lowered blood pressure in both animal models, despite normal or suppressed plasma renin angiotensin activities [23–25]. In support of these observations, Longnecker *et al.* demonstrated that saralasin-dilated arterioles in the spontaneous hypertensive rat with normal plasma renin activity [26].

Although several different explanations have been proposed for these observations, a likely possibility is that these agents inhibited the local generation of angiotensin II in the vessel wall. Implicit in this hypothesis is that local tissue concentrations of angiotensin II may be substantially higher than the plasma levels. This may explain the discrepancy between the receptor-binding affinity of angiotensin and the plasma concentration as reviewed earlier in this paper.

Distribution and localization of renin angiotensin in blood vessels

If vascular wall renin-angiotensin systems contribute to the control of vascular tone, it would be important to know which blood vessels contain this local system. Renin-like activities have been demonstrated in aorta and mesenteric arteries [20, 27]. We have observed renin-like activities in renal, carotid and coronary arteries [28]. Rosenthal and co-workers also reported the detection of renin-like activity in the veins [29]. Thus, renin appears to be present in most, if not all, blood vessels. Angiotensin-converting enzyme is present throughout the vasculature, localized especially to the endothelium. Immunoreactive angiotensins and angiotensin receptors have also been found in various vascular sites [28]. Taken together, these data suggest that a local renin-angiotensin system may be present in most blood vessels.

Let us examine the cellular distribution of vascular renin angiotensin. The vast majority of angiotensin receptors are located on vascular smooth muscle cells of the arterial medial layer. Angiotensin II receptors may also be present on noradrenergic nerve endings that innervate the blood vessel as well as on vascular endothelial cells. Although direct evidence is lacking, one would expect the vasovasorum to contain angiotensin II receptors as well. Angiotensin-converting enzyme is known to be present principally on endothelial cells. In addition, some data suggests that vascular smooth muscle cells may contain an angiotensin-converting enzyme [28]. What about the distribution of renin? Using polyclonal and monoclonal antirenin antibodies, we performed immunohistochemical studies on dog and mouse tissues [28, 30]. In the aorta of both species, intense staining with antirenin antibody can be appreciated in the entire blood vessel wall. Part of the staining is in the interstitial areas, probably due to entrapment of plasma renin. In addition, cellular staining can be seen in both the intimal and medial layers of the aorta. In large- and medium-size arteries, immunostaining with antirenin antibody is primarily seen in the intimal area and in the outer two-thirds of the medial periadventitial regions. It is interesting to consider that the former regiori is composed principally of endothelial cells and the latter region contains vascular smooth muscle cells, vasovasorum as well as sympathetic nerve endings. In small arteries and arterioles, the entire thickness of the blood vessel wall is stained positively (Fig. 1).

To examine further which vascular cells contain renin and whether renin is synthesized in situ in the blood vessel, we studied cultured endothelial and smooth muscle cells [31–33]. We chose to study cultured cells because the cell population is nearly homogenous, and the problem of contamination by plasma components is largely circumvented, especially when serum is removed from growth media for two days prior to assay of the cells. Cultured bovine and canine aortic vascular smooth muscle cells as well as cultured rat mesenteric arterial cells contained immunoreactive renin [31, 32]. Immunoreactive renin was also demonstrated in cultured bovine aortic endothelial cells [33]. Using pulse-labeling with ^{35}S-methionine, we were able to demonstrate that renin was synthesized in situ by both smooth muscle and endothelial cells. In addition, these cells also contain angiotensinogen, angiotensin-converting enzyme and angiotensins. In summary, components of the renin-angiotensin system appear to be localized in both endothelial and smooth muscle cells of the blood vessel supporting the possibility of local angiotensin production by an endogenous system.

Evidence of local production and secretion of angiotensin by blood vessels

In the blood vessel wall, the presence of immunoreactive angiotensin can be interpreted as due to local synthesis, uptake and/or entrapment from plasma [34]. Support for local production of angiotensin independent of plasma angiotensin is obtained from experiments of bilateral nephrectomy. Aguirela *et al.* reported that immunoreactive angiotensin II persisted in the plasma 48 hours after bi-nephrectomy in the rat, at which time plasma renin activity was undetectable [35]. Fei and co-workers measured arterial and venous blood levels of angiotensin I in the sleep, and observed that concentrations of angiotensin I in venous blood are higher than those in the arterial blood [36]. These findings have been interpreted to reflect production of angiotensin I in peripheral tissues, given the extensive conversion and degradation of angiotensin I by the peripheral vasculature. Recently, Campbell reviewed the kinetic data for AI and AII metabolism in peripheral vascular beds of sheep and man [37], and concluded that local productions of angiotensin I and angiotensin II have to take place in the peripheral tissues to account for the venous-arterial differences *in vivo*. Our studies on cultured vascular endothelial cells provide further insight into this issue. Using high-performance liquid chromatography and radioimmunoassay, we have identified angiotensinogen, renin and angiotensin inside these cells [38]. Our experi-

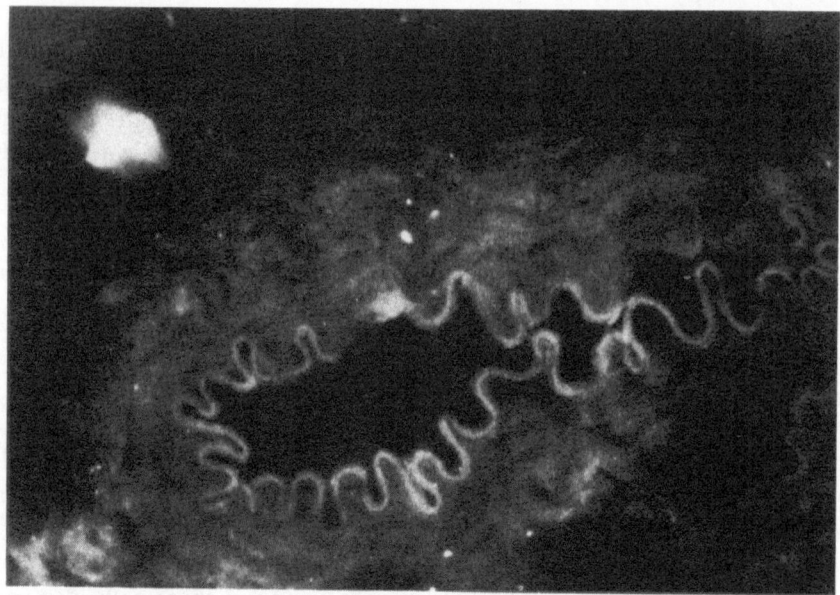

Figure 1. Immunofluorescent staining of a small- to medium-size artery in the mouse kidney with antirenin antibody. No positive staining in the intima, media as well as periadventitial area.

ments demonstrated that endothelial cells secrete angiotensins II and III. Taken together, the data suggest that a renin-angiotensinogen reaction takes place intracellularly in the blood vessel wall, resulting in the production of angiotensins which are subsequently secreted extracellularly where these vasoactive peptides exert their actions.

Physiological significance of vascular renin-angiotensin system

The observations that angiotensins may be synthesized and secreted by vascular cells may have important physiological, pathophysiological and pharmacological implications. Vascular renin angiotensin may accumulate in the blood vessel wall in concentrations that exceed those of plasma. Local angiotensins may exert a variety of autocrine or paracrine influences on vascular tone (Fig. 2). Local angiotensin may stimulate vasoconstriction by activating its receptors on vascular smooth muscle cells. Accumulation of angiotensin in the region of noradrenergic nerve endings (especially in the outer medial layers) may increase sympathetic vascular tone by facilitating catecholamine release from nerve endings [39–41]. Vascular angiotensin may also influence endothelial prostacyclin synthesis which may result in vasodilatation [42]. Recently, Nishimura and co-workers observed that Sar^{1}Val^5 angiotensin II may relax chicken aorta by the release of a endothelial-derived relaxant-like factor [18]. Support for the physiological relevance of local vascular angiotensin on the control of blood pressure and vascular tone is

POSSIBLE INFLUENCES OF VASCULAR ANGIOTENSIN:

ENDOTHELIAL - SMOOTH MUSCLE CELL INTERACTION

A.

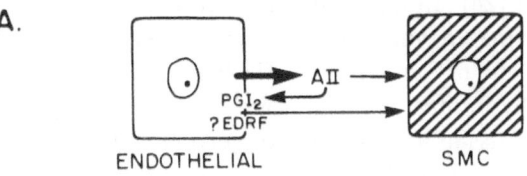

ENDOTHELIAL   SMC

SMOOTH MUSCLE CELL - CELL INTERACTION

B.

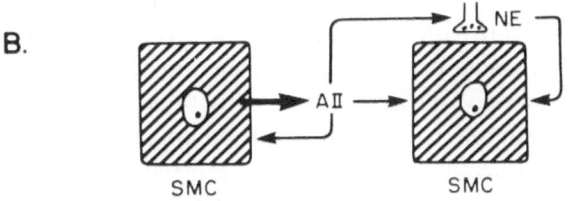

SMC   SMC

Figure 2. Possible mechanisms of action of vascular renin angiotensin.
A. Endothelial cells release angiotensin II (AII) which stimulates autocrine secretion of prostacyclin (PGI$_2$) and possibly endothelial-derived relaxant factor (EDRF). These vasoactive agents influence the contractile state of the vascular smooth muscle.
B. Smooth muscle cell (SMC) releases angiotensin II (AII) which stimulates autocrine contraction. AII may also produce a paracrine influence on smooth muscle tone by activating AII receptors on adjacent SMC or by facilitating norepinephrine (NE) release by sympathetic nerve ending.

derived from experiments measuring renin angiotensin in vascular tissues of hypertensive animals and from studies of inhibitors of the renin-angiotensin system in animals and man. Asaad and Antonaccio [23] observed that in spontaneously hypertensive rats with normal plasma renin levels, the systolic blood pressure correlated closely with the concentration of renin in the aorta but not in the plasma. In these rats, chronic captopril administration significantly decreased systemic blood pressure. In another experimental hypertension model with suppressed plasma renin concentration, that is, the chronic phase of two-kidney one-clip hypertension, prolonged saralasin infusion corrected the hypertension [25]. Recently, Okamura extended the above observation to include measurements of vascular angiotensin-converting enzyme activity and angiotensin II generation in the chronic phase of this model of hypertension [24]. These investigators demonstrated that during the chronic phase of rat 2-kidney 1-clip hypertension, when plasma renin activity is almost normal, vascular renin-angiotensin activity is increased. This is documented by increases in angiotensin-converting enzyme activity of vascular tissues and in the constrictor response of isolated arteries to angiotensin I. Their data suggests that increased angiotensin II concentration is present in the vascular tissues and may be responsible for chronic hypertension. The dissociation of vascular and circulating renin-angiotensin activities supports the postulate that a local system exists in blood vessels which contributes to the control of vascular tone [24]. Indeed, Okamura and co-workers demonstrated that angiotensin-converting enzyme inhibitor (enalapril) and angiotensin II antagonist (sarcosine[1] isoleucine[8] angiotensin II) lowered blood pressure in the chronic 2-kidney 1-clip hypertensive rats despite near normal plasma renin level [24]. The importance of tissue angiotensin-converting enzyme, rather than the serum counterpart, in determining long-term response to angiotensin-converting enzyme inhibitors has been suggested by several investigators [43–45]. In these studies, the magnitude and duration of blood pressure reduction appeared to correlate better with the inhibition of angiotensin-converting enzyme activity in certain critical tissues than with the inhibition of serum enzyme activity. For example, hours after a single dose of angiotensin-converting enzyme inhibitor (when serum angiotensin-converting enzyme activity as well as the pressor response to exogenous angiotensin I had returned to normal) blood pressure remained reduced. The duration of the antihypertensive response paralleled the suppression of aortic and kidney angiotensin-converting enzyme activities but not serum angiotensin-converting enzyme.

Additional support for the importance of noncirculating renin angiotensin is provided by studies using renin inhibitory peptide which induced depressor responses in human subjects with normal plasma renin activity [46]. Similarly, the statine-containing renin inhibitory peptide lowered blood pressure in dogs with completely suppressed plasma renin activity [47]. Its effect on blood pressure appears to be dissociated from plasma renin inhibition. Finally, it has been well documented that angiotensin-converting enzyme inhibitors, e.g. captopril can lower blood pressure in some patients with normal or low plasma renin activity.

Possible influence of vascular renin angiotensin on resistance and conduit arteries (Fig. 3)

Given the widespread distribution of renin angiotensin in the vascular tree, let us consider the vascular responses to blockade of vascular renin angiotensin. Longnecker *et al.* demonstrated that saralasin administration resulted in significant dilation of arterioles in the spontaneously hypertensive rats [26]. Saralasin has also been shown to cause vasodilation of small- and medium-size vessels. It is well accepted that the depressor response to inhibition of renin angiotensin is due to relaxation of resistance vessels. Data of Safar and co-workers add another dimension of the renin angiotensin effect on the vasculature. These investigators observed that the compliance and diameter of brachial and carotid arteries in man increased with captopril [48–50]. The increase in diameters occurred without a necessary detectable reduction in systemic blood pressure suggesting a direct

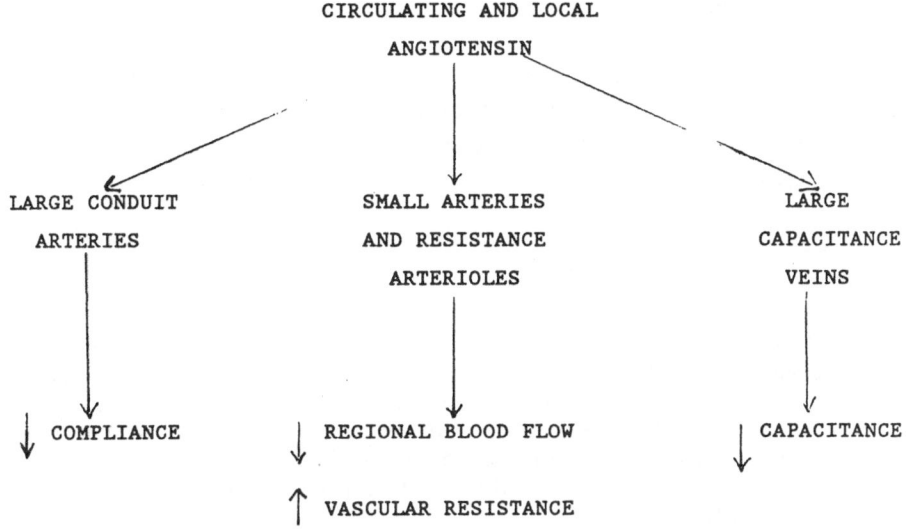

Figure 3. Possible effects of vascular renin-angiotensin system inhibition on small resistance and large conduit vessels and veins.

effect of angiotensin on the arterial wall. This observation raises the possibility that the local renin angiotensin activity in the aorta and large arteries can influence the conduit and buffering functions of these vessels. This interesting effect of renin-angiotensin inhibition on increases in arterial compliance may have beneficial influence in arterial impedance and ventricular afterload. In addition, the possibility of hypertensive arterial wall injury, which is believed to play a role in the genesis of atherosclerosis may also be reduced.

Summary

The renin-angiotensin system affects blood pressure and regional blood flow through endocrine, paracrine and autocrine influences. The circulating renin-angiotensin system is activated for acute cardiovascular homeostasis. The recent demonstration of a local renin-angiotensin system in the blood vessel wall and its activation in chronic hypertension have led us to speculate that the local production of angiotensin is involved with tonic control of vascular resistance. In addition to producing arteriolar constriction, arterial wall renin angiotensin may influence the compliance of large conduit arteries. Although direct data are lacking, vascular angiotensin production could occur in the veins and may influence capacitance vessels and preload.

162

Acknowledgement

The author is indebted to Ms. Sarah Curwood for preparing and editing this manuscript. Supported in part by NIH grants R01 HL35610, P01 HL19259 and a grant from R.J. Reynolds Industry, Inc. The author is an Established Investigator of the American Heart Association.

References

1. Mendelsohn FAO (1985): Editorial review: Localization and properties of angiotensin receptors. J Hypertension 3: 307–316.
2. Lin S-Y, Goodfriend TL (1970): Angiotensin receptors. Am J Physiol 218: 1319–1328.
3. Devynck M-A, Pernollet M-G, Meyer P, Fermandjian S, Fromageot P (1973): Angiotensin receptors in smooth muscle cell membranes. Nature New Biol 245: 55–58.
4. Le Morvan P, Faliac D (1975): Characterization of the angiotensin receptor in guinea pig aorta. J Pharmacol Exp Ther 195: 167–175.
5. Penit J, Faure M, Jard S (1983): Vasopressin and angiotensin II receptors in rat aortic smooth muscle cells in culture. Am J Physiol 244: E72–E82.
6. Wright GB, Alexander RW, Ekstein LS, Gimbrone Ma Jr (1982): Sodium, divalent cations and guanine nucleotides regulate the affinity of rat mesenteric artery. Circ Res 40: 462–469.
7. Toda N (1984): Endothelium-dependent relation induced by angiotensin II and histamine in isolated arteries of dog. Br J Pharmac 81: 301–307.
8. Yamaguchi K, Nishimura H (1986): Endothelium-dependent relaxation of fowl aorta induced by angiotensin II. Fed Proc 54: 869 (Abst).
9. Ichikawa I, Brenner BM (1984): Glomerular action of angiotensin II. Am J Med 76: 43–49.
10. Gavras H, Liang CS, Brunner HR: Redistribution of regional blood flow after inhibition of the angiotensin-converting enzyme. Cir Res 43 (Suppl I): 159–163.
11. Creager MA, Halperin J, Bernard D, Faxon D, Melidossian C, Gavras H, Ryan TJ (1981): Acute regional circulatory and renal hemodynamic effects of converting-enzyme inhibition in patients with congestive heart failure. Circulation 64: 483–489.
12. Dzau VJ, Creagen MA (1986): Neurohormonal mechanisms in heart failure. Heart Failure 2: 3–5.
13. Hricik DE, Browning PJ, Kopelman RI, Goorno WE, Madias NE, Dzau VJ (1983): Captopril-induced functional renal insufficiency in patients with bilateral renal-artery stenosis or renal-artery stenosis in solitary kidney. N Engl J Med 308: 373–376.
14. Textor SC, Novick AC, Mujais SK (1983): Response of the stenosed and contralateral kidneys to Sar-1-Thr-8-AII in human renovascular hypertension. Hypertension 5: 796–804.
15. Aguilera G, Catt K (1981): Regulation of vascular angiotensin II receptors in the rat during altered sodium intake. Circulation Res 49: 751–758.
16. Hollenberg NK, Chenitz WR, Adams DR, Williams GH (1974): Reciprocal influence of salt intake on adrenal glomerulosa and renal vascular response to angiotensin II in normal man. J Clin Invest 54: 34–42.
17. Gunther S, Gimbrone MA Jr, Alexander RW (1980): Regulation by angiotensin II of its receptors in resistance blood vessels. Nature 287: 230–232.
18. Foidart J, Sraer J, Delarue F, Mahieur P, Ardaillou R (1980): Evidence for mesangial glomerular receptors for angiotensin II linked to mesangial cell contractility. FEBS Lett 121: 333–339.
19. Swales JD, Thurston H (1973): Generation of angiotensin II of peripheral vascular level: studies using angiotensin II antisera. Clin Sci Mol Med 45: 691–700.
20. Dzau VJ (1984): Vascular wall renin-angiotensin pathway in control of the circulation: A

hypothesis. Am J Med 77 (4A): 31–36.

21. Rozenthal J, Boucher R, Rojo Ortega JM, Genest J (1969): Renin activity in aortic tissue of rats. Can J Physiol Pharmacol 47: 53–56.

22. Basso N, Taquin AC (1971): Effect of bilaterial nephrectomy on renin activity of blood vessel walls. Acta Physiol 210: 8–14.

23. Assad MM, Antonaccio MJ (1982): Vascular wall renin in spontaneously hypertensive rats; potential relevance to hypertension maintenance and antihypertensive effect by captopril. Hypertension 4: 487–493.

24. Okamura T, Myazaki M, Inagami T, Toda N (1986): Vascular renin-angiotensin system in two-kidney, one clip hypertensive rats. Hypertension 8: 000–000.

25. Riegger AJG, Lever AF, Millar JA, Morton JJ, Slack B (1977): Correction of renal hypertension in the rat by prolonged infusion of saralasin inhibitors. Lancet 2: 1317–1319.

26. Longnecker DE, Durieux ME, Donovan KR, Miller ED, Peach MJ (1984): Saralsin dilates arterioles in SHR but not WKY rats. Hypertension 6 (Suppl I): I-106–I-110.

27. Desjardins-Gaisson S, Gutkowska J, Gracia R, Genest J (1981): Renin substrate in rat mesenteric artery. Can J Physiol Pharmacol 58: 528–532.

28. Dzau VJ (unpub. observation).

29. Rosenthal JH, Pfeifle B, Michailov ML, Pschorr J, Jacob ICM, Dahlheim H (1984): Investigations of components of the renin-angiotensin system in rat vascular tissue. Hypertension 6: 383–390.

30. Molteni A, Dzau VJ, Fallon JT, Haber E (1984): Monoclonal antibodies as probes of renin gene expression. Circulation 70 (Suppl II): II-196 (abstract).

31. Re R, Fallon JT, Dzau VJ, Quay SC, Haber E (1982): Renin synthesis by canine aortic smooth muscle cells in culture. Life Sci 30: 99–106.

32. Dzau VJ (1984): Vascular renin-angiotensin: A possible autocrine or paracine system in control of vascular function. J Cardiovasc Pharmacol 6: S377–S382.

33. Lilly LS, Pratt RE, Alexander RW, Larson DM, Ellison KE, Gimbrone MA, Dzau VJ (1984): Renin expression by vascular endothelial cells in culture. Cir Res 57: 312–318 (E-38).

34. Loudon M, Bing RF, Thurston H, Swales JD (1983): Arterial wall uptake of renal renin and blood pressure control. Hypertension 5: 629–634.

35. Aguirela G, Schirar A, Baukai A, Gatt KJ (1981): Circulating angiotensin II and adrenal receptors after nephrectomy. Nature 289: 507–509.

36. Fei DTW, Scoggins BA, Tregear GW, Coghlan JP (1981): Angiotensin I, II and III in sheep: A model of angiotensin production and metabolism. Hypertension 3: 730–737.

37. Campbell DJ (1985): The site of angiotensin production. J Hypertension 3: 199–207.

38. Kifor I, Roth T, Dzau VJ (1985): Cultured vascular cells synthesize and secrete angiotensins. Circulation 72: III-420.

39. Malik KU, Nasjletti A (1976): Facilitation of adrenergic transmission by locally generated angiotensin II in rat mesenteric arteries. Circ Res 38: 26–30.

40. Zimmerman BG (1981): Adrenergic facilitation by angiotensin: Does it serve a physiological function? Clin Sci 60: 343–348.

41. Kawasaki H, Cline WH Jr, Su C (1984): Involvement of the vascular renin-angiotensin system in beta adrenergic receptor-mediated facilitation of vascular neurotransmission in spontaneously hypertensive rats. J Pharmacol Exp Ther 231: 23—32.

42. Gimbrone RW, Alexander RW (1975): Angiotensin II stimulation of prostaglandin production in cultured human vascular endothelium. Science 189: 219–220.

43. Unger T, Ganten D, Lang RE, Scholkens BA (1985): Persistent tissue converting enzyme inhibition following treatment with Hoe498 and MK421 in spontaneously hypertensive rats. J Cardiovasc Pharmacol 7: 36–41.

44. Unger T, Ganten D, Lang RE, Scholkens BA (1984): Is tissue converting inhibition a determinant of the antihypertensive efficacy of converting enzyme inhibitors? Studies with the two

164

different compounds, Hoe398 and MK421, in spontaneously hypertensive rats. J Cardiovasc Pharmacol 6: 872–880.

45. Cohen L, Kurz KD (1982): Angiotensin converting enzyme inhibition in tissues from spontaneously hypertensive rats after treatment with captopril or MK-421. J Pharm Exp Therap 220: 1.

46. Haber E, Zusman R, Burton J, Dzau VJ, Barger AC (1983): Is renin a factor in the etiology of essential hypertension? Hypertension 5 (Suppl V): V-8–V-15.

47. Blaine EH, Schorn TW, Boger J (1984): Statine-containing renin inhibitor. Dissociation of blood pressure lowering and renin inhibition in sodium-deficient dogs. Hypertension 6: I-11–I-118.

48. Safar ME, Bouthier JA, Levenson J, Simon A (1983): Peripheral large arteries and the response to antihypertensive treatment. Hypertension 4 (Suppl III) III-63–III-68.

49. Simon ACh, Levenson J, Bouthier JA, Safar ME (1984): Captopril induced changes of large arteries in essential hypertension. Regional hemodynamics following captopril therapy. Am J Med 76 (5B): 71–76.

50. Safar ME, Laurent St, Bouthier JA, London GM (1986): Comparative effects of captopril and isosorbide dinitrate on the arterial wall of hypertensive human brachial arteries. J Cardiovasc Pharmacol 8: 1257–1261.

Part IV

Regional circulations

The coronary circulation in hypertensive left ventricular hypertrophy

PIERRE A. WICKER and ROBERT C. TARAZI†

There is ample evidence to suggest that the coronary circulation may be inadequate in hypertensive heart disease. Patients with elevated blood pressure, particularly those with left ventricular hypertrophy (LVH), may develop symptoms suggestive of myocardial ischemia such as angina pectoris or ST-T segment depression during exercise [1, 2]. Myocardial infarction is more severe in hypertensive humans and animals [3, 4] and the size of the infarcted area is larger in hypertensive dogs with LVH [5]. Moreover, these coronary abnormalities may contribute to the increased risk of cardiac complications or sudden death in hypertensive patients with electrocardiographic and possibly echocardiographic evidence of LVH [6, 7]. Advances in our understanding of the effects of hypertensive LVH on the coronary circulation will therefore provide crucial and clinically relevant information. This question assumes even further significance in view of recent developments regarding the possibility of reversing hypertensive LVH [8].

A large body of data is available on coronary blood flow changes in hypertensive LVH. However, the adequacy of myocardial oxygen supply depends not only on the amount of flow delivered to the heart but also on diffusion between capillaries and tissue. Despite its important physiological role, this microcirculatory aspect of the coronary circulation has never been thoroughly investigated, essentially because of methodological limitations. For similar reasons, studies of the coronary circulation in human hypertension are scarce. Current techniques for measuring coronary blood flow in mass are invasive and cannot be either ethically justified or repeated easily. Thus the following review mainly focuses on animal studies, from which most of our knowledge originates.

I. Coronary circulation during the development of hypertensive left ventricular hypertrophy

A. Coronary blood flow studies

a) Resting coronary blood flow
Resting coronary blood flow per unit mass of LV myocardial tissue has been reported to be normal in most experimental and clinical studies (Tables 1 and 2). In hypertensive LVH, resting coronary blood flow remains autoregulated by myocardial oxygen needs, as it is in normal conditions. This conclusion is substantiated by studies showing a correlation between coronary blood flow and myocardial oxygen consumption whether the latter was measured directly or estimated indirectly from its main determinants [14, 22].

Since oxygen supply matches oxygen needs under baseline conditions, resting flow determinations do not provide any information as to whether a hypertrophied ventricle is at a greater risk of ischemia. The same conclusion applies to the transmural distribution of coronary flow (endo/epi ratio). This ratio, which can be measured in animals only, remains normal in hypertensive LVH with a perfusion gradient favoring the subendocardial layers (endo/epi ratio greater than one) (Table 1). In a few studies, however, the endo/epi ratio was slightly less than that measured in control animals [12, 18], although the difference was not significant. This pattern of resting flow distribution probably reflects variations in myocardial oxygen needs between the various myocardial layers and therefore shall not be considered as evidence for subendocardial ischemia.

b) Coronary reserve in hypertensive left ventricular hypertrophy [26–28]
Myocardial ischemia develops when oxygen supply is no longer equal to oxygen needs, either because of an increase in myocardial consumption or a reduction in flow secondary to a decrease in perfusion pressure. In both situations, the coronary circulation responds by vasodilation. It has therefore been proposed to study the coronary circulation after the administration of vasodilatory stimuli, in order to assess its ability to dilate and to provide an adequate myocardial perfusion under these conditions. The 'maximal' coronary flow or the 'minimal' coronary resistance per unit mass following these maneuvers have been termed coronary flow and coronary vasodilator (or resistance) reserve, respectively. Two different types of stimuli have been proposed to determine coronary reserve. Most studies have used a pharmacological approach with potent coronary vasodilators, such as adenosine, dipyridamole, or carbochrome. Physiological interventions have been less commonly utilized. They include exercise, cardiac pacing or ischemia elicited by a transient coronary occlusion. Finally, it is also possible to assess coronary reserve in isolated hearts, an experimental situation in which coronary vessels are nearly maximally dilated.

Table 1. Resting coronary blood flow, its transmural distribution (endo/epi ratio) and coronary resistance in experimental left ventricular hypertrophy.

Author	(Ref)	Animal/Model	LVCBF/unit mass		LVCR/ unit mass
			Total	endo/epi	
Breull	[9]	RAT/1K-1C, DOCA	↓	–	↑
Breull	[9]	RAT/2K-1C, SHR	NS	–	↑
Mueller	[10]	DOG/1K-1C	NS	NS	↑
Bache	[11]	DOG/1K-1W	NS	NS	↑
Marcus	[12]	DOG/2K-2C	NS	NS	↑
Wangler	[13]	RAT/SHR	NS	NS	NS
Ely	[14]	DOG/1K-1W	NS	NS	–
Kobayashi	[15, 16]	RAT/2K-1C, SHR-SP	NS	–	–
Yamamoto	[17]	RAT/DOCA	NS	NS	↑
Tomanek	[18]	RAT/SHR	NS	NS	NS
	[19]	DOG/1K-1C	NS	NS	↑
Wicker	[20, 21]	RAT/2K-1C	NS or ↑	NS	↑

LVCBF: Left ventricular coronary blood flow.
LVCR: Left ventricular coronary resistance.

1K-1C, 2K-1C, 2K-2C: one kidney - one clip, two kidney - one clip, two kidney - two clip Goldblatt hypertension; 1K-1W: one kidney - one wrapped Page Hypertension; DOCA = Doca salt hypertension; SHR: Spontaneously hypertensive rats; SP: Stroke prone.

NS = not statistically different from controls.

↑ or ↓ : Significantly greater or lower than controls.

–: not reported.

Table 2. Resting left ventricular coronary blood flow and coronary resistance in hypertensive patients with and without left ventricular hypertrophy.

Author	(Ref)	Patients	LVCBF/ unit mass	LVCR/ unit mass
Nichols	[22]	LVH (+116%), AP, no CAD	↓	↑
Nichols	[22]	no LVH, AP, no CAD	NS	NS
Bing	[23]	LVH?, CAD?	NS	–
Rowe	[24]	LVH?, CAD?	NS	↑
Opherk	[1]	LVH (+62%), AP, no CAD	NS	↑
Strauer	[25]	LVH (+33% to +109%), with or without CAD	↑	↑

LVH: left ventricular hypertrophy.
AP = angina pectoris; CAD = Coronary artery disease.
All other abbreviations as in Table 1.

1) Coronary Vasodilator Reserve

With one exception, coronary vasodilator reserve ('minimal' coronary resistance/ unit mass) has consistently been found to be reduced in experimental hypertensive LVH (Table 3). This basic agreement is remarkable in view of the various species, models of hypertrophy, and types of vasodilatory stimuli used. Moreover, similar observations have been made in man. In the only two clinical studies so far published, Strauer *et al.*, and Opherk *et al.*, have reported that post-dipyridamole minimal coronary resistance/g of tissue was elevated in hypertensive patients with LVH [1, 25].

Table 3. Coronary total or transmural (endo/epi) flow reserve and coronary vasodilator reserve in experimental left ventricular hypertrophy.

Author	(Ref)	Animal/Model	Coronary Flow Reserve		Coronary Vasodilator Reserve
			Total	endo/epi	
Pharmacological Dilatation[1]					
Mueller	[10]	DOG/1K-1C	NS	NS	↓
Marcus	[12]	DOG/2K-1C	↓	NS	↓
Wangler	[13]	RAT/SHR 7 mos	NS	↑	↓
		3,15 mos	NS	↑	NS
Kobayashi	[15, 16]	RAT/2K-1C, SHR-SP	NS	–	–
Yamamoto	[17]	DOG/DOCA	NS	NS	↓
Tomanek	[18]	RAT/SHR	NS	NS	↓
	[19]	DOG/1K-1C	NS	NS	↓
Wicker	[20, 21]	RAT/2K-1C	NS	NS or ↓	↓
Exercise					
Bache	[11]	DOG/1K-1W	NS	NS	NS
Ischemia (Transient Coronary Occlusion)[2]					
Peters	[29]	RAT/SHR 3,7 mos	↓	–	–
		15 mos	NS	–	–
Isolated hearts[2]					
Klepzig	[30]	RAT/SHR	–	–	↓
Friberg	[31]	RAT/SHR	↓	–	–
Buttrick	[32]	RAT/2K-1C	↓	–	–

[1] Pharmacological dilatation induced by adenosine: (ref. 10, 12, 19). dipyridamole: (ref. 13, 17, 18), and carbochrome: (ref. 15, 16, 20, 21).

[2] Minimal LV coronary resistance (LV coronary vasodilator reserve) was not measured or reported in these studies (except ref 30). However, maximal LV coronary flow was either similar to controls or decreased despite an increased or a similar coronary perfusion pressure respectively. This suggests that coronary vasodilator reserve was reduced.

All abbreviations as in Table 1.

i) Factors modulating coronary vasodilator reserve. Although in the vast majority of studies it has been concluded that coronary vasodilator reserve is limited in hypertensive LVH, the extent of this reduction is by no means identical. Various factors, such as the species, the duration, and the severity of hypertrophy may modulate the consequences of cardiac hypertrophy on the coronary circulation. Coronary vasodilator reserve is usually more depressed in humans than in animals [1, 25] (Table 3). Apart from an obvious species difference, this contrast between experimental and clinical situations may also be related to a greater degree of hypertrophy noted in these clinical studies. The effects of hypertrophy duration are controversial at the present time. Some studies have reported an improvement in coronary vasodilator reserve when hypertension was present for more than one year in spontaneously hypertensive rats (SHR) [13, 29]. However, another study could not document such an amelioration [31].

ii) Structural and functional basis for the diminished coronary vasodilator reserve. Theoretically, the elevation in minimal coronary resistance/unit mass of tissue can either be related to an increase in cardiac mass without associated changes in the coronary vasculature or to an intrinsic alteration in the ability of the coronary resistance vessels, i.e. the coronary arterioles, to dilate. Computation of the minimal coronary resistance for the entire LV, as proposed by Mueller *et al.* [10], provides an important conceptual background to interpret the effects of LVH on the coronary circulation as it allows separation of the role of changes in LV mass from that of alterations in the coronary resistance vessels. With only one exception [12], minimal total coronary resistance following pharmacological dilation has consistently been found to be unchanged in hypertensive LVH [10, 13, 15–21]. These results suggest that the total size of the coronary resistance bed does not keep pace with the development of hypertrophy [26]. The exact reasons for this lack of growth are not completely understood, but are probably related to structural or functional alterations of the coronary circulation. One simple explanation may be that the coronary resistance vessels do not proliferate and that their individual vasodilatory capacity remains unchanged. One recent study indicates that arteriolar density, the number of arterioles/unit cross-sectional area of tissue, does diminish in a model of pressure overload hypertrophy induced by aortic banding [33], thus lending support to this hypothesis. However, there have been no reported studies of this in hypertensive LVH, and whether vascular rarefaction (relative to mass) also occurs in hypertension remains speculative. A decrease in the vasodilatory capacity of each individual coronary resistance vessel constitutes a more likely explanation. Various histological studies have demonstrated an increase in the thickness of the media or in the wall-to-thickness ratio of coronary arteries from hypertensive patients [34, 35] and animals [36, 37]. According to Folkow's hypothesis [38], these structural alterations will lead to an increased resistance at maximal dilation. Other lines of indirect evidence derived from experiments in isolated hearts [39] or studies of the right ventricular coronary circulation [18, 40] also favor the responsibility of structural alterations in the diminution in coronary vasodilator reserve. However, other anatomical studies in dogs with renal hypertension [19] or in hypertensive patients [1] could not document any significant changes in the coronary artery wall-to-lumen ratio. These observations led us to postulate that the coronary vasodilatory capacity may also be impaired because of functional factors. Although many functional factors can potentially alter coronary vasomotricity, the sympathetic nervous system and the renin hypertensive system are the most likely candidates. These two systems have been involved in the development and maintenance of hypertension [41, 42] and stimulation of their activity can cause coronary vasoconstriction or limit pharmacologically induced coronary vasodilation [43, 44]. However, preliminary observations from our laboratory suggest that the renin angiotensin system does not significantly affect coronary reserve, at least in renal hypertensive rats (Wicker P, unpublished observations).

2) Coronary flow reserve

In most of the studies summarized in Table 3, coronary flow reserve in hypertensive animals is unchanged as compared to their controls. The reasons for the maintenance of a normal coronary flow reserve can be easily understood by analyzing the relationship between coronary flow reserve and its determinants, that is peripheral pressure, total LV coronary resistance and LV mass [20, 27]. Since minimal coronary resistance for the entire LV is unchanged, coronary perfusion pressure will set maximal total flow and the ratio between perfusion pressure and LV mass will thus determine coronary flow reserve, i.e. total flow/LV mass. Thus, in hypertensive LVH, coronary flow reserve remains normal because, in most of the experimental models so far studied, cardiac hypertrophy is usually appropriate to the increased load and the pressure/mass ratio is normal. The role of an appropriate balance between arterial pressure and LV mass in determining coronary flow reserve was further substantiated by two studies in which we dissociated blood pressure from LV mass either by therapeutic manipulations in renal hypertensive rats or by using strains with divergent degrees of cardiac hypertrophy and hypertension [16, 20]. A significant correlation was found between the pressure/LV mass ratio and pharmacologically induced coronary flow reserve either in renal hypertensive rats (Fig. 1) or in rats with a genetically determined pressure/mass ratio [16].

Studies of the transmural coronary flow reserve have yielded more viable results, particularly in rats (Table 3). Most investigations, however, have reported a normal endo/epi ratio following pharmacological vasodilation or exercise.

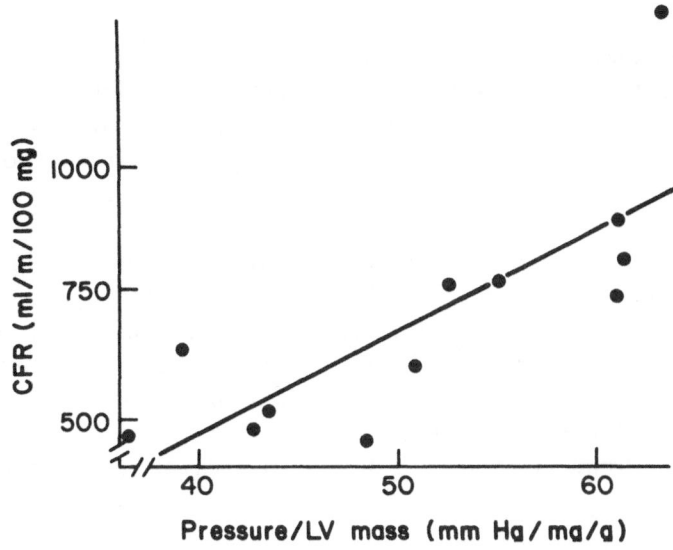

Figure 1. Correlation between coronary flow reserve and the ratio of coronary pressure to left ventricular mass. n = 12, r = 0.76, p<0.01.

B. Coronary microcirculation

Among the various parameters that can be measured to characterize the terminal coronary bed, capillary density and intercapillary distance have been the most widely investigated, since they determine tissue oxygenation according to the Krogh model [45]. The mean anatomical capillary density, which is defined as the number of capillaries/mm^2 of tissue cross-sectional area, has been found to be either reduced, particularly in the subendocardial layers [18, 19, 46–52] or unchanged [19, 47, 49, 50, 53]. Accordingly, the mean distance between capillaries is either increased [50, 54] or normal [53, 54]. Studies in SHR suggest that the duration of hypertrophy and/or the age of the animal are important factors in modulating the response of the capillary bed to hypertension. In SHR younger than 2–3 months, epicardial capillary density and intercapillary density remain normal despite a mild degree of hypertrophy [49, 50, 53]. With the development of hypertrophy, capillary density significantly declines until cardiac mass reaches a plateau [46, 48–50, 52). Surprisingly, epicardial capillary density may increase and then normalize following a long period of stable hypertrophy in SHR [49, 50]. This favorable course of events, however, could not be confirmed in the same model by other investigators [54]. Apart from these divergences, most studies agree that capillary growth lags behind the increase in LV mass, particularly in the subendocardial layers, during the stable phase of hypertrophy either in SHR or in other models of hypertension [18, 19, 46–52, 54]. That the capillary bed does not proliferate – or shows little growth – in pressure overload hypertrophy has also been demonstrated by studies using autoradiographic techniques [55] or by the fact that the capillary-to-fiber ratio remains unchanged [14, 47]. Another potential important variable governing tissue oxygenation is the heterogeneity of capillary spacing [56]. Cellular hypoxia occurs when peri-mitochondrial PO_2 reaches 0 mm Hg. Such a low PO_2 will be observed in those areas most remote from the capillary vessels [56]. Thus, the presence and degree of tissue hypoxia will be more influenced by the relative proportion of capillaries with long inter-capillary distances than by the overall mean intercapillary distance [56]. Assuming a log-normal distribution for the distance between capillaries, Rakusan *et al.* found that the variability of intercapillary spacing was significantly higher in SHR, particularly in older animals [54]. These initial obervations need to be confirmed by future studies. However, they already provide an attractive explanation for the frequent occurrence of areas of focal necrosis in hypertrophied hearts [57].

II. The coronary circulation in hypertensive left ventricular hypertrophy. Therapeutic aspects

A. Pharmacological treatment

a) Coronary blood flow studies
1) Resting coronary blood flow. Resting coronary blood flow has been reported to be decreased [58], unchanged [20, 59] or increased [15, 60] in hypertensive animals following chronic treatment with various antihypertensive drugs and reversal of LVH. The response to these antihypertensive medications results from a complex interplay between the direct vascular effects of any particular drug and its indirect effects on coronary resistance secondary to changes in myocardial oxygen consumption. A precise delineation of the relative importance of these mechanisms would require simultaneous measurements of myocardial oxygen consumption and/or an evaluation of its main determinants. Such studies have not been reported so far. A more complete discussion of these problems can be found in ref. 61.

2) Coronary reserve. In one of the few studies of coronary reserve following reversal of left ventricular hypertrophy with antihypertensive medications, we found that captopril decreased substantially both blood pressure and LV mass in renal hypertensive rats [20]. Total coronary flow reserve remained within normal limits because 1) minimal total LV coronary resistance remained unchanged and 2) blood pressure and LV mass varied in parallel so that the pressure/mass ratio remained normal. Consequently, mean coronary resistance/unit mass of tissue (coronary vasodilator reserve), which was elevated in untreated rats, returned to normal or near normal levels after captopril therapy [20]. Similar observations have been made following chronic treatment with other classes of antihypertensive agents, such as calcium entry blockers [15], vasodilators [18, 30], or beta blocking drugs [30]. To account for this improvement in coronary reserve, a direct pharmacological vasodilatory effect on the coronary vessels cannot be excluded. This possibility is likely in the case of hydralazine since, in a study by Tomanek *et al.*, minimal coronary resistance/g of tissue or for the whole left ventricle was markedly decreased both in SHR and WKY treated with this medication [18]. Such a mechanism, however, was not likely in our study of captopril since very similar results were obtained after treatment with nephrectomy in renal hypertensive rats, in which any potential pharmacological influence of captopril was excluded [20].

Besides a direct pharmacological coronary effect, two other mechanisms may potentially account for the improvement in coronary vasodilator reserve:
1) an increase in the number of arterioles/unit mass and 2) a reversal of the structural arteriolar abnormalities observed in untreated hypertensive LVH. No data are available on arteriolar density. Regarding the second possibility, one report suggests that the increased wall-to-lumen ratio tends to regress with blood pressure control [18]. However, these morphological observations were not quantitated and more studies are needed before any definite conclusion can be drawn.

b) Coronary microcirculation

Few data are available on the coronary microcirculation following pharmacological antihypertensive therapy and LVH reversal and only the SHR model has been evaluated so far. Studies by Tomanek *et al.* in young adult SHR indicate that mean capillary density was either improved or prevented from deteriorating during the developmental phase of hypertrophy by a treatment with alphamethyldopa [48] or a combination of hydralazine, reserpine, and hydrochlorothiazide [62]. Hydralazine alone, however, failed to influence mean capillary density [18]. Changes in capillary density during the development and reversal of hypertrophy are inversely related to changes in myocyte size and in cardiac mass [48–50, 62], suggesting that the improvement in capillary density was not due to capillary proliferation but resulted from a decrease in muscle cell volume per unit mass. Whatever the exact mechanism is, the observation of an inverse relationship between myocyte size and capillary density may offer potentially important therapeutic implications. Drugs that control blood pressure without a simultaneous reduction in cardiac mass will not alter mean capillary density; on the contrary, medications that regress cardiac hypertrophy will also improve capillary density regardless of their antihypertensive effects.

B. *Nonpharmacological treatment*

Various studies indicate that physical training may promote myocardial vascularity, particularly in rodents. In normal rats and also in dogs, capillary density and coronary vasodilator reserve have been found to be improved following conditioning by swimming or running [63]. These observations led us [21] and others [32, 52] to postulate that exercise, when superimposed on hypertension, could protect the coronary circulation against some of the deleterious effects of cardiac hypertrophy. Unfortunately, results of these studies have not been consistent. On one hand, Crisman *et al.* [52] have reported a normalization in capillary density in SHR conditioned by running. On the other hand, Buttrick and co-workers as well as our group could not document any improvement in either coronary flow or coronary vasodilator reserve in renal hypertensive rats following a swimming program [21, 32]. These contradictory observations are preliminary and obviously the nature of the effects of exercise on myocardial perfusion in hypertensive LVH deserves further investigations. Chronic exercise is now widely accepted as a nonpharmacological approach to treat hypertension. Moreover, some studies suggest that physical training may improve cardiac function in hypertensive animals [64]. These beneficial effects cannot be fully understood without some information on the changes that the coronary circulation undergoes in similar circumstances.

III. Clinical implications

Because of the dependency of chronic flow reserve on the level of coronary perfusion pressure in relation to the perfused mass, hypertensive hearts may theoretically be more susceptible to develop ischemia when aortic pressure is acutely or chronically decreased without any concomitant change in LV mass. However, myocardial consequences of a reduction in aortic pressure may prove to be complex, as any fall in pressure will also decrease LV stress and myocardial oxygen requirements, thereby diminishing the severity of ischemia or even preventing its occurrence. However, large increments in the other two major determinants of myocardial oxygen consumption, heart rate, and contractility, may offset the beneficial consequences of a decrease in blood pressure on oxygen requirements. Because the reduction in blood pressure will hamper blood supply, ischemia may ensue. This could be the case during acute exercise in hypertensive patients treated with antihypertensive medications that control resting and exercise blood pressure without any concomitant LVH regression. However, in the absence of data in man, these extrapolations on the role of the pressure/mass ratio from animal studies to the clinical arena must remain speculative at the present time.

In addition, the consequences of these coronary abnormalities on tissue oxygenation may become far more important when hypertensive LVH is associated with other pathological states that also alter oxygen supply, such as coronary artery disease. In this situation, resting vasodilation will maintain an adequate supply but at the expense of the coronary reserve, and further increments in myocardial requirements may not be met. This mechanism can partially account for the greater severity of coronary artery disease in patients or animals with hypertensive LVH [3–5].

Conclusions

A large body of knowledge, mostly from animal studies, is currently available on the coronary circulation in hypertensive LVH. However, as pointed out many times in this review, much remains to be learned. Obviously, most of these experimental observations have to be extended to clinical situations, particularly during reversal of left ventricular hypertrophy. The current development of noninvasive methods for measuring coronary blood flow in man holds promise in that matter, as these techniques will allow repeated measurements in asymptomatic hypertensive patients. Also, investigations of the anatomical and functional characteristics of the coronary microcirculation, which are potentially as relevant as flow measurements in terms of tissue oxygenation, are in their infancy because of methodological difficulties. Despite these technical limitations, this area should be more often explored. Finally, studies directly linking these coronary abnormalities to the development of ischemia are needed, as the consequences of these alterations on myocardial metabolic supply are more often assumed than demonstrated. Answers to these questions will significantly improve our understanding of hypertensive heart disease and ultimately translate into improved patient care.

References

1. Opherk D, Mall G, Zebe H, Schwarz F, Weihe E, Manthey J, Kubler W (1984): Reduction of coronary reserve: a mechanism for angina pectoris in patients with arterial hypertension and normal coronary arteries. Circulation 69: 1–7.
2. Harris CN, Aronow WS, Parker DP, Kapaln MA (1973): Treadmill stress test in left ventricular hypertrophy. Chest 63: 353–357.
3. Kannel WB, Sorlie P, Castelli WP, McGee D (1980): Blood pressure and survival after myocardial infarction: The Framingham Study. Am J Cardiol 45: 326–330.
4. Koyanagi S, Eastham C, Marcus ML (1982): Effects of chronic hypertension and left ventricular hypertrophy on the incidence of sudden cardiac death after coronary artery occlusion in conscious dogs. Circulation 65: 1192–1197.
5. Koyanagi S, Eastham CL, Harrison DG, Marcus ML (1982): Increased size of myocardial infarction in dogs with chronic hypertension and left ventricular hypertrophy. Circ Res 50: 55–62.
6. Kannel WB (1983): Prevalence and natural history of electrocardiographic left ventricular hypertrophy. Am J Med 75 (Suppl 3A): 4–11.

7. Casale PN, Milner M, Devereux RB, Zullo G, Harshfield G, Pickering TG, Spitzer MC, Laragh JH (1985): Value of echocardiographic left ventricular mass in predicting cardiovascular morbid events in hypertensive men. Circulation 72 (Suppl III): III-130 (Abstr).

8. Tarazi RC, Foud FM (1984): Reversal of cardiac hypertrophy in humans. Hypertension 6 (Suppl III): III-140-III-146.

9. Breull W, Redel D, Dahners H, Schotte J, Flohr H (1973): Myocardial blood flow in left ventricular hypertrophy. Bibl Anat 11: 174-179.

10. Mueller TM, Marcus ML, Kerber RE, Young JA, Barnes RW, Abboud FM (1978): Effect of renal hypertension and left ventricular hypertrophy on the coronary circulation in dogs. Circ Res 42: 543-549.

11. Bache RJ, Vrobel TR (1979): Effects of exercise on blood flow in the hypertrophied heart. Am J Cardiol 44: 1029-1033.

12. Marcus ML, Mueller TM, Eastham CL (1981): Effects of short- and long-term left ventricular hypertrophy on coronary circulation. Am J Physiol 241: H358-H362.

13. Wangler RD, Peters KG, Marcus ML, Tomanek RJ (1982): Effects of duration and severity of arterial hypertension and cardiac hypertrophy on coronary vasodilator reserve. Circ Res 51: 10-18.

14. Ely SW, Sun C-W, Knabb RM, Gidday JM, Rubio R, Berne RM (1983): Adenosine and metabolic regulation of coronary blood flow in dogs with renal hypertension. Hypertension 5: 943-950.

15. Kobayashi K, Tarazi RC (1983): Effect of nitrendipine on coronary flow and ventricular hypertrophy in hypertension. Hypertension 5 (Suppl II): II-45-II-51.

16. Kobayashi K, Tarazi RC, Lovenberg W, Rakusan K (1984): Coronary blood flow in genetic cardiac hypertrophy: Am J Cardiol 53: 1360-1364.

17. Yamamoto J, Tsuchiya M, Saito M, Ikeda M (1985): Cardiac contractile and coronary flow reserves in dioxycorticosterone acetate-salt hypertensive rats. Hypertension 7: 569-577.

18. Tomanek RJ, Wangler RD, Bauer CA (1985): Prevention of coronary vasodilator reserve decrement in spontaneously hypertensive rats. Hypertension 7: 533-540.

19. Tomanek RJ, Palmer PJ, Pfeiffer GL, Schreiber KL, Eastham CL, Marcus ML (1986): Morphometry of canine coronary arteries, arterioles, and capillaries during hypertension and left ventricular hypertrophy. Circ Res 58: 38-46.

20. Wicker P, Tarazi RC, Kobayashi K (1983): Coronary blood flow with reversal of cardiac hypertrophy. Am J Cardiol 51: 1744-1749.

21. Wicker P, Tarazi RC: Effects of exercise on the coronary circulation in conscious rats with renovascular hypertension. Submitted for publication.

22. Nichols AB, Sciacca RR, Weiss MB, Blood DK, Brennan DL, Cannon PJ (1980): Effect of left ventricular hypertrophy on myocardial blood flow and ventricular performance in systemic hypertension. Circulation 62: 329-340.

23. Bing RJ, Hammond MM, Handelsman JC, Powers SR, Spencer FC, Eckenhoff JE, Goodale WT, Hafkenschiel JH, Kety SS (1949): The measurement of coronary blood flow, oxygen consumption, and efficiency of the left ventricle in man. Am Heart J 38: 1-24.

24. Rowe GG, Castillo CA, Maxwell GM, Crumpton CW (1961): A hemodynamic study of hypertension including observations on coronary blood flow. Ann Intern Med 54: 405-412.

25. Strauer BE (1979): Ventricular function and coronary hemodynamics in hypertensive heart disease. Am J Cardiol 44: 999-1006.

26. Marcus ML, Mueller TM, Gascho JA, Kerber RE (1979): Effects of cardiac hypertrophy secondary to hypertension on the coronary circulation. Am J Cardiol 44: 1023-1028.

27. Wicker P, Tarazi RC (1982): Coronary blood flow in left ventricular hypertrophy: a review of experimental data. Eur Heart J 3 (Suppl A): 111-118.

28. Hoffman JIE (1984): Maximal coronary flow and the concept of coronary vascular reserve. Circulation 70: 153-159.

29. Peters KG, Wangler RD, Tomanek RJ, Marcus ML (1984): Effects of long-term cardiac hypertrophy on coronary vasodilator reserve in SHR rats. Am J Cardiol 54: 1342–1348.
30. Klepzig M, Strauer BE (1985): Coronary reserve in spontaneously hypertensive rats, the influence of vessel diameter and antihypertensive therapy. J Am Coll Cardiol 5: 487. (Abstr).
31. Friberg P, Nordlander M, Lundin S, Folkow B (1985): Effects of ageing on cardiac performance and coronary flow in spontaneously hypertensive and normotensive rats. Acta Physiol Scand 125: 1–11.
32. Buttrick PM, Schaible TF, Scheuer J (1986): Combined effects of hypertension and conditioning on coronary vascular reserve in rats. J Appl Physiol 60: 275–279.
33. Breisch EA, White FC, Nimmo L, Bloor CM (1985): The interrelationship of coronary vascular structure and flow during pressure overload hypertrophy. Circulation 72 (Suppl III): III–76, (Abstr).
34. Naeye RL (1967): Arteriolar abnormalities with chronic systemic hypertension. A quantitative study. Circulation 35: 662–670.
35. Schneeweiss A, Sherf L, Lehrer E, Lieberman Y, Neufeld HN (1982): Segmental study of the terminal coronary vessels in coarctation of the aorta: A natural model for study of the effect of coronary hypertension on human coronary circulation. Am J Cardiol 49: 1996–2002.
36. Yamori Y, Mori C, Nishio T, Ooshima A, Horie R, Ohtaka M, Soeda T, Saito M, Abe K, Nara Y, Nakao Y, Kihara M (1979): Cardiac hypertrophy in early hypertension. Am J Cardiol 44: 964–969.
37. Anversa P, Melissari M, Tardini A, Olivetti G (1984): Connective tissue accumulation in the left coronary artery of young SHR. Hypertension 6: 526–529.
38. Folkow B, Karlstrom G (1984): Age- and pressure-dependent changes of systemic resistance vessels concerning the relationships between geometric design, wall distensibility, vascular reactivity and smooth muscle sensitivity. Acta Physiol Scand 122: 17–33.
39. Noresson E, Hallback M, Hjalmarsson A (1977): Structural 'resetting' of the coronary vascular bed in spontaneously hypertensive rats. Acta Physiol Scand 101: 363–365.
40. Wicker P, Tarazi RC (1985): Right ventricular coronary flow in arterial hypertension. Am Heart J 110: 845–850, 1985.
41. Nabel EG, Gibbons GH, Dzau VJ (1985): Pathophysiology of experimental renovascular hypertension. Am J Kidney Dis 5: A111–A119.
42. Abboud FM (1982): The sympathetic system in hypertension. State-of-the-Art review. Hypertension 4 (Suppl II): II–208–II–225.
43. Vlahakes GJ, Baer RW, Uhlig PN, Verrier EI, Bristow JD, Hoffmann JIE (1982): Adrenergic influence in the coronary circulation of conscious dogs during maximal vasodilation with adenosine. Circ Res 51: 371–384.
44. Gavras H, Liang C-S, Brunner HR (1978): Redistribution of regional blood flow after inhibition of the angiotensin-converting enzyme. Circ Res 43 (Suppl I): I–59–I—63.
45. Kreuzer F (1982): Oxygen supply to tissues: The Krogh model and its assumptions. Experientia 38: 1415–1426.
46. Lund DD, Romanek RJ (1978): Myocardial morphology in spontaneously hypertensive and aortic-constricted rats. Am J Anat 152: 141–152.
47. Anversa P, Loud AV, Giacomelli F, Wiener J (1978): Absolute morphometric study of myocardial hypertrophy in experimental hypertension. II. Ultrastructure of myocytes and interstitium. Lab Invest 38: 597–609.
48. Tomanek RJ, Davis JW, Anderson SC (1979): The effects of alpha-methyldopa on cardiac hypertrophy in spontaneously hypertensive rats: ultrastructural, stereological, and morphometric analysis. Cardiovasc Res 13: 173–182.
49. Tomanek RJ, Hovanec JM (1981): The effects of long-term pressure-overload and aging on the myocardium. J Mol Cell Cardiol 13: 471–488.
50. Tomanek RJ, Searls JC, Lachenbruch PA (1982): Quantitative changes in the capillary bed

during developing, peak, and stabilized cardiac hypertrophy in the spontaneously hypertensive rat. Circ Res 51: 295–304.

51. Michel JB, Ossondo M, Barres D, Camilleri JP (1984): Effets de l'hypertrophie myocardique experimentale du rat sur la microcirculation coronaire. Arch Mal Coeur 77: 1172–1175.

52. Crisman RP, Rittman B, Tomanek RJ (1985): Exercise-induced myocardial capillary growth in the spontaneously hypertensive rat. Microvasc Res 30: 185–194.

53. Anversa P, Melissari M, Beghi C, Olivetti G (1984): Structural compensatory mechanisms in rat heart in early spontaneous hypertension. Am J Physiol 246: H739–H746.

54. Rakusan K, Hrdina PW, Turek Z, Lakatta EG, Spurgeon HA, Wolford GD (1984): Cell size and capillary supply of the hypertensive rat heart: quantitative study. Basic Res Cardiol 79: 389–395.

55. Ljungqvist A, Unge G (1973): The proliferative activity of the myocardial tissue in various forms of experimental cardiac hypertrophy. Acta Path Microbiol Scand, Section A, 81: 233–240.

56. Turek Z, Rakusan K (1981): Lognormal distribution of intercapillary distance in normal and hypertrophic rat heart as estimated by the method of concentric circles: Its effect on tissue oxygenation. Pfluegers Arch 391: 17–21.

57. Buchner F (1971): Qualitative morphology of heart failure. Light and electron microscopic characteristics of acute anc chronic heart failure. Methods Achiev Exp Pathol 5: 60–120.

58. Nishiyama K, Nishiyama A, Pfeffer MA, Frohlich ED (1978): Systemic and regional flow distribution in normotensive and spontaneously hypertensive young rats subjected to lifetime β-adrenergic receptor blockade. Blood Vessels 15: 333–347.

59. Pegram BL, Ishise S, Frohlich ED (1982): Effect of methyldopa, clonidine, and hydralazine on cardiac mass and haemodynamics in Wistar Kyoto and spontaneously hypertensive rats. Cardiovasc Res 16: 40–46.

60. Kobrin I, Sesoko S, Pegram BL, Frohlich ED (1984): Reduced cardiac mass by nitrendipine is dissociated from systemic or regional haemodynamic changes in rats. Cardiovasc Res 18: 158–162.

61. Wicker P, Fouad FM, Tarazi RC: Effects of antihypertensive treatment on left ventricular hypertrophy and coronary blood flow. IN: Cardiology, Parmley W (ed), J.B. Lippincott Co, Philadelphia. In Press.

62. Tomanek RJ (1979): The role of prevention or relief of pressure overload on the myocardial cell of the spontaneously hypertensive rat. A morphometric and stereologic study. Lab Invest 40: 83–91.

63. Scheuer J (1982): Effects of physical training on myocardial vascularity and perfusion. Circulation 66: 491–495.

64. Schaible TF, Ciambrone GJ, Capasso JM, Scheuer J (1984): Cardiac conditioning ameliorates cardiac dysfunction associated with renal hypertension in rats. J Clin Invest 73: 1086–1094.

Carotido-cerebral circulation in patients with sustained essential hypertension

M.E. SAFAR, ST. LAURENT & J.A. BOUTHIER

In normal subjects, cerebral blood flow is autoregulated, i.e. blood flow may be maintained constant despite wide changes in perfusion pressure [1]. Intrinsic mechanisms participate to the autoregulatory process, due to changes in the caliber of cerebral arterioles and small arteries, which respond to an increase in perfusion pressure by constriction and to a decrease in perfusion pressure by dilatation. In man there is a lower and an upper limit of cerebral blood flow auto-regulation: (i) below a given level of perfusion pressure (about 50–70 mm Hg), autoregulatory vasodilatation is inadequate and flow decreases, and (ii) beyond a certain pressure (about 130 mm Hg) autoregulatory vasoconstriction is offset, resulting in an increase in cerebral blood flow [1].

In patients with hypertension, the absolute value of cerebral blood flow is maintained within normal range (about 50 ml/min/100 g), while the autoregula-tion plateau is modified. The upper and lower limits of autoregulation are shifted to the right on the blood pressure axis in proportion to the severity of hyperten-sion [1]. From this finding, it results that, while hypertensive patients can tolerate without discomfort very high blood pressures, cerebral hypoperfusion might result from rapid blood pressure reduction below the lower limit of autoregula-tion.

Since common carotid arteries contribute the major share of cerebral blood flow [2], the study of carotid hemodynamics is likely to be an important subject in the fields of hypertension. In addition to its conduit function, the carotid circula-tion has two others special features in hypertension: (i) the arterial wall of the carotid bifurcation contains baroreceptor endings which are greatly involved in the regulation of blood pressure [3], and (ii) the initial portion of the carotid artery represents an elective site of atherosclerotic lesions which play a particular role in the genesis of cerebral ischemic attacks [4]. In the present chapter, the methods for the evaluation of common carotid parameters in man are described and applied to the following problems: (i) common carotid parameters in men with uncomplicated essential hypertension, (ii) relationship between baroreflex mechanisms and the carotid arterial wall, (iii) common carotid parameters in patients with stenosis of the internal carotid artery, and (iv) effect of antihypertensive drugs on the common carotid artery circulation.

Noninvasive evaluation of common carotid artery parameters in man

The methodologic basis for the evaluation of common carotid artery parameters in man is to measure independently the internal diameter (D) and the mean blood flow velocity (V) of the artery using pulsed Doppler systems [5, 6, 7]. Then blood flow is calculated as $3.14 \, D^2/4 \times V$ according to a cylindrical model of the carotid artery.

The zero-crossing velocimeter used for the investigation of the common carotid circulation operates at a frequency of 8 MHz and has two original features in addition to its pulsed emission: (i) on adjustable range gated time system and (ii) a double transducer probe which provides a bidimensional blood velocity measurement that minimizes considerably the errors introduced by the observation angle between the ultrasonic beam and the vessel axis.

Briefly, each of the two transducers acts alternatively as emitter and receiver. Between the emitted pulses, the transducer operates as a receiver and an electronic gate selects the signals reflected at a given time from the emission. This time represents the time delay of the reception. The reception duration can also be selected. Adjustments of time delay and reception duration are made using constant steps of half a microsecond. With such a system, it is possible to determine exactly the distance, d, between the red cells of the blood column and the transducer, according to the echographic relation $d = C/2 \times t$, where C is the ultrasound speed in tissues and t the reception time. The time delay and the duration reception respectively represent the depth and the thickness of the sample volume along the ultrasound beam axis. Using this procedure, it is possible to determine the diameter of the vessel and the cross-sectional blood flow velocity.

The double tranducer system overcomes the difficulty of measuring the angle between the ultrasonic beam and the vessel axis. The probe contains two tranducers set at a known angle one to the other; in the present system, this is 120°. Probe position is adjusted until two successive velocities, one from each transducer, are equal in absolute value. So the angle between each ultrasonic beam and the vessel axis is equal to 60°. In such conditions, the error for the determination of angle is less than 2%. Validation of Doppler determinations has been performed using hydraulic test devices, as detailed elsewhere [7].

In practice, the probe position is adjusted so that the two velocity curves, successively recorded for a duration of ten cardiac cycles, are equal in terms of absolute values. Then with the probe properly placed and maintained by a flexible arm, arterial walls are located by changing the time delay step by step. Thus, the interval between the successive waves corresponds to the step advance of the time delay. Knowing the difference in distance between the distal and proximal walls, and the angle between the ultrasonic beam and the vessel axis, arterial diameter is calculated. Cross-sectional blood velocity is measured with the time delay adjusted to the depth of the proximal wall of the artery and the duration reception to its diameter. Since the calibration voltage of the apparatus corresponds to a velocity of 38 cm/sec for an incidence angle of 60°, mean velocity is easily calculated by electronic integration of the velocity curve and expressed as the mean value of ten successive cardiac cycles for each transducer.

Usually, after a rest period of 20 minutes, measurements are carried out with the patient in the supine position. The head is tilted backward and the examination is performed in a quiet and semi-darkened room, at a constant temperature of 20° C. The position of the carotid artery is determined by palpation along the medial edge of the sterno-cleidomastoid muscle. After the carotid bifurcation has been located by continuous wave Doppler assessment, the pulsed Doppler probe is placed on the common carotid artery 3 cm proximal to the carotid bifurcation (Fig. 1) [5]. The common carotid artery is studied rather than the internal carotid artery since the internal and the external carotid arteries may be difficult to distinguish with conventional Doppler systems. Also, as concerns the probe transducer incidence angle, the precision of the axis of the common carotid artery in the neck is fairly constant, while the configurations of the internal and external carotid arteries give a high degree of variability. An ultrasonic gel is used as a coupling medium between the probe and the skin. The Doppler signals are monitored by a loud speaker throughout the examination. The velocity signals are recorded on a Siemens apparatus with rapid speed. All measurements of diameter and blood flow velocity are repeated at least twice for each common carotid artery and the values used are the mean of these determinations. Indices of reproducibility of the method have been published elsewhere [7, 5, 6]. Normal values in healthy subjects between 45 and 75 years are 0.653 ± 0.011 cm (± 1 standard error of the mean) (ranges: from 0.560 to 0.780 cm) for diameter, 19.4 ± 1.0 cm/sec (ranges: from 15 to 31 cm/sec) for blood velocity, and 380 ± 15 ml/mn (ranges: from 250 to 520 ml/min) for blood flow [5]. In normal subjects, no significant difference may be observed between the right and the left common carotid artery [5].

Common carotid artery parameters in sustained essential hypertension

Studies of the common carotid circulation in hypertensive humans have been performed in ambulant male subjects with mild to moderate essential hypertension in comparison with age-matched healthy volunteers [5]. All treatments were discontinued at least 3 weeks before the investigation. Sustained hypertension was documented on the basis of the averaging of three successive supine diastolic blood pressure between 95 to 114 mm Hg during the untreated ambulant period.

184

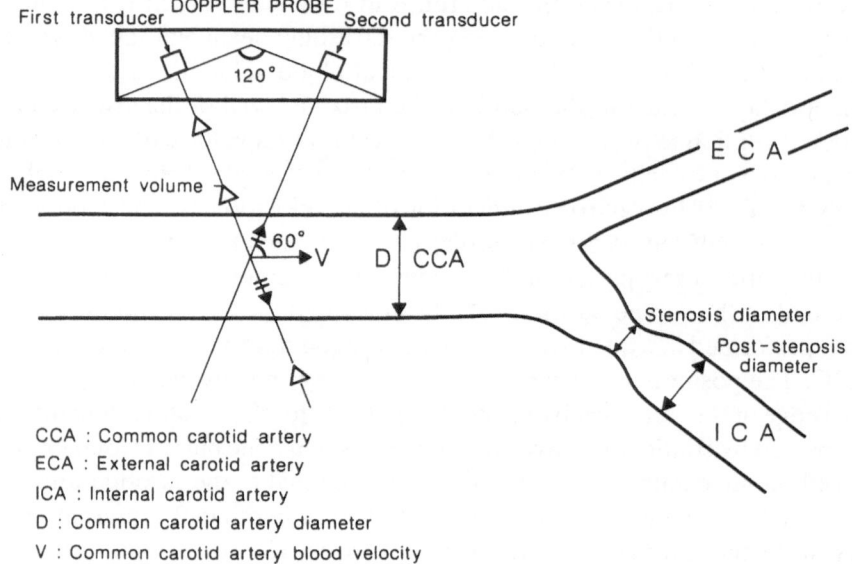

Figure 1. Determination of common carotid parameters using pulsed Doppler systems in patients with stenosis of the internal carotid artery. The sites of diameter measurements are represented by arrows; when the velocity signals recorded from each transducer are equal in absolute value, the angle between the ultrasonic beam emitted by each transducer and the vessel axis is equal to half the angle between the two transducers, i.e. 60°; the crossing of the common carotid arterial lumen by a small measurement volume is schematized along the ultrasound beam of one transducer.

No patient had hemiplegia or another neurological or cardiac complication. Continuous Doppler examination of extracranial cerebral arteries was assessed to be within the normal range both in controls and in patients with hypertension [5].

In subjects younger than 45 years, arterial diameter was 0.639 ± 0.014 cm in hypertensives and 0.651 ± 0.015 cm in controls. Blood velocity was respectively 19.7 ± 0.9 cm/sec and 21.2 ± 0.9 cm/sec and blood flow 385 ± 20 ml/min and 410 ± 23 ml/min. For all these parameters, no significant difference was observed between normal subjects and hypertensives. Vascular resistance in the carotid circulation was significantly increased in hypertensives (341 ± 19 mm Hg · min/l versus 235 ± 14 mm Hg · min/l; $p<0.01$). In subjects older than 45 years, arterial diameter was similar in hypertensives and normotensives (0.665 ± 0.018 cm and 0.653 ± 0.011 cm). Blood velocity and blood flow were reduced in hypertensives: respectively 15.6 ± 0.6 cm/sec versus 19.4 ± 2.0 cm/sec ($p<0.005$) and 321 ± 14 versus 385 ± 15 ml/min ($p<0.001$). Vascular resistance was strikingly increased in hypertensive patients (392 ± 20 mm Hg · min/l versus 267 ± 14 mm Hg · min/l; $p<0.001$) [5].

Table 1 summarizes the hemodynamic changes according to age in normotensive and hypertensive subjects [5]. In controls, no modification is observed in the diameter, blood velocity, blood flow and vascular resistance with age. On the other hand, a decrease in blood velocity and blood flow of the common carotid artery is noticed in the older group of patients with hypertension as compared to the younger patients.

Finally, the study indicates that the arterial diameter of common carotid artery remains within the normal range whatever age and the blood pressure level may be. This finding contrasts with the elevated brachial artery diameter previously described in patients with sustained hypertension [8]. No modification of arterial diameter was observed with aging although previous publications have reported an increase of the size of the thoracic aorta with age [9]. Thus it appears that the common carotid artery diameter in men with sustained essential hypertension may be considered as abnormal for the blood pressure level. Such a finding implies intrinsic modifications of the arterial wall, due either to a change in vasomotor tone or to an increased thickness of the arterial wall [5, 1, 9]. In favor of the latter hypothesis, histological studies of human hypertensive carotid arteries have shown an elevated incidence of tetraploid cells and DNA, indicating an increased mass of arterial smooth muscle [10].

While there is no change of blood velocity or blood flow of common carotid artery in younger patients with hypertension, clinical data point to a decrease in flow in hypertensive patients older than 45 years [5]. This reduction in flow reflects an increase in vascular resistance and therefore indicates a decrease in the cross-sectional area of small arteries which is more pronounced in older than in younger hypertensives.

In conclusion, both small and large arteries are modified in the carotid circulation of patients with sustained essential hypertension. Modifications of small

Table 1. Hemodynamic changes with age of common carotid artery parameters in normotensive and hypertensive subjects (see text) (with permission) [5].

	Normal Subjects		Hypertensive patients	
	Younger (n = 17)	Older (n = 21)	Younger (n = 17)	Older (n = 21)
Arterial diameter (cm)	0.651 ± 0.015	0.653 ± 0.11	0.639 ± 0.014	0.665 ± 0.018
Blood velocity (cm/sec)	21.2 ± 0.9	19.4 ± 1.0	19.7 ± 0.7	15.6 ± 0.6* * *
Volume flow (ml/min)	410 ± 23	385 ± 15	385 ± 20	321 ± 14* * *
Vascular resistance (mm Hg · min/l)	235 ± 14	267 ± 14	341 ± 19	392 ± 20

* * * $p < 0.005$ (older versus younger).

arteries in the carotido-cerebral circulations have been extensively studied in the literature [1, 4, 11]. As regards large vessels, the abnormalities in the cushioning function of the carotid arteries may have many practical implications, in particular for modifications of arterial wall tension and shear stress (Table 2) [9–11].

Common carotid artery and baroreflex mechanisms in hypertensive humans

An important feature of carotid hemodynamics concerns the role of the arterial wall in mediating baroreceptor afferent nerve activity [12, 13, 14]. The arterial wall of the carotid sinus contains a high content of connective tissue (especially elastin) and very little vascular muscle. This region also exhibits low circumferential stiffness. Baroreceptor nerve activity unquestionably is associated with wall deformation since restricting wall distension with plaster casts abolishes baroreceptor-mediated reflexes [15].

In normal animals, the nerve endings respond either to tensile deformation or to tensile stress. Bergel and coworkers [12, 13, 16] reported that carotid sinus nerve discharge was linearly related to sinus diameter, even at high pressures and large diameters. However, at large diameters, the wall becomes exceedingly stiff, so that an elevation in pressure produces little change in diameter. Although such data suggest that receptors respond to deformation rather than to stress under such conditions, it is not possible to tell with certainty from observations at large diameters whether the receptor endings respond to deformation or to stress at physiological pressures and/or at more moderate dimensions.

Table 2. Carotid bifurcation shear stress (dynes/cm^2) (by permission) [26]. 'At the apex of the flow divider and along the inner wall of the carotid sinus, shear stress is high and is accentuated at peak systolic flow rates due to the very high velocity gradient at the vessel wall. Along the outer wall of the carotid sinus, shear stress is very low, principally due to the low flow velocities at this location. In the internal carotid artery beyond the carotid sinus, outer wall shear stress is again restored to common carotid levels. Along the inner wall of the distal internal carotid artery, calculated wall shear stress at Re 1200 is 565 dynes/cm^2, which exceeded the value for shear stress previously reported to cause endothelial damage' [9] (by permission) [26].

	Mean Flow (Re400)	Peak Flow (Re1200)
Common Carotid	10 ± 1	29 ± 3
Carotid sinus		
Inner Wall	23 ± 5	203 ± 61
Outer Wall	0 ± 2	− 2 ± 2
Internal Carotid		
Inner Wall	50 ± 10	565 ± 170
Outer Wall	39 ± 8	50 ± 10

± standard error of the mean.

Although similar problems may be posed in hypertension in man, it is generally admitted that the resetting of baroreceptors observed during the established phase of the disease is related to modifications of the arterial wall of the blood vessel containing receptors [2, 3]. Indeed, reduced arterial compliance is a common feature of patients with hypertension and has been shown to be highly correlated with baroreflex sensitivity [17]. However, more direct evidence for an active effect of the carotid artery on the baroreflex mechanisms in hypertensive humans has been provided by pharmacological studies [18]. The hemodynamic effects of a dihydralazine-like substance (cadralazine) [19] have been investigated on the common carotid artery of patients with sustained essential hypertension. Four hours after oral administration of cadralazine (20 mg), blood pressure decreased markedly and heart rate was significantly enhanced, reflecting the activation of the autonomic nervous system. Diameter, blood flow velocity and blood flow of the common carotid artery were not significantly modified. On the other hand, vascular resistance and tangential tension (i.e. the product between mean arterial pressure and the radius of the artery) were slightly decreased. However, the most important result was the significant correlation observed between the change in tangential tension and the change in heart rate (Fig. 2): the greater the decrease in tangential tension, the greater the increase in heart rate [18].

Since no direct stimulating effect of hydralazine and derivatives on the isolated heart has been previously reported [19], the change in heart rate can be used as an index of sympathetic activation. Thus the relationship between the changes in heart rate and in tangential tension after cadralazine suggests that cadralazine-induced sympathetic activation is related to modifications of the carotid artery hemodynamics and that the carotid system participates actively in the baroreflex mechanisms observed in hypertensive humans [18].

Common carotid artery parameters in patients with stenosis of the internal carotid artery

Most ischemic cerebral vascular disease results from arterial narrowing or occlusion. Hypertension is the most important risk factor associated with stroke [20]. In particular, it promotes the development of atherosclerosis in the extracranial and intracranial arteries. In the former case, atherosclerosis and superimposed thrombotic disease usually occur either at the origin of the internal carotid artery or at the bifurcation of the common carotid artery [4]. For that reason, the study of carotid parameters proximal to a given stenosis of the internal carotid artery may be relevant for the investigation of normotensive and hypertensive patients.

Common carotid blood flow has been studied in patients with internal carotid artery stenosis [21]. In all cases, the stenosis was strictly unilateral, as judged by arteriography. No associated occlusion was observed in the remaining carotido-

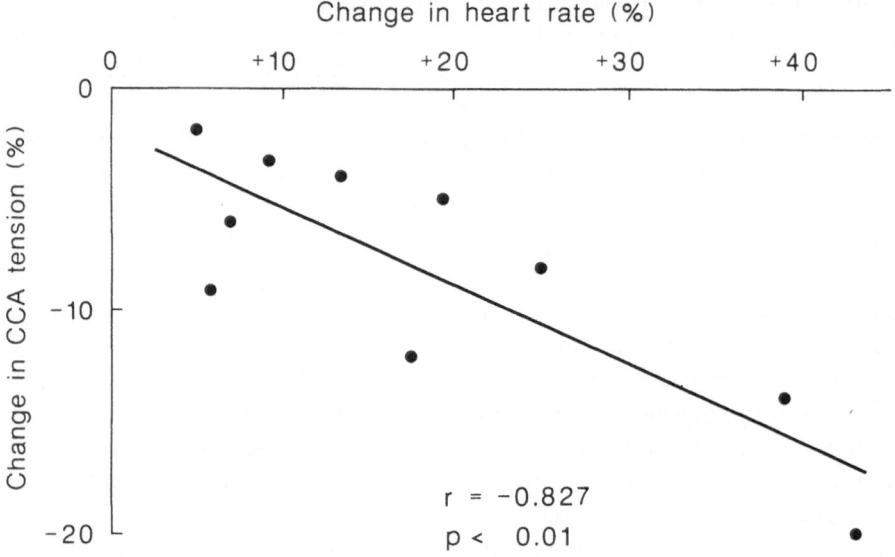

Figure 2. Acute administration of cadralazine in patients with sustained essential hypertension: relationship between the change in heart rate and the change in tangential tension of the common carotid artery (CCA) personal data.

cerebral circulation. The group consisted of 19 males and 5 females. Their age ranged between 45 and 75 years. All treatment was discontinued at least 15 days before the study. Fifteen patients presented a carotid bruit, 9 patients had had a transient ischemic attack. 7 patients suffered from ischemic heart disease and 2 from arterosclerosis obliterans of the lower limbs. Table 3 summarizes the individual arterial parameters in patients with unilateral stenosis of the internal carotid artery [21]. On the uninvolved side, mean values of arterial diameter, blood velocity and blood flow remained within the normal range. In comparison, the involved side exhibited a significant reduction in arterial diameter, blood velocity and, in particular, blood flow.

Fig. 3 shows the values of common carotid artery blood flow of the involved side as a function of the degree of stenosis appraised on conventional arteriography. From 40% to 80% diameter stenosis, blood flow was reduced (mean value: 250 ml/min) and remained nearly constant. After 80% diameter stenosis, blood flow decreased abruptly. A strong negatively curvilinear relationship results from this hemodynamic pattern, as previously shown in experimental studies [9].

In order to evaluate the role of hypertension in stenosis of the internal carotid artery, patients with stenosis of the internal carotid artery were divided into two groups: those with normal blood pressure and those with elevated blood pressure. Comparison of normotensives and hypertensives indicated that arterial diameter and blood flow velocity were nearly similar while blood flow was more

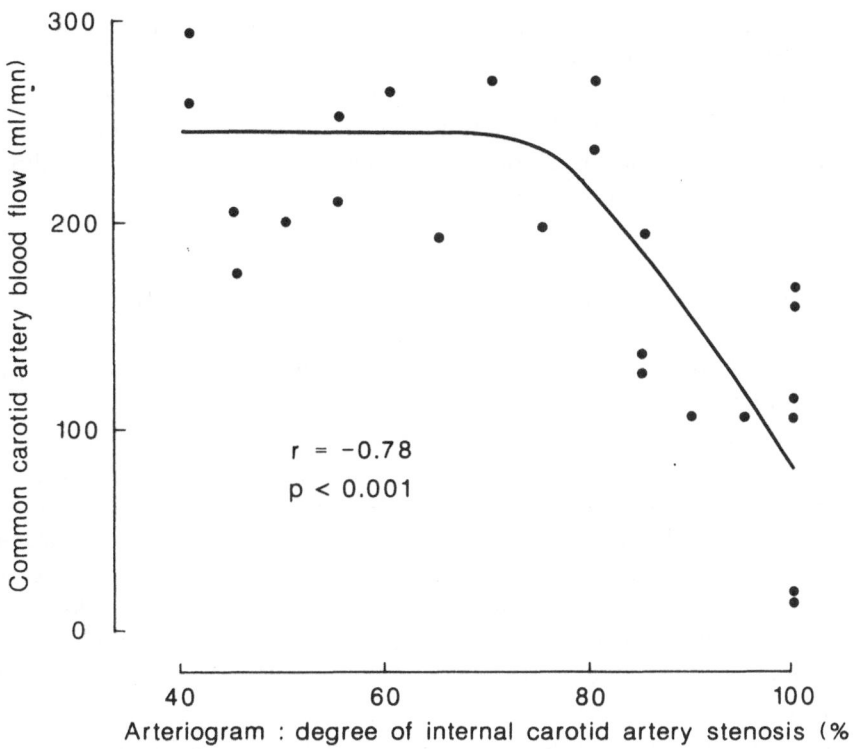

Figure 3. Patients with unilateral stenosis of the internal carotid artery: relationship between the degree of stenosis judged by arteriography and the homolateral common carotid artery blood flow (with permission) [21].

reduced in hypertensives. Vascular resistance was more elevated in hypertensives than in normotensives. Figure 4 depicts the value of common carotid blood flow in normotensives and hypertensives, as function of the degree of stenosis of the internal carotid artery. Common carotid blood flow is expressed as the ratio between blood flow of the involved side on blood flow of the uninvolved side. Both in normotensives and in hypertensives, blood flow and the degree of

Table 3. Normotensives patients with unilateral stenosis of the internal carotid artery (24 subjects) (by permission) [21].

	Uninvolved Side	Involved Side
Arterial Diameter (cm)	0.610 ± 0.017	0.508 ± 0.026* * *
Blood Flow Velocity (cm/sec)	19.9 ± 0.86	14.7 ± 0.92* * *
Blood Flow (ml/min)	350 ± 16	188 ± 14* * *

± standard error of the mean.
* * * p<0.001.

stenosis are inversely related: the higher the degree of stenosis, the lower the ratio and the more reduced the blood flow of the involved side. However, the ratio was lower in hypertensives than in normotensives at any degree of stenosis.

Thus, significant stenosis of the internal carotid artery is responsible for severe ischemia in the carotid circulation, with higher reductions in blood flow in patients with hypertension.

Vasodilating antihypertensive drugs and the common carotid artery circulation

Since the hemodynamic pattern of the carotido-cerebral circulation in essential hypertension involves both resistive and capacitative arterial vessels, it appeared important to evaluate the effect of vasodilating antihypertensive drugs on the carotid circulation taking into account both small and large arteries [22].

For this purpose, hemodynamic measurements were performed before and 2 to 4 hours after oral administration of three vasodilating drugs: captopril, a classical converting-enzyme inhibitor [23], isosorbide dinitrate, a nitroglycerine-like substance, and nitrendipine, an available calcium-entry blocker [24]. Doses were respectively 75 mg, 20 mg and 20 mg in order to produce the same blood pressure reduction for similar values in baseline blood pressure in the three subgroups of patients [22].

Figure 5 summarizes the dominant observations of the investigation. Captopril produced both a dilatation of small (decrease in vascular resistance) and large (increase in arterial diameter) arteries. Isosorbide dinitrate dilated predominantly the common carotid artery diameter, but no significant change in the cross-sectional area of arterioles was observed. Nitrendipine markedly decreased vascular resistance (dilatation of small arteries), but no change in the common

Table 4. Patients with unilateral stenosis of the internal carotid artery: common carotid parameters of the involved side in normotensive and hypertensive patients (personal data).

	Normotensive (n = 14)	Hypertensives (n = 10)
Diameter (cm)	0.528 ± 0.020	0.520 ± 0.040
Blood flow velocity (cm/sec)	14.3 ± 1.2	13.2 ± 1.3
Blood flow (ml/min)	212 ± 67	167 ± 26*
Vascular resistance (mm Hg · sec/ml)	28.0 ± 3.2	43.1 ± 4.8* * *

± 1 standard error of the mean.
Legend:
* $p < 0.05$.
* * *$p < 0.001$.

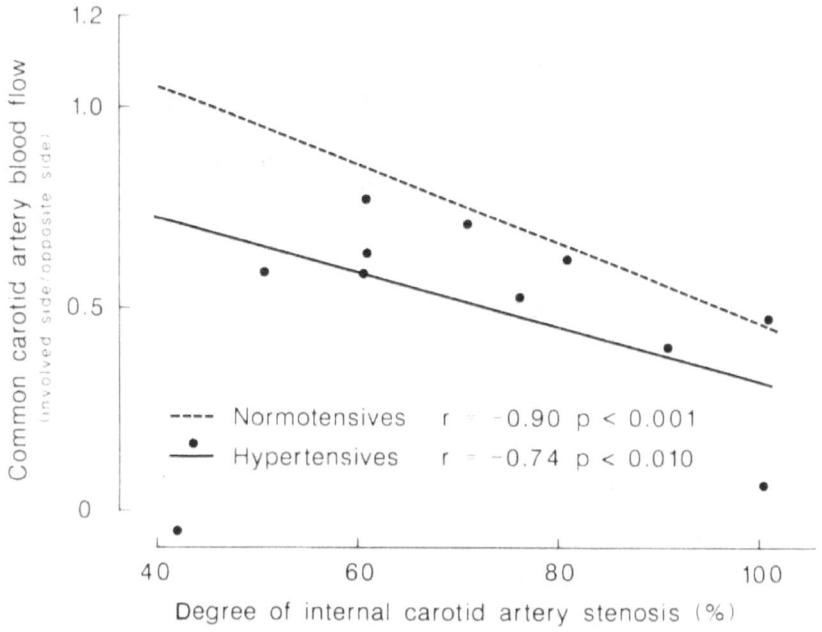

Figure 4. Patients with unilateral stenosis of the internal carotid artery: relationship between the degree of stenosis judged by arteriography and the common carotid blood flow represented as the ratio between the involved side versus the uninvolved side (see text). Notice that normotensives and hypertensives may be represented by two different curves, so that, at any degree of stenosis, blood flow is more reduced in hypertensives that in normotensives (with permission [27]).

carotid artery caliber occurred [22]. Thus, vasodilating drugs acted differently on small and large arteries. Only captopril dilated both small and large vessels.

It has been reported that the pressure distal to the narrowing of the vessel in patients with arterial stenosis of the internal carotid artery was influenced by two different parameters: the importance of arteriolar dilatation and the degree of stenosis [25]. Poststenotic pressure is decreased when arterioles dilate and is enhanced when the large artery diameter increases, mainly at the site of the stenosis. From this observation, it ensues that antihypertensive drugs causing exclusively arteriolar vasodilatation may reduce the pressure distal to the stenosis of the internal carotid artery, while drugs causing a preferential dilatation of large carotido-cerebral arteries should preserve the poststenotic pressure better. In that regard, it is important to notice that dilatation of the internal carotid artery obtained by surgery in patients with stenosis of the internal carotid artery improved significantly the blood flow of the common carotid artery both in normotensive and hypertensive subjects (Fig. 6). Such findings suggest that vasodilating drugs causing dilatation of both small and large arteries could be a better choice to improve cerebro-vascular circulation in patients treated for hypertension.

In conclusion, the present study has shown that the common carotid circulation

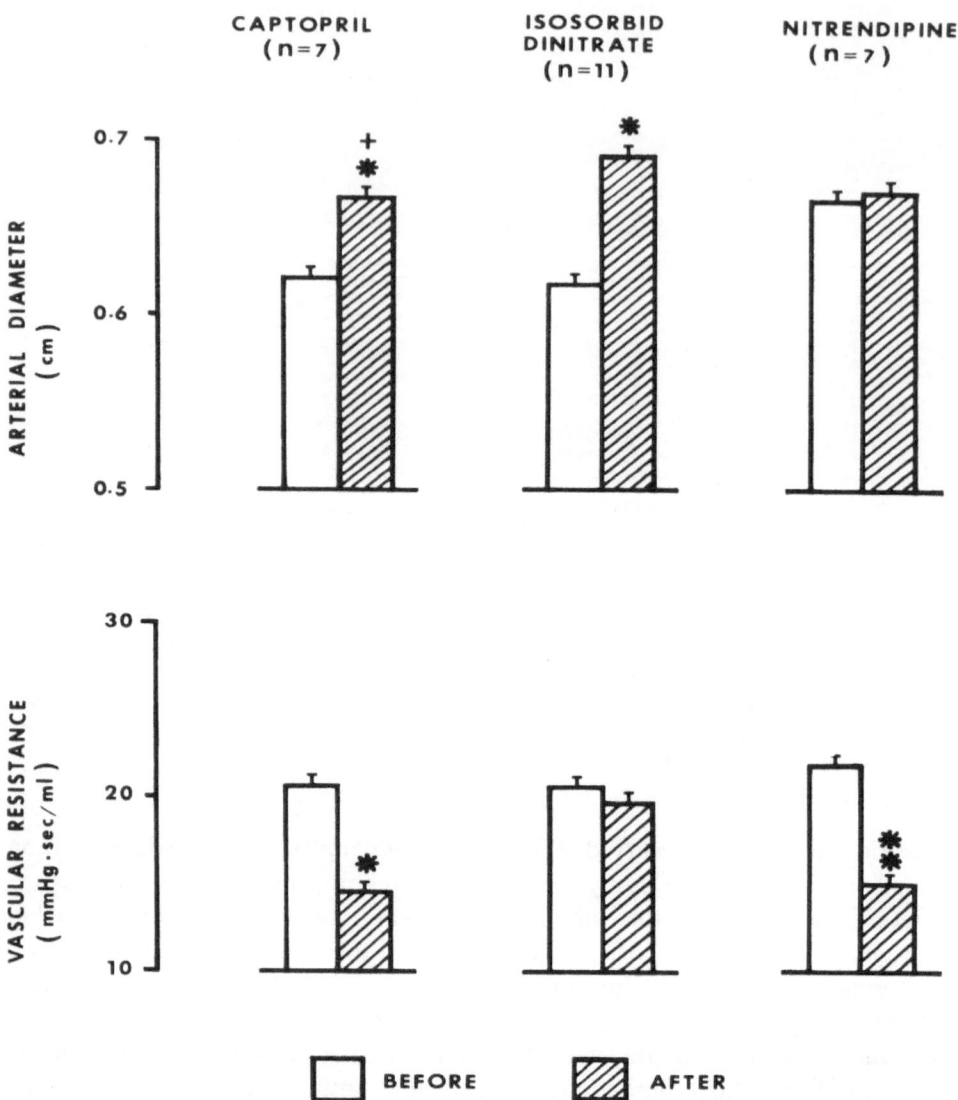

Figure 5. Summary of the hemodynamic effects of captopril, isosorbide dinitrate and nitrendipine on the common carotid artery diameter (used as an index of large vessels) and on vascular resistance (used as an index of the cross-sectional area of small vessels) in patients with essential hypertension. For explanations, see text (by permission) [22].
Legend:
* p<0.05.
+ * p<0.02.
* * * p<0.01.

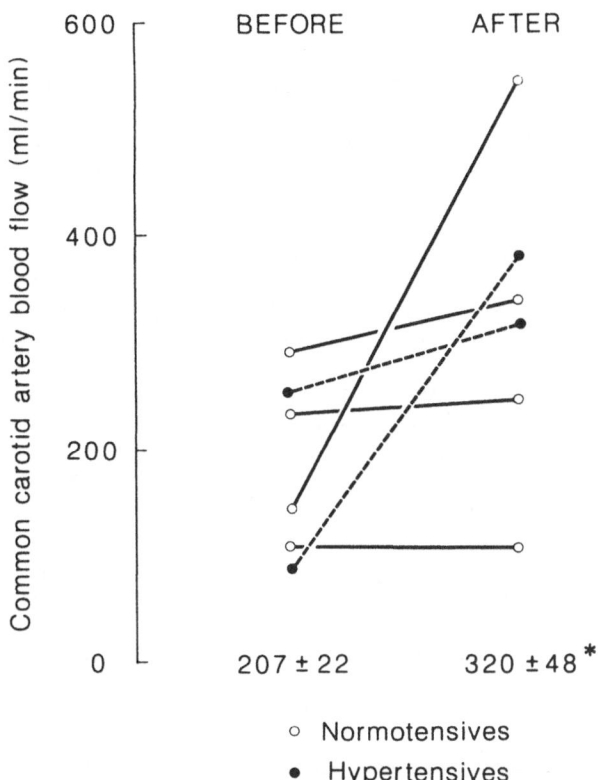

Figure 6. Patients with unilateral stenosis of the internal carotid artery: common carotid blood flow before and after surgical treatment (with permission [27]).
* p<0.05.

is modified in patients with essential hypertension with changes in both small (increase in vascular resistance) and large arteries (normal arterial diameter despite elevated blood pressure). Larges vessels are probably involved actively in the modifications of the baroreflex mechanisms observed in hypertension. Evaluation of common carotid parameters may be useful for the evaluation of the degree of narrowing observed in patients with stenosis of the internal carotid artery. In such patients, common carotid blood flow is more altered in hypertensive than in normotensive patients. Finally, the study of carotid parameters may be extremely relevant in clinical pharmacology. In the carotid circulation, vasodilating drugs may dilate either small arteries or large arteries or both, with possible implications in the choice of antihypertensive drugs to preserve the carotido-cerebral circulation.

References

1. Barry DI, Lassen NL (1984): Cerebral blood flow autoregulation in hypertension and effects of antihypertensive drugs. J Of Hypertension 2 (suppl. 3): 519–526.
2. Olson RM, Looke JP (1975): Human carotid artery diameter and flow by a non-invasive technique. Medical Instrumentation 9: 99–102.
3. Gribbin B, Pickering RG, Sleight P, Peto R (1971): Effect age and high blood pressure on baroreflex sensitivity in man. Circul Res 29: 424–431.
4. Kister JP, Ropper AH, Heros RC (1984): Therapy of ischemic cerebral vascular disease due to atherothrombosis. New Engl J Med 311: 27–33.
5. Bouthier J, Benetos A, Simon A, Levenson J, Safar M (1985): Pulsed Doppler evaluation of diameter, blood velocity and blood flow of common carotid artery in sustained essential hypertension. J Cardio Vas Pharmacol (suppl. 2): S28–S32.
6. Fitzgerald DE, O'Shaughnessy AM, Kreveny JT (1982): Pulsed Doppler: determination of blood velocity and voluic flow in normal and diseased common carotid arteries in man. Cardiovasc Res 16: 220–224.
7. Levenson JA, Peronneau PA, Simon ACh. Safar ME (1981): Pulsed Doppler determination of diameter, blood flow velocity and volumic flow of brachial artery in man. Cardiovasc Res 15: 164–170.
8. Safar ME, Peronneau PA, Levenson JA, Toto-Moukouo JA, Simon ACh (1981): Pulsed Doppler: diameter, blood flow velocity and volumic flow of the brachial artery in sustained essential hypertension. Circulation, 63: 393–400.
9. O'Rourke MF (1982): Arterial function in health and disease. Ed. Churchill Livingstone, Edinburgh, London, Melbourne, and New York, pp 53–64.
10. Schwartz SM (1984): Hypertension as a vascular response to injury. Hypertension 6 (suppl III): III*33–III*37.
11. Cox RH (1979): Comparison of arterial wall mechanisms in normotensive and spontaneously hypertensive rats. Heart Circ Physiol 6 (2): H159–H167.
12. Bergel DH (1960): The visco-elastic properties of the arterial wall. Ph D Thesis, University of London.
13. Bergel DH, Brooks DE, McDermott AJ, Robinson JJ, Sleight P (1976): Comparison of the mechanical properties of the carotid sinus and adjacent common carotid artery and the effects of noradrenaline. J Of Physiol 263: 266–275.
14. Dobrin PB, Rovick AA (1969): Influence of vascular smooth muscle on contractile mechanics and elasticity of arteries. Am J of Physiol 217: 1644–1651.
15. Hauss WH, Kreuziger H, Asteroth H (1949): Uber die reizung der pressorrezeptorem-im Sinus caroticus beim Humd. Z Kreislaufforsch 38: 28–33.
16. Peveler RC, Bergel DH, Robinson JL, Sleight P (1983): The effect of phenylephrine upon arterial pressure, carotid sinus radius and baroreflex sensitivi'y in the conscious greyhound. Clinical Science 64: 455–461.
17. Randall Os, Elser MD, Bulloch GF, Maisel AS, Ellis CN, Zweifler AJ, Julius S (1976): Relationship of age and blood pressure to baroreflex sensitivity and arterial compliance in man. Clin Science 51: 357–360.
18. Laurent S, Safar ME, London GM, Levenson JA, Simon AC. Diameter, velocity and blood flow of the common carotid artery before and after vaso dilatation in essential hypertension (unpublished data).
19. Catalano M, Parini J, Libretti A (1983): Cadralazine (ISF 2469): Dose related antihypertensive activity after single oral administration to patients. Eur J Clin Pharmacol 24: 157–161.
20. Kannel WB, Dawber TR, Sorlie P, Wolf PA (1976): Components of blood pressure and risk of atherothrombotic braim infraction: the Framingham study. Stroke 7: 327–331.
21. Benetos A, Simon A, Levenson J, Lagneau P, Bouthier J, Safar M (1986): Pulsed Doppler: an

evaluation of diameter, blood velocity and blood flow of the common carotid artery in patients with isolated unilateral stenosis of the internal carotid artery. Stroke 16: 969–972.

22. Bouthier JD, Benetos A, Simon ACh, Levenson JA, Safar ME (1986). Hemodynamic effects of vaso-dilating drugs on the common carotid and the brachial circulations of patients with essential hypertension. Brit J Clin Pharmacol 21: 137–142.

23. Vidt DG, Bravo EL, Fouad FM (1982): Captopril N Engl J Med 306: 214–219.

24. Spivack C, Ocken S, Frishman WH (1983): Calcium antagonists: clinical use in the treatment of systemic hypertension. Drugs 25: 154–177.

25. Young DF, Cholvin NR, Roth RC (1976): Pressure drop across artificially induced stenoses in the femoral arteries in dogs. Circ Res 36: 735–743.

26. Zarins CK, Giddens DP, Glagov S (1983): Atherosclerotic plaque distribution and flow velocity profiles in the carotid bifurcation in 'Cerebro vascular Insufficiency'. Bergon JJ and Yao JST (edit). Grune & Stratton, pp 19–26.

27. Benetos A, Safar ME, Laurent St, Bouthier JD, Lagreau PL, Hugue Ch (1986): Common carotid blood flow in patients with hypertension and stenosis of the internal carotid artery. J Clin Hypertension 1: 44–54.

Renal circulation in essential hypertension

P.W. DE LEEUW and W.H. BIRKENHÄGER

Introduction

Among the various organs which could play a role in the pathogenesis of essential hypertension, the kidney ranks high. This may be inferred from the observation that many experimental procedures which affect the kidney can readily produce hypertension. Furthermore, it is difficult if not impossible to construct a hypothetical pathogenesis of hypertension without attributing to the kidney a central role. Admittedly, the kidney is one of the main targets of the hypertensive disease and renal abnormalities which have been observed in essential hypertension often seem to be a consequence of the disease rather than its cause. However, it is conceivable that such abnormalities may contribute not only to the maintenance of hypertension, but also to progression of the disease.

Current theories on blood pressure regulation emphasize the relation between arterial pressure and urinary sodium excretion [1–3]. An increase in arterial pressure causes increased losses of sodium and water, which results in a fall in arterial pressure until it reaches a level where the output of sodium and water again equals intake. According to this view, the relation between arterial pressure and sodium output must be altered, in a sense that an abnormally high renal perfusion pressure is required for the excretion of a given amount of sodium, if hypertension is to persist. Thus, sodium balance is achieved at the expense of increased arterial pressure. Of course, it is difficult to get direct evidence for this in man, but it may be worthwhile to consider some aspects of renal function which are more readily accessible. In particular, this applies to the study of renal haemodynamics.

Renal blood flow in essential hypertension

Although renal blood flow is reduced in most patients with essential hypertension [4–8], it is sometimes normal [8–12] and in a minority of patients it even appears to be increased [13–17]. It is of interest that in young subjects at risk of developing hypertension, renal blood flow may also be remarkably high [18–19]. The reason for these divergent haemodynamic patterns is not yet clear. Although it has been suggested that high renal flow rates would be due to an increased cardiac output [15, 20], such a mechanism has not been uniformly accepted [18, 19, 21]. It seems, therefore, that an increase in renal perfusion is due to some unknown stimulus and may represent, for instance, a compensation for a genetic abnormality in glomerular filtration [18]. According to Williams and co-workers subjects who exhibit high flow rates through the kidney do, indeed, form a separate subgroup characterized by other abnormalities as well [22]. Despite the lack of an explanation these findings are important because they suggest that renal ischaemia may not always be the prime mover in essential hypertension. However, even when renal blood flow was increased, calculated renal vascular resistance was already elevated [19]. In fact, in all studies where hypertensives were found to have normal renal blood flow, resistance in the kidney must have been enhanced as well.

When interpreting renal blood flow data one has to take into account that age is an important modulator of renal perfusion. In normal man renal flow declines with age, particularly over the age of 40 years [4, 5, 9, 23–26]. In patients with essential hypertension, the decrease in renal flow with age appears to be exaggerated [12, 26–28]. Moreover, renal blood flow is inversely related to the height of blood pressure [9–11, 26–29]. In the study of Reubi et al. [29] the latter relationship was not found when only cases of benign hypertension were considered; this discrepancy may be due to a lack in standardization of sodium intake or to differences in patient selection.

Another point to be emphasized is the fact that renal blood flow not only changes as a result of local alterations in vascular tone but is also affected by systemic blood flow. In other words, despite the presence of vascular abnormalities, the kidney could still exhibit a relatively high flow rate in relation to cardiac output. Hence, renal blood flow is only acceptable as a measure of (selective) renal vascular changes when it is expressed as a fraction of cardiac output. In our own series [28] the renal fraction of cardiac output appeared to be normal in the younger age groups and to decline significantly with age, indicating that preferential renal vascular involvement probably is a secondary phenomenon. Other studies in hypertensive patients have also revealed a lower renal fraction in comparison to normotensives, this being due to diminished renal blood flow rather than to changes in cardiac output [30–32]. London et al. analysed renal blood flow in relation to cardiac output and age in normotensives and hypertensives; they found parallel relationships between renal flow and cardiac index in both groups, but the intercept was lower in the hypertensive group [26]. They concluded that a 'normal' value for renal blood flow may be found in a large proportion of hypertensive patients, especially the younger ones, but for a given cardiac output renal blood flow in such patients is still lower than in control subjects. In addition, the investigators showed that the renal fraction displayed a significant inverse relationship with age in the hypertensives, whilst such a relationship was absent in the normotensives. Thus, it may be concluded that a rise in renal vascular resistance is an early but also a progressive marker of essential hypertension. The downward trend of renal blood flow and the steady increase in renal vascular resistance with time has been derived mainly from cross-sectional data, but in a follow-up study on 26 patients with essential hypertension we have been able to confirm this pattern [28, 33].

The reduction in renal blood flow is most prominent in the cortical region of the kidney as shown by xenon-washout studies [6, 17, 31, 33, 34]. However, while normals exhibit a fall in cortical perfusion with age [25, 31, 34], such a relationship is less easy to demonstrate in hypertensives. In our own series [34] we found only a weak effect of age, while Case *et al.* [35] did not find any effect at all. On the other hand, cortical flow is already clearly reduced in the majority of hypertensives at an early stage [17]. Thus, in the initial phases of hypertension vascular tone in the renal cortex seems to be exaggerated. It is still elusive whether this is a cause or the result of the hypertensive process but with others [17] we believe that the abnormality occurs sufficiently early to be of causative potential in the pathogenesis of essential hypertension.

At this point the obvious question is: what is the nature of the increased renal resistance? Although structural narrowing of the arterioles may contribute to the rise in renal resistance once hypertension is established, there is little to suggest that such a mechanism is operative in the initial stages. On the contrary, there is ample evidence that arteriolar resistance is not fixed since it can readily be reduced by pyrogens [8], saline loading [31, 33, 36–38] or pharmacological agents [26, 34, 39]. Therefore, the enhanced impedance to flow in the kidney must at least in part have a functional basis. In this respect one may think of the renin-angiotensin system or the adrenergic system which could be overactive or of vasodilator mechanisms which are deficient. Alternatively, all these systems may operate on a normal level, but sensitivity (or response) of the renal vasculature is abnormal.

Role of the renin-angiotensin system

In order to implicate a role for the renin-angiotensin system in the regulation of renal vascular tone, two requirements should be fulfilled. Firstly, one should demonstrate that angiotensin, indeed, is able to constrict the renal vessels and secondly, if angiotensin participates in renal vasoconstriction, one should be able to reverse its effects by ablation experiments.

From what is known, it would seem reasonable to assume that angiotensin II has the potential to produce renal vasoconstriction. Earlier studies on the renal response to infused angiotensin II in man are difficult to interpret because pressor doses of the agent were used [40–43], but a fall in renal blood flow was the uniform finding. However, even subpressor doses of angiotensin II raise vascular resistance in the kidney as was first shown by Statius van Eps [44] and later confirmed by Ljungman [45]. In the latter study changes did not reach statistical significance in normotensives, while they did in the hypertensives. This may indicate that sensitivity to angiotensin II is greater in hypertensives than in normals. Since clearance techniques were used to measure renal flow, the theoretical possibility remains that in the studies cited above angiotensin had some direct effect on intrarenal transport of the indicator. However, even more convincing data were presented by Hollenberg and co-workers, who infused angiotensin II in incremental doses into the renal artery of normal subjects and measured renal blood flow by means of the xenon washout technique [46]. In doses which did not produce systemic effects, angiotensin II clearly reduced mean renal flow as well as cortical flow in a dose-dependent way. In patients with essential hypertension the renal response to angiotensin is even enhanced: both a significant reduction in threshold dose and a steeper slope relating drug dose to response have been found [47]. Thus, there is compelling evidence that exogenous angiotensin II has an intrarenal vasoconstrictor action, making this compound a potential candidate as a cause of impaired renal perfusion in hypertension. However, these studies do not yet prove that endogenous angiotensin contributes to renal vascular tone. The classic way to approach this problem is to perform ablation experiments. In a strict sense such investigations are impossible, even in experimental animals, because the kidney is both source and target of the hormone. Therefore, we have to make do with pharmacological interruption of the renin-system which, of course, has obvious disadvantages. The most important tools that are available at present are the angiotensin analogues which compete with angiotensin for its receptors and, more recently, the inhibitors of angiotensin converting-enzyme.

In normal man administration of an angiotensin antagonist or a converting-enzyme inhibitor has little effect on renal blood flow when the renin-angiotensin system is suppressed by a liberal sodium diet. Under these conditions renal perfusion may even fall either as a consequence of partial agonistic activity of the analogue [48, 49] or secondary to a fall in blood pressure. On the other hand, when the renin system is activated usually a striking increase in renal blood flow is observed [49–51]. In patients with essential hypertension administration of converting-enzyme inhibitors invariably increases renal blood flow and in this group the response is even potentiated [52]. Also, when renal blood flow increases only marginally, a fall in renal vascular resistance is readily demonstrated [53–55]. Moreover, sodium intake modulates the effect of the converting-enzyme inhibitor captopril differently in hypertensives and in normals. Thus, in normals on a liberal sodium diet captopril does not augment renal flow, while it does in hypertensives on a similar diet [51]. We have found that the inhibitor enalaprilic acid also increases renal blood flow (Fig. 1) but only at doses which completely

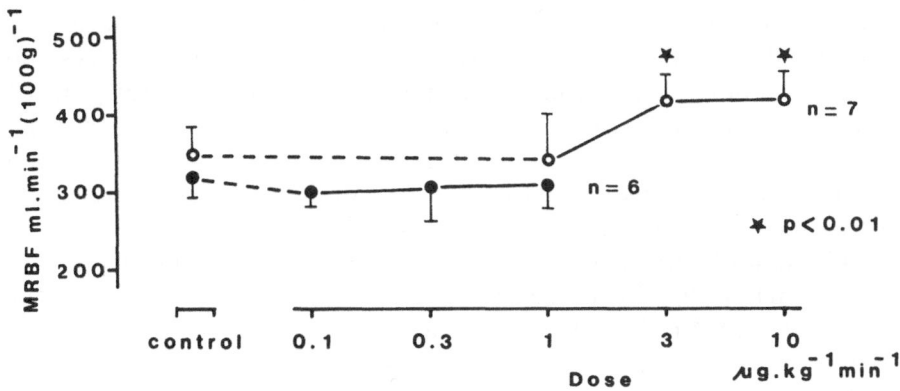

Figure 1. Effect of the converting-enzyme inhibitor enalaprilic acid on mean renal blood flow (MRBF) in two groups of patients receiving incremental doses of the drug. Only at the two highest doses renal blood flow increased.

suppress plasmatic converting-enzyme [56].

With the proviso that no pharmacologic agent is entirely specific, the accumulated data point to an important role of endogenous angiotensin in the regulation of renal vascular resistance. It also seems that the hypertensive kidney is more sensitive to this substance than the normotensive one. Unfortunately, we are not yet able to answer the question whether it is circulating angiotensin or intra-renally formed angiotensin which is the most important regulator of renal vascular tone.

Role of the adrenergic system

Although it is frequently assumed that the sympathetic nervous systems plays a major part in the pathophysiology of essential hypertension, data about adrenergic participation in renal vasoconstriction are only beginning to emerge. What was discussed for angiotensin also applies to the adrenergic system; that is, it should not only be proven that adrenergic stimulation can increase renal resistance, it should also be demonstrated that blockade of neurons or receptors can reverse this process.

Indeed, the renal circulation responds to noradrenaline both in normotensives and in hypertensives [57, 58] and various manoeuvres which activate the sympathetic system also reduce renal flow [59–64]. In our own study we found that isometric (handgrip) exercise in 5 hypertensive patients reduced renal blood flow from an average of $302\,ml\,min^{-1}\,(100\,g)^{-1}$ to an average of $250\,ml\,min^{-1}\,(100\,g)^{-1}$, indicating that (neurogenic) vasocontriction had taken place in the kidney [63]. Likewise, mental stress has a profound impact on renal flow. For instance, Hollenberg found that confrontation with a non-vertal IQ-test depressed mean renal blood flow by an average of 80 ml min^{-1} (100 g)$^{-1}$ in 15 patients with essential hypertension. Several studies have now shown that a major disturbing stimulus evokes an accentuated renal vascular response in hypertensives, which is in contrast to the reaction seen in normotensives [7, 60–62]. It should be emphasized, however, that this was not always the case [64]. Normotensive subjects whose parents have hypertension may frequently display a renal response that resembles that of patients with hypertension. On this basis Hollenberg argues that the renal effects of neurogenic stimulation are not a consequence of high blood pressure, but rather a factor present at the initiation of this disorder.

It is not yet clear what mediates the renal vascular response to a neurogenic stimulus, but arguments have been presented for a direct effect rather than an indirect one, for instance via angiotensin [60]. Consistent with this view are the observations on a fall in renal vascular resistance brought about by the administration of drugs with a central sympatholytic action or with peripheral alpha-adrenoceptor blocking properties [26, 39, 65–69]. At least the renal vasoconstriction related to isometric exercise requires the functional presence of alpha-1 receptors, although in this context alpha-2 receptors may even be more important [63, 70]. The same may be true for resting vascular tone in the kidney [39, 63] (Fig. 2).

Role of vasodilator systems

Many uncertainties exist regarding the potential impact of prostaglandins on renal blood flow. Since these substances are local rather than circulating hormones it is extremely difficult to prove that they play a regulating role. Moreover, current techniques are not adequate enough to measure prostaglandins in blood or urine. Despite these drawbacks London and co-workers measured plasma prostaglandins E$_2$ and F$_{2\alpha}$ in 13 men with either borderline or sustained essential hypertension [71]. They were able to show a significant positive relationship between log values of PGE$_2$ and renal plasma flow. The same appeared true for the ratio between PGE$_2$ and PGF$_{2\alpha}$, whereas a non-significant inverse relationship was found between PGF$_{2\alpha}$ and renal plasma flow. The correlations were independent of age or the level of arterial pressure. On the basis of these findings the authors speculated about a possible role of renal prostaglandins on the regulation of renal flow, at least in hypertensives. The observation that prostaglandin-synthetase inhibitors impair blood flow through the kidney [72] may be in line with the hypothesis of London. However, too few data are presently available to implicate deficient production of PGE$_2$ or enhanced release of PGF$_{2\alpha}$ as a pathogenetic mechanism in essential hypertension. With respect to the

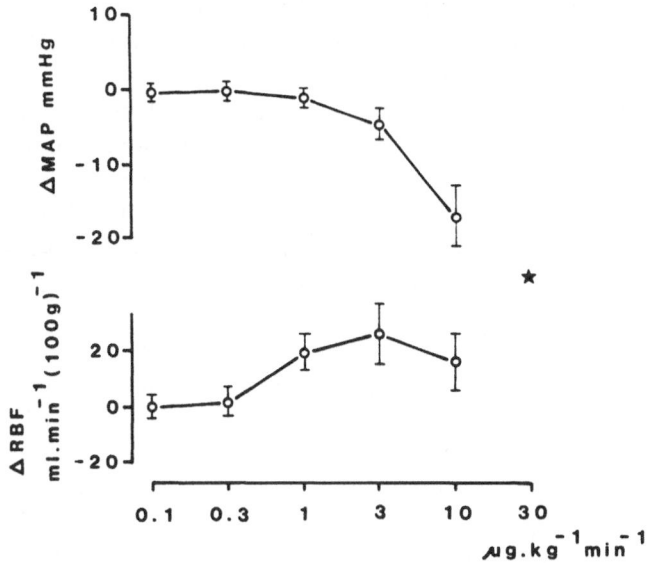

Figure 2. Changes in mean arterial pressure (MAP) and in renal blood flow (RBF) during infusion of incremental doses of the alpha-1 antagonist doxazosin. Note that only a small increase in renal blood flow ensued.

kallikrein-kinin system there are no certainties either. Levy *et al.* found both in normotensives and in hypertensives a positive relationship between urinary kallikrein excretion and renal blood flow [73]. When kallikrein excretion was substituted by the ratio between urinary kallikrein and supine plasma renin activity a similar relationship emerged. Although such data may point to an important regulating role of kinins, again too few data are available to substantiate this.

Several other vasodilating systems such as for instance dopamine or the atrial natriuretic factor may be involved as determinants of renal perfusion but at present the relevant information is too scanty.

Impact on glomerular filtration

Glomerular filtration rate is well maintained in essential hypertension until a late stage of the disease; a rapid decline of glomerular filtration rate is often seen in the malignant phase. In our own series glomerular filtration appeared to be largely maintained around an average normal value of 70 ml min^{-1} m^{-2} as long as renal plasma flow did not fall below 300 ml min^{-1} m^{-2}; at lower flow rates filtration declined but even then proportionally less than the decrement in plasma flow [28]. Filtration fraction, therefore, increased as blood pressure rose and renal blood flow fell. Although an elevated filtration fraction is a common finding in essential hypertension, this variable may be normal especially in the early stages of the disease [9, 28, 29].

In view of the reduction in renal cortical blood flow, the raised filtration fraction in essential hypertension could be the consequence of a shift in blood flow from areas with relatively low filtration to regions where it is relatively high. There are no data on regional differences in filtration fraction in man, but studies in experimental animals indicate that filtration fraction in the cortex is either not different from whole-kidney filtration or perhaps somewhat higher [74].

Alternative explanations for an increased filtration fraction could be increased effective filtration pressure or enhanced permeability of glomerular capillaries. The force causing filtration is the head of pressure transmitted to the glomerular capillaries from the systemic circulation, and this is opposed by the oncotic pressure.

Variations in glomerular hydrostatic pressure may result from changes in systemic hydrostatic pressure but also from changes in the resistance of the small renal arteries, the afferent and efferent arterioles, and the veins. Thus, glomerular pressure cannot be estimated in a direct way from the arterial pressure in the systemic circulation. Micropuncture studies in rats and monkeys have shown that filtration is highly flow-dependent, in the sense that changes in renal blood flow tend to be associated with parallel changes in glomerular filtration. If this is true for man as well, then a rise in filtration fraction, associated with the fall in blood flow through the kidney must imply an absolute or relative increase in glomerular hydrostatic pressure. Indeed, there is evidence that hydrostatic pressure in the proximal tubules is raised in essential hypertension [37]. It may therefore be assumed that glomerular capillary hydrostatic pressure is elevated as well. Moreover, Parving et al. [75] found a positive correlation between systemic arterial pressure and albuminuria (measured by radioimmunoassay) in patients with benign hypertension and 'normal' renal function, which was also interpreted as evidence for increased filtration pressure.

The two studies mentioned here suggest that it is transmission of an elevated systemic pressure which causes intraglomerular hydrostatic pressure to go up. Such an hypothesis has also been put forward by others [36, 76]. However, Willassen and Ofstad [72] failed to observe differences in wedged renal venous pressure between normotensives and hypertensives. Although this is in contrast with the findings of Lowenstein [37], it should be emphasized that Willassen and Ofstad's patients had higher values of renal blood flow and, hence, may not have had renal vascular abnormalities as severe as the patients in other studies [36, 37, 76]. Nevertheless, the discrepancy should alert that there may be another mechanism involved. From recent data it would appear that the efferent arteriole plays a pivotal role in the regulation of glomerular filtration rate. Constriction of the efferent arteriole raises glomerular hydrostatic pressure and this in itself may be sufficient to maintain filtration under conditions of a reduced blood supply.

Evidence, albeit indirect, for the participation of such a mechanism has come from studies where the renal effects of converting-enzyme inhibitors have been investigated. The results hint at angiotensin II as the modulator of filtration, in particular when renal blood is impaired [78, 79]. However, those results usually have been obtained under somewhat extreme conditions and there is as yet no compelling evidence that angiotensin II-mediated efferent arteriolar constriction is the crucial factor in the maintenance of filtration rate in essential hypertension.

Except for an increased hydrostatic pressure, alterations in glomerular capillary permeability could be involved. According to Bianchi the primary defect in hypertension would be a reduction in the ultrafiltration coefficient [18]. To compensate for this abnormality the organism would tend to increase renal blood flow in order to deliver a greater amount of plasma to the glomeruli. The finding of increased blood supply in some young subjects at risk of developing hypertension is certainly in support of such a view [18]. It is further assumed that later, when the capacitance of the renal vascular bed is put to limits, the higher plasma flow through the kidneys cannot be maintained and the compensation for the reduced ultrafiltration coefficient shifts to an increase in effective filtration pressure and hence hypertension develops. It should be emphasized, however, that a normal glomerular filtration rate with reduced plasma flow could equally well result from an increased ultrafiltration coefficient. Clearly, further studies are necessary to elucidate the exact mechanisms involved.

Conclusions

The possibility that the renal vasculature plays an important role in the pathogenesis of essential hypertension still receives a lot of attention. An increase in renal vascular resistance is demonstrable in all patients with essential hypertension. Total renal blood flow declines in an accelerated way as compared to physiological senescence and this is particularly evident in the outer cortial region. Blood flow measurements in this area correlate surprisingly well with angiographic assessments of vascular abnormalities [35, 80–82]. Although the nature of the increased vascular resistance is still elusive, there is compelling information that implicates both the sympathetic nervous system and angiotensin II. It is not known whether these two pressor mechanisms attack the kidney at the same site. A rise in efferent arteriolar resistance produced by angiotensin may be the explanation for the observation that glomerular filtration rate is kept within normal limits up to a stage of vascular complications. It is not excluded that the adrenergic system acts preferably at the level of the afferent arterioles. Wherever it comes into play, it is likely that alpha-2 adrenoceptors are the mediators of the vascular responses.

Regardless of the initiating factors it may be envisaged that hypertension, from an early phase, is accompanied by accelerated destruction of renal arterioles and glomeruli. The remaining afferent arterioles, as a consequence of the high systemic pressure, may be mechanically dilated resulting in hyperperfusion of intact glomeruli. Thus, in 'intact' nephrons glomerular filtration rate may be disproportionally high as compared to flow. Along this line of thought, the apparent normality of whole-kidney glomerular filtration rate would in fact be the result of two deviations from normal: an increased single nephron filtration rate in a decimated number of glomeruli. Such a change would fit the angiographical description by Ljunquist [83].

References

1. Borst JGG, Borst-de Geus A (1963): Hypertension explained by Starling's theory of circulatory homeostasis. Lancet 1: 677–82.
2. Ledingham JM (1971): The etiology of hypertension. Practitioner 207: 5–19.
3. Guyton AC, Coleman TC, Cowley AW, Scheel KW, Manning RD, Norman RA (1974): Arterial pressure regulation. Overriding dominance of the kidneys in long-term regulation and in hypertension. In: Laragh JH, ed. Hypertension Manual, vol. 111. New York: Yorke Medical Books, Dun-Donnelley Publ Corp: 111–34.
4. Smith HW (1951): The kidney. New York: Oxford Med Publ.
5. Leeuw PW de (1978): Vasoregulation and renal function in essential hypertension. Rotterdam: Erasmus Universiteit, 255 pp. Dissertation.
6. Hollenberg NK, Mangel R, Fung HYM (1976): Assessment of intrarenal perfusion with radioxenon: a critical review of analytical factors and their implications in man. Sem Nucl Med 6: 193–216.
7. Brod J, Fencl V, Hejl Z, Jirkan J, Ulrych M (1962): General and regional haemodynamic pattern underlying essential hypertension. Clin Sci 23: 339–49.
8. Goldring W, Chasis H (1944): Hypertension and hypertensive disease. New York: The Common Wealth Fund.
9. Pedersen EB, Kornerup HJ (1976): Renal haemodynamics and plasma renin in patients with essential hypertension. Clin Sci Mol Med 50: 409–14.
10. Pedersen EB (1977): Effect of sodium loading and exercise on renal haemodynamics and urinary sodium excretion in young patients with essential hypertension before and during propranolol treatment. Acta Med Scand 201: 365–73.
11. Pedersen EB (1978): Abnormal renal haemodynamics during exercise in young patients with mild essential hypertension without treatment and during long-term propranolol therapy. Scand J Clin Lab Invest 38: 567–71.
12. Bauer JH, Brooks CS, Burch RN (1982): Renal function and haemodynamic studies in low- and normal-renin essential hypertension. Arch Intern Med 142: 1317–23.
13. Bello CT, Sevy RW, Harakal C (1965): Varying hemodynamic patterns in essential hypertension. Am J Med Sci 250: 24–35.
14. Bello CT, Sevy RW, Harakal C, Hillyer PN (1967): Relationship between clinical severity of disease and hemodynamic patterns in essential hypertension. Am J Med Sci 253: 194–208.
15. Kioschos JM, Kirkendall WM, Valenca MR, Fitz EA (1967): Unilateral renal hemodynamics and characteristics of dye-dilution curves in patients with essential hypertension and renal disease. Circulation 35: 229–49.
16. Hollenberg NK, Merrill JP (1970): Intrarenal perfusion in the young 'essential' hypertensive: a subpopulation resistant to sodium restriction. Trans Assoc Am Physicians 83: 93–101.
17. Hollenberg NK, Borucki LJ, Adams DF (1978): The renal vasculature in early essential hyperten-

sion: evidence for a pathogenetic role. Medicine (Baltimore) 57: 167–78.

18. Bianchi G, Cusi D, Gatti M et al (1979): A renal abnormality as a possible cause of 'essential' hypertension. Lancet 1: 173–7.

19. Leeuw PW de, Kho TL, Birkenhäger WH (1981): Hemodynamic and endocrinologic data in early essential hypertension. In: Onesti G, Kim KE, eds. Hypertension in the young and the old. New York: Grune and Stratton: 57–62.

20. Messerli FM, Carvalho JGR de, Christie B, Frohlich ED (1978): Systemic and regional hemodynamics in low, normal and high cardiac output borderline hypertension. Circulation: 441–8.

21. Tuck MCL, Sullivan JM, Hollenberg NK, Dluhy RG, Williams GH (1973): Hemodynamic and endocrine response patterns in young patients with normal renin essential hypertension. Clin Res 21: 505.

22. Williams GH, Tuck ML, Sullivan JM, Dluhy RG, Hollenberg NK (1982): Parallel adrenal and renal abnormalities in young patients with essential hypertension. Am J Med 72: 907–14.

23. Davies DF, Shock NW (1950): Age changes in glomerular filtration rate, effective renal plasma flow and tubular excretory capacity in adult males. J Clin Invest 29: 496–507.

24. Wesson LG (1969): Physiology of the human kidney. New York: Grune and Stratton.

25. Hollenberg NK, Adams DF, Solomon HS, Rashid A, Abrams HL, Merrill JP (1974): Senescence and the renal vasculature in normal man. Circ Res 34: 309–16.

26. London GM, Safar ME, Sassard JE, Levenson JA, Simon AC (1984): Renal and systemic hemodynamics in sustained essential hypertension. Hypertension 6: 743–54.

27. Safar ME, Chau NP, Weiss YA, London GM, Milliez PL (1976): Cardiac output in essential hypertension. Am J Cardiol 38: 332–6.

28. Leeuw PW de, Kho TL, Falke HE, Birkenhäger WH, Wester A (1978): Haemodynamic and endocrinological profile of essential hypertension. Acta Med Scand; suppl 622.

29. Reubi FC, Weidmann P, Hodler J, Cottier PT (1978): Changes in renal function in essential hypertension. Am J Med 64: 556–63.

30. Bolomey AA, Michie AJ, Michie C, Breed ES, Schreiner GE, Lauson HI (1949): Simultaneous measurements of effective renal blood flow and cardiac output in resting normal subjects and patients with essential hypertension. J Clin Invest 28: 10–7.

31. Kolsters G (1976): De bloedsomloop door de nieren bij essentiële hypertensie. Rotterdam, Erasmus Universiteit, 190 pp. Dissertation.

32. Taquini AC, Villamil MF, Aramendia P, Riva IJ de la, Fermoso JD (1962): Effect of postural changes on cardiac and renal function in hypertensive subjects. Am Heart J 63: 78–85.

33. Birkenhäger WH, Leeuw PW de, Schalekamp MADH. Control mechanisms in essential hypertension. Amsterdam: Elsevier Biomedical Press, 1982.

34. Leeuw PW de, Birkenhäger WH (1982): Renal response to propranolol treatment in hypertensive humans. Hypertension 4: 125–31.

35. Case DB, Casarella WJ, Laragh JH, Fowler DL, Cannon PJ (1978): Renal cortical blood flow and angiography in low- and normal-renin essential hypertension. Kidney Int 13: 236–44.

36. Schalekamp MADH, Krauss XH, Schalekamp-Kuyken MPA, Kolsters G, Birkenhäger WH (1971): Studies on the mechanism of hypernatriuresis in essential hypertension in relation to measurements of plasma renin concentration, body fluid compartments and renal function. Clin Sci 41: 219–31.

37. Lowenstein J, Beranbaum ER, Chasis H, Baldwin DS (1970): Intrarenal pressure and exaggerated natriuresis in essential hypertension. Clin Sci 38: 359–74.

38. Leeuw PW de, Birkenhäger WH (1983): Renal blood flow in hypertension: relationship to sodium excretion and adrenergic activity. NZ Med J 96: 851–2.

39. Hollenberg NK, Adams DF, Solomon H, Chenitz WR, Burger BM, Abrams HL, Merrill JP (1975): Renal vascular tone in essential and secondary hypertension. Medicine (Baltimore) 54: 29–44.

40. Bock KD, Krecke HJ (1958): Die Wirkung von synthetischem Hypertensin II auf die PAH- und

Inulin-Clearance, die renale Hämodynamik und die Diurese beim Menschen. Klin Wschr 36: 69–74.

41. Bono E de, Le GDJ, Mottram FR, Pickering GW, Brown JJ, Keen H, Peart WS, Sanderson PH (1963): The action of angiotensin in man. Clin Sci 25: 123–57.

42. Louis WJ, Doyle AE (1965): The effects of varying doses of angiotensin on renal function and blood pressure in man and dogs. Clin Sci 29: 489–504.

43. Brod J, Hejl Z, Hornych A, Jirke J, Slechta V, Burianová B (1969): Comparison of haemodynamic effects of equipressor doses of intravenous angiotensin and noradrenaline in man. Clin Sci 36: 161–72.

44. Statius van Eps LW, Smorenberg-Schoorl ME, Zürcher-Mulder A, Birkenhäger WH, Vries LA de (1962): Vergelijking van de orthostatische water- en zoutretentie met die welke ontstaat bij toediening van angiotensine, noradrenaline en aldosteron. Ned Tijdschr Geneeskd 106: 2184–90.

45. Ljungman S (1982): Renal function, sodium excretion and the renin-angiotensinaldosterone system in relation to blood pressure. Acta Med Scand; Suppl 663.

46. Hollenberg NK, Solomon HS, Adams DF, Abrams HL, Merrill JP (1972): Renal vascular responses to angiotensin and norepinephrine in normal man. Circ Res 31: 750–7.

47. Hollenberg NK, Adams DF (1976): The renal circulation in hypertensive disease. Am J Med 60: 773–84.

48. Hoogdalem P van, Donker AJM, Leenen FHH (1978): Angiotensin II blockade before and after marked sodium depletion in patients with hypertension. Clin Sci Mol Med 54: 75–83.

49. Hollenberg NK, Williams GH, Burger B, Ishikawa I, Adams DF (1976): Blockade and stimulation of renal, adrenal and vascular angiotensin II receptors with 1-sar, 8-ala angiotensin II in normal man. J Clin Invest 57: 39–46.

50. Hollenberg NK, Williams GH, Taub KJ, Ishikawa I, Brown C, Adams DF (1977): Renal vascular response to interruption of the renin-angiotensin system in normal man. Kidney Int 12: 285–93.

51. Hollenberg NK, Meggs LG, Williams GH, Katz J, Garnic JD, Harrington DP (1981): Sodium intake and renal responses to captopril in normal man and essential hypertension. Kidney Int 20: 240–5.

52. Williams GH, Hollenberg NK (1977): Accentuated vascular and endocrine response to SQ 20881 in hypertension. N Engl J Med 1977: 184–8.

53. Kiowski W, Brummelen P van, Hulthén L, Amann FW, Bühler FR (1982): Antihypertensive and renal effects of captopril in relation to renin activity and bradykinin-induced vasodilation. Clin Pharmacol Ther 31: 677–84.

54. Dunn FG, Oigman W, Ventura HO, Messerli FH, Kobrin I, Frohlich ED (1984): Enalapril improves systemic and renal hemodynamics and allows regression of left ventricular mass in essential hypertension. Am J Cardiol 53: 105–8.

55. Ventura HO, Frohlich ED, Messerli FG, Kobrin I, Kardon MB (1985): Cardiovascular effects and regional blood flow distribution associated with angiotensin converting enzyme inhibition (captopril) in essential hypertension. Am J Cardiol 55: 1023–6.

56. Leeuw PW de, Es PN van, Looman M, Birkenhäger WH (1985): Renal response to converting enzyme blockade. J Hypertension 3 (suppl 3): S295–6.

57. Gombos EA, Hulet WH, Bopp P, Goldring W, Baldwin DS, Chasis H (1962): Reactivity of renal and systemic circulations to vasoconstrictor agents in normotensive and hypertensive subjects. J Clin Invest 41: 203–17.

58. Lowenstein J, Steinmetz PR, Effros RM, Meester M de, Chasis H, Baldwin DS, Gomez DM (1967): The distribution of intrarenal blood flow in normal and hypertensive man. Circulation 35: 250–4.

59. Hollenberg NK, Epstein M, Basch RI, Merrill JP, Hickler RB (1969): Renin secretion in the patient with hypertension. Circ Res 24/25 (suppl 1): I–113–22.

60. Hollenberg NK, Williams GH, Adams DF (1981): Essential hypertension: abnormal renal vascular and endocrine responses to a mild psychological stimulus. Hypertension 3: 11–7.

61. Pfeiffer JB, Wolff HG, Winter OS (1950): Studies in renal circulation during periods of life stress and accompanying emotional reactions in subjects with and without essential hypertension; observations on the role of neural activity in regulation of renal blood flow. J Clin Invest 29: 1227–42.

62. Wolf S, Pfeiffer JB, Ripley HS, Winter OS, Wolff HG (1948): Hypertension as a reaction pattern to stress: summary of experimental data on variations in blood pressure and renal flow. Ann Intern Med 29: 1056–76.

63. Leeuw PW de, Bos R de, Es PN van, Birkenhäger WH (1985): Effect of sympathetic stimulation and intrarenal alpha-blockade on the secretion of renin by the human kidney. Eur J Clin Invest 15: 106–70.

64. Bello CT, Sevy RW, Ohler EA, Papacostas CA, Bucher RM (1960): Renal hemodynamic responses to stress in normotensive and hypertensive subjects. Circulation 22: 573–82.

65. Falch DK, Quist Paulsen A, Ødegaard AE, Norman N (1979): Central and renal circulation, renin and aldosterone in plasma during prazosin treatment in essential hypertension. Acta Med Scand 206: 489–94.

66. Leeuw PW de, Wester A, Willemse PJ, Birkenhäger WH (1980): Effects of prazosin on plasma noradrenaline and plasma renin concentrations in hypertensive subjects. J Cardiovasc Pharmacol 2 (suppl 3): S361–72.

67. Kobrin I, Amodeo C, Ventura HO, Messerli FH, Frohlich ED (1985): Immediate hemodynamic effects of urapidil in patients with essential hypertension. Am J Cardiol 55: 722–5.

68. Chrysant SG (1983): Autonomic, systemic, and renal hemodynamic actions of trimazosin in hypertensive patients. Am Heart J 106: 1243–50.

69. Thananopavarn C, Golub MS, Eggena P, Barrett JD, Sambhi MP (1982): Clonidine, a centrally acting sympathetic inhibitor, as monotherapy for mild to moderate hypertension. Am J Cardiol 49: 153–8.

70. Leeuw PW de, Es PN van, Bos R de, Birkenhäger WH (1986): Acute renal effects of doxazosin in man. Br J Clin Pharmacol 21 (suppl 1): 41s–3s.

71. London GM, Hornych A, Safar ME, Levenson JA, Simon AC (1982): Plasma prostaglandins PGE_2 and $PGF_{2\alpha}$, total effective vascular compliance and renal plasma flow in essential hypertension. Nephron 32: 118–24.

72. Clive DM, Stoff JS (1984): Renal syndromes associated with non-steroidal anti-inflammatory drugs. N Engl J Med 310: 563–72.

73. Levy SB, Lilley JJ, Frigon RP, Stone R (1977): Urinary kallikrein and plasma renin activity as determinants of renal blood flow. The influence of race and dietary sodium intake. J Clin Invest 60: 129–38.

74. Nissen OI (1966): The filtration fractions of plasma supplying the superficial and deep venous drainage area of the cat kidney. Acta Physiol Scand 68: 275–85.

75. Parving HH, Mogensen CE, Jensen HA, Evrin PE (1974): Increased urinary albumin excretion rate in benign essential hypertension. Lancet 1: 1190–2.

76. Schalekamp MADH, Krauss XH, Kolsters G, Schalekamp MPA, Birkenhäger WH (1973): Renin suppression in hypertension in relation to body fluid volumes, patterns of sodium excretion and renal haemodynamics. Clin Sci Mol Med 45 (suppl 1): 283s–6s.

77. Willassen Y, Ofstad J (1980): Renal sodium excretion and the peritubular capillary physical factors in essential hypertension. Hypertension 2: 771–9.

78. Levens NR, Peach MJ, Carey RM (1981): Role of the intrarenal renin-angiotensin system in the control of renal function. Circ Res 48: 157–67.

79. Leeuw PW de, Birkenhäger WH. Physiological effects of angiotensin II on the kidney. Handbook of Hypertension, vol 8; in press.

80. Hollenberg NK, Epstein M, Basch RI, Merrill JP (1969): 'No man's land' of the renal vasculature: an arteriographic and hemodynamic assessment of the interlobar and arcuate arteries in essential and accelerated hypertension. Am J Med 47: 845–54.

81. Gatta A, Merkel C, Pessina AC, Milani L, Sacerdoti D, Zuin R (1982): Renal haemodynamics in essential hypertension assessed by 133-Xenon washout and selective renal angiography. Angiology 33: 818–24.
82. Arlart IP, Rosenthal J (1984): Peripheral renal vascular disease in essential hypertension: hemodynamic, angiographic, and endocrine assessment. Cardiovasc Intervent Radiol 7: 221–8.
83. Ljunquist A (1963): The intrarenal arterial pattern in the normal and diseased human kidney; a micro-angiographic and histologic study. Acta Med Scand; suppl 40.

Hepato-splanchnic circulation in human hypertension

Y.A. WEISS, G.H. LONDON and M.E. SAFAR

Under normal conditions, the hepato-splanchnic circulation receives a large portion of the cardiac output (about 25%), contains a substantial fraction of the blood volume (about 20%) and provides a major share of the total body lymph flow and transvascular protein flux [1]. Therefore, hypertension-induced changes in the vasculature of this region can play a significant role in systemic hemodynamics.

Although experimental studies [1] have suggested that abnormalities of the splanchnic circulation are important and even might be an initiating factor in hypertension [2], little research has been done on hepatic and splanchnic blood flow in hypertension in man. The present report summarizes the methods used for the evaluation of hepatic blood flow in humans with applications to the pathophysiology and clinical pharmacology of essential hypertension.

Methods for the measurement of hepatic blood flow in hypertension

Measurements of hepatic blood flow (HBF) are based on the general equation of clearances [3]. For any substance cleared from the circulation by the liver, the hepatic clearance (HC) is such that:

$$HC = HBF \times E$$

in which E denotes hepatic extraction (arterio-venous difference in concentration divided by arterial concentration of the substance). When hepatic extraction is nearly complete (E = 1, with hepatic venous concentration nearly zero), hepatic blood flow equals hepatic clearance [3]. In other cases, invasive techniques requiring catheterization of hepatic veins are used to evaluate E [4] and hepatic blood flow is calculated as HC/E.

In the most classical method [4], two catheters are inserted into the antecubital veins for infusion and blood sampling. A catheter is introduced into the hepatic vein by the Seldinger technique under fluoroscopic control. Estimation of the hepatic blood flow uses a plasma concentration plateau of freshly prepared indocyanine green (ICG) [4, 5]. This plateau is obtained in 30 min by means of an intravenous bolus of 20 mg followed by constant infusion of the dye at a rate of 0.6 mg/min. The infusion pump and the syringe are calibrated after each procedure. Six paired peripheral and hepatic venous samples are taken at 5-min intervals. ICG concentrations are determined with a Beckman spectrophotometer. Hepatic blood flow (HBF) in milliliter per minute is calculated from the formula:

$$HBF = Q/(P - V)(1 - Ht)$$

where Q is the ICG infusion rate, P and V are the peripheral and hepatic venous concentrations of the dye and Ht is the hepatic venous hematocrit. HBF is usually corrected for body surface area. The reproducibility of the method is $4 \pm 2\%$.

In order to avoid hepatic catheterizations, clearance of indocyanine green is often evaluated instead of real hepatic blood flow [6]. Fractional clearance is calculated using the method of the least squares for the natural logarithmic values of the serum concentration. Subsequently, the fractional clearance is multiplied by the plasma volume to obtain plasma clearance of indocyanine green. This value is corrected for the total body hematocrit to obtain the total blood clearance. In patients with normal hepatic function, the clearance seems to parallel closely any changes in total liver blood flow [6]. However, indocyanine green clearance consistently underestimates total hepatic blood flow [3], an error which is not observed with substances having more reproducible values of hepatic extraction ratio [5].

Many compounds, by virtue of quite elevated hepatic extraction ratios, can be considered to have flow-dependent hepatic clearances which are highly sensitive to changes in hepatic blood flow. Previous studies with aldosterone [7], lignocaine and oxyphenylbutazone [8] have determined the relationship between changes in hepatic blood flow and total clearance of these substances. A high hepatic extraction ratio of (dl) propranolol has been shown in monkeys and in dogs [9]. A nearly complete extraction has also been postulated to occur in man at relatively low drug concentration [9], suggesting that propranolol might be added to the list of the flow-dependent drugs. Indeed, a high hepatic ratio of both (d) and (dl) propranolol has been observed in hypertensive men (Fig. 1) [5]. A highly significant relationship has been shown between hepatic blood flow measured from ICG clearance and hepatic extraction and the total clearance of propranolol. A decrease in hepatic blood flow is produced by the beta-adrenergic receptor blockade due to (dl) propranolol. On the other hand, (d) propranolol has no hemodynamic effect. The slope of the relationship between hepatic blood flow measured from the ICG method and (d) propranolol clearance is 1.05 ± 0.27 (Fig. 2) [5]. Such a result provides evidences that the (d) propranolol and not (dl)

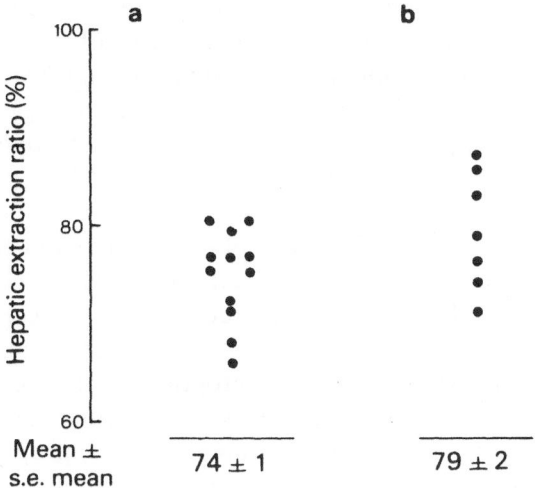

Figure 1. Hepatic extraction ratios of (dl) (a) and (d) (b) propranolol in individual hypertensive patients (with permission) [5].

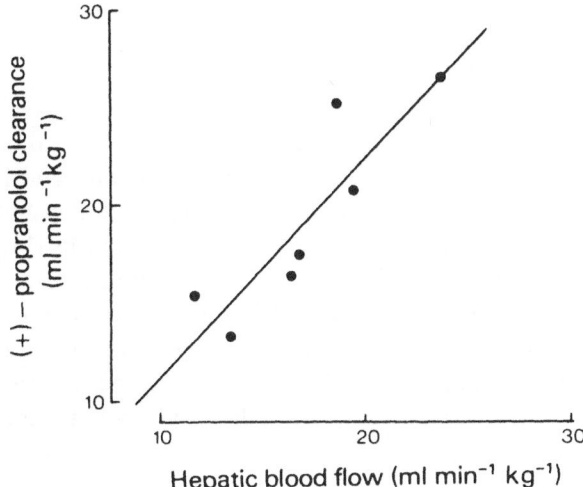

Figure 2. Relationship between hepatic blood flow and (d) propranolol total plasma clearance. The equation is $y = 1.06x + 1.16$ ($y = ax + b$). Note that the b value is not significantly different from zero. $r = 0.86$, $P < 0.01$ (with permission) [5].

propranolol total plasma clearance constitutes a safe method for the estimation of hepatic blood flow without catheterization in men with normal liver function.

In clinical practice, (d) propranolol is administered intravenously until steady-state concentrations are achieved. The bolus size (0.27 mg/kg) and the continuous infusion rate (0.08 mg/kg/h) are based on classical kinetic data [10]. In all cases, higher initial levels decline rapidly within 30–45 min to the predetermined concentration which is maintained during the infusion period. The reproducibility of the determination is $6 \pm 3\%$. Propranolol is often assayed fluorometrically by using Shand *et al.* methods [11]. Propranolol concentrations are determined both in blood and plasma. The blood plasma ratio is 0.90 ± 0.03 [12].

The bolus technique may be used with propranolol as a simpler procedure than the plateau technique [11]. A bolus of (d) propranolol (0.2 mg/kg) is administered intravenously in 30 s. Blood samples are taken before and 5, 10, 15, 20, 30, 60, 120 and 180 min after propranolol administration. The (d) propranolol clearance is calculated from the disappearance curve of (d) propranolol. Since the feathering technique does not indicate significant differences in the results between the one-compartment and two-compartment models, only the one-compartment model is widely used for the calculation of (d) propranolol clearance. The reproducibility of the determination is $8 \pm 2\%$.

Hepatic blood flow in hypertensive humans

The splanchnic vascular bed has not been extensively studied in patients with sustained essential hypertension. Both Culbertson *et al.* and Brod *et al.* (12–13) reported an increase in estimated splanchnic resistance in hypertension. It decreased after splanchnicectomy but only for a few months [14]. Thus splanchnic blood flow is generally normal [13–15] (Table 1), although some work has shown it to be slightly decreased in subjects with renovascular hypertension [16].

In patients with borderline hypertension and elevated cardiac output, Messerli *et al.* [6] found that the ICG and hippuran clearances varied in parallel with cardiac output, with no evidence of redistribution between these two major

Table 1. Regional haemodynamics (by permission) [15].

	Normal Subjects	Borderline Hypertension	Sustained Hypertension
Lower limb blood flow (ml/min/100 g)	2.03 ± 0.17	$3.06 \pm 0.28^*$	1.9 ± 0.18
Renal blood flow (ml/min/m²)	894 ± 32	853 ± 37	$751 \pm 27^*$
Hepatic blood flow (ml/min/m²)	930 ± 56	973 ± 50	885 ± 31

Results are means $\pm$ 1 SEM. Significance of differences:
* $p < 0.01$ in comparison with normal subjects.

circulations. No comparison with control subjects was performed. When hepatic, renal and lower limb blood flows are considered together in borderline hypertension and compared to normal subjects (Table 1), it appears that the increased cardiac output is dominantly related to an increase in lower limbs and muscle blood flow [5]. Since the increased lower limb blood flow is associated with a normal hepatic blood flow, as measured from the (d) propranolol clearance, an interesting interpretation of the redistribution of cardiac output may be proposed in borderline hypertension. On the basis of animal experiments, Caldini *et al.* [17] proposed that the circulation functioned as though it were two semi-independent circuits in parallel, one chiefly comprising the splanchnic bed, having a long time-constant for venous drainage, and the other, chiefly the muscles, a short time-constant for the venous drainage. If applicable to man, this observation is relevant to the hemodynamic results of patients with borderline hypertension and elevated cardiac output. A redistribution of blood flow could occur at the hepato-splanchnic level with an arteriolar constriction of the splanchnic bed and an increase in muscle blood flow, resulting in a faster average venous return to the heart by means of the shorter time-constant pathway.

Hepatic blood flow and humoral and fluid volume abnormalities in human hypertensives

The splanchnic vascular system is unusual in having two capillary systems, the intestinal and the hepatic. The liver possesses a double blood supply from the portal vein under low peripheral pressure and from the hepatic artery in which the perfusion pressure equals systemic arterial pressure. This anatomic situation explains why splanchnic blood flow is equal to hepatic blood flow if no significant collateral circulation exists [1, 3, 16]. In subjects with normal liver function, collaterals are usually absent or meaningless and the two terms hepatic and splanchnic blood flow can be used interchangeably, as it is the case in patients with hypertension. In this section, the relationships of hepatic blood flow will be analyzed on the basis of three parameters: plasma renin activity, plasma aldosterone and fluid volumes in hypertension.

In contrast with patients with essential hypertension, patients with reno-vascular hypertension (RAS) exhibit a normal or slightly elevated cardiac output associated with an even lower hepatic blood flow [16]. This finding must be interpreted in hypertensive patients with RAS, where circulating pressor substances might produce vasoconstriction in the splanchnic vascular bed, thereby diminishing hepatic blood flow. This possibility is supported by the decrease in splanchnic blood flow which has been produced by angiotensin II infusion in animal [18] and in normotensive humans with or without liver disease [19]. A decrease in splanchnic blood flow was also found in experimental renal hypertension in the rat [20]. Finally, in normal subjects [11] and in patients with RAS [21], plasma renin activity and hepatic blood flow are negatively related, a finding which is never observed in patients with essential hypertension [21].

In patients with hypertension, the level of hepatic blood flow may be especially important in the view of the metabolism of aldosterone and other steroids, which are inactivated to a large degree by the liver [7]. Previous investigations [22] have indicated that the mean metabolic clearance rate of aldosterone measured by a constant infusion technique was lower in patients with essential hypertension than in healthy subjects. In addition, a marked decrease in the metabolic clearance rate of aldosterone has also been reported [23] in patients with renal arterial stenosis, which partially normalized after corrective surgery. However, more recent studies in large populations of patients with essential hypertension have shown that hepatic blood flow, evaluated from the (d) propranolol clearance, was invariably normal, showing no correlation with plasma aldosterone [11].

Structural or neurohumoral influences could lead to a reduction in vascular capacity. This would increase cardiac filling pressure as blood is translocated centrally and the resulting elevation of cardiac output and hence hepatic blood flow has been implicated as an early step in the development of several forms of hypertension [1, 2, 24]. Since the splanchnic circulation contains approximately 22% of total blood volume, changes in the venous capacity in this region could contribute to this process. A shift in the pressure-volume curve of ileal veins toward the pressure axis in dogs with one-kidney, one-wrap perinephritic hypertension has been described [1]. As reported elsewhere [24], venous compliance is reduced in essential hypertension, mainly in its splanchnic compartment. Reduction in splanchnic compliance may contribute to maintain or increase cardiac output and hence hepatic blood flow [24]. On the other hand, reduced venous compliance favors a shift of intravascular volume toward interstitial fluid volume [24]. In that condition, it seems logical that a negative relationship is observed between hepatic blood flow and the ratio between plasma volume and interstitial fluid volume in hypertension: the greater the reduction in the venous compliance, the higher the hepatic blood flow, the more substantial the shift of intravascular volume toward the interstitial space (Fig. 3).

Antihypertensive drugs and hepatic blood flow

Studies of the effect of antihypertensive drugs on hepatic blood flow are few. Most of them involve only indocyanine green blood clearance which has been found to be reduced after nitroglycerin and unchanged after hydralazine [25].

Hepatic blood flow measured using hepatic venous catheterization is decreased after administration of (dl) propranolol [5] and captopril [26] but unchanged after pindolol [27]. The finding of decreased hepatic blood flow after drug administration might be a relevant subject at least for two reasons = (i) reduction in hepatic blood flow might predispose to further impairment in drinkers and patients with

.PLASMA VOLUME / INTERSTITIAL VOLUME

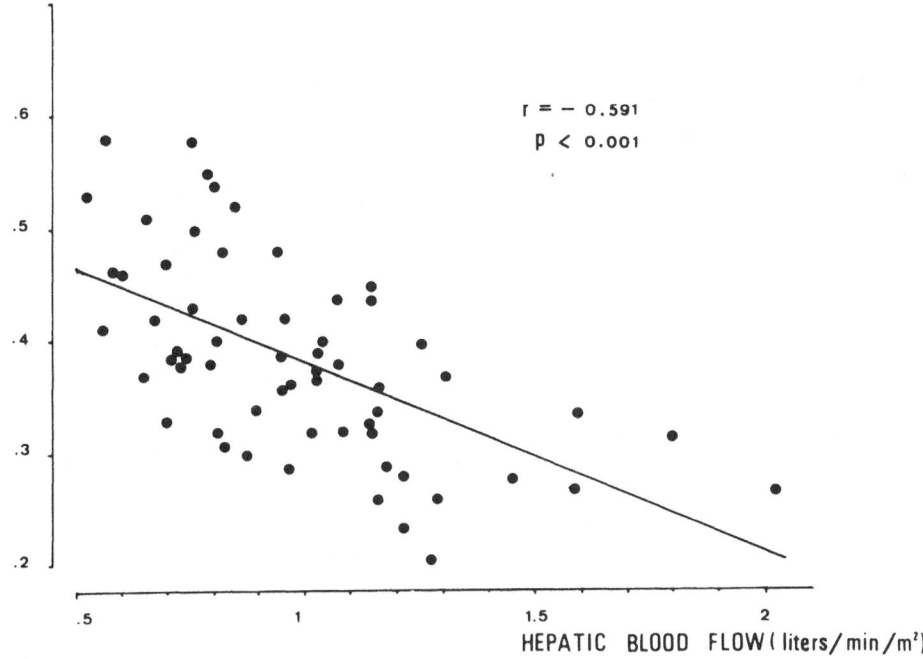

Figure 3. Patients with sustained essential hypertension: relationship between hepatic blood flow and the ratio between plasma volume and interstitial fluid volume (personal data).

abnormalities of liver function [28], and (ii) a persistent decrease in hepatic blood flow might also be expected to decrease systemic elimination of drugs that have a high hepatic extraction such as the anti-arrhythmic agents, lidocaine and verapamil, as well as the lipid-soluble beta-adrenoreceptor antagonists and opiate analgesics [29]. For such reasons, the direct evaluation of hepatic extraction of drugs might be particularly relevant in the fields of hypertension. While the hepatic extraction of dl propranolol is $74 \pm 1\%$ [5], the value is $23 \pm 4\%$ with pindolol (Fig. 4) [30, 31, 32]. From these determinations, it has been shown that total body clearance of propranolol nearly equals hepatic clearance [5, 32, 33]. On the other hand, total clearance of pindolol has been shown to be the sum of both the renal and non-renal clearances in equal parts [27–31]. In addition, the non-renal clearance of pindolol was found to equal the hepatic clearance directly measured from the hepatic extraction ratio and hepatic blood flow [27–31]. Such findings are particularly relevant for the treatment of hypertensive patients with renal insufficiency.

218

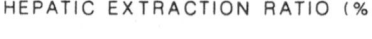

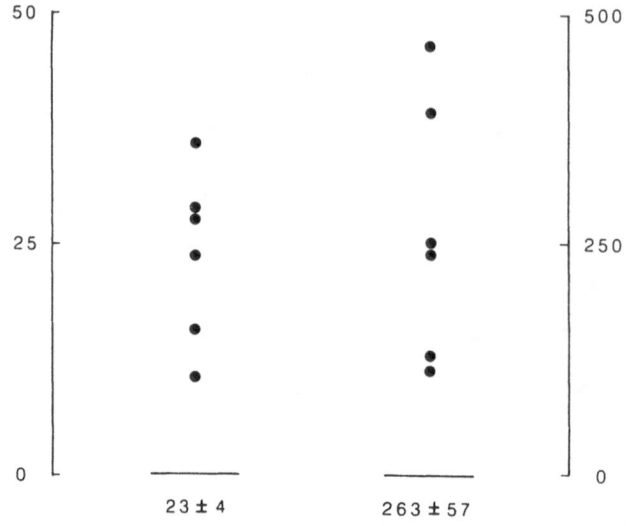

HEPATIC EXTRACTION RATIO (%)   HEPATIC CLEARANCE (ml/min)

23 ± 4   263 ± 57

Figure 4. Hepatic extraction ratio and hepatic clearance of pindolol in six hypertensive patients with unilateral renal artery stenosis (with permission) [31].

References

1. Nyhof RA, Laine GA, Meininger GA, Granger HJ (1983): Splanchnic circulation in hypertension. Federation Proc 42: 1690–1693.
2. Simon G, Pamnani MB, Dunkel JF, Overbeck HW (1975): Mesenteric hemodynamics in early experimental renal hypertension in dogs. Circul Res 36: 791–798.
3. Benhamou JP, Sicot C, Erlinger S (1971): Exposés de physiologie et de physiopathologie hépatique. La Presse Médicale, 79: 185–191.
4. Caesar J, Shaldon S, Chiandussi L, Guevara L, Sherlock S (1961): The use of indocyanin green in the measurement of hepatic blood flow. Clin Sci 21: 43–57.
5. Weiss YA, Safar ME, Lehner JP, Levenson JA, Simon A, Alexandre JM (1978): (+)-propranolol clearance, an estimation of hepatic blood flow in man. Br J Clin Pharmacol 5: 457–460.
6. Messerli FH, De Carvalho JGR, Christie B, Frohlich ED (1978): Systemic and regional hemodynamics in low, normal and high cardiac output borderline hypertension. Circulation 58: 441–448.
7. Tait JF, Bougas J, Little B, Tait SAS, Flood C (1965): Splanchnic extraction and clearance of aldosterone in subjects with minimal and marked cardiac dysfunction. J Clin Endocrin Metab 25: 219–225.
8. Stenson RE, Constantino RT, Harrison DC (1971): Interrelationship of hepatic blood flow, cardiac output and blood levels of lidocaine in man. Circulation 43: 205–211.
9. Nies AS, Evans GH, Shand DG (1972): The hemodynamic effects of beta-adrenergic blockade on the flow-dependent hepatic clearance of propranolol J Pharmacol Exp Ther 184: 716–722.
10. Weiss YA, Safar ME, Chevillard C, Frydman A, Simon A, Lemaire P, Alexandre JM (1976): Comparison of the pharmacokinetics of intravenous dl-Propranolol in borderline and permanent hypertension. Europ J Clin Pharmacol 10: 387–393.

11. Safar ME, Simon ACh, Dard SA, Parlier HR, Pauleau NE, Vincent ML, Sassard JE (1982): Aldosterone in sustained essential hypertension. Clinical Endocrinology 16: 77–88.

12. Brod J (1960): Essential hypertension. Hemodynamic observations with a bearing on its pathogenesis. Lancet 1: 773–778.

13. Culbertson JW, Wilkins RW, Ingelfinger FJ, Bradley SE (1951): The effect of the upright posture on hepatic blood flow in normotensive and hypertensive subjects. J Clin Invest 30: 305–311.

14. Wilkins RW, Culbertson JW, Rymut AA (1957): The hepatic blood flow in resting hypertensive patients before and after splanchnicectomy. J Clin Invest 31: 529–531.

15. Temmar MM, Safar ME, Levenson JA, Totomoukouo JM, Simon ACh (1981): Regional blood flow in borderline and sustained essential hypertension. Clincial Science 60: 653–658.

16. Messerli FH, Genest J, Nowaczynski W, Kuchel O, Honda M, Latour Y, Dumont G (1975): Splanchnic blood flow in essential hypertension and in hypertensive patients with renal artery stenosis. Circulation 51: 1114–1119.

17. Caldini P, Permutt S, Waddel JA, Riley RL (1974): Effect of epinephrine on pressure, flow and volume relationship in the systemic circulation of dogs. Circulation Research 34: 602–623.

18. Bashour FA, McClelland R, Nafrawi A (1963): Effects of angiotensin and splanchnic circulation and liver in dogs. L Lab Clin Med 62: 857–865.

19. Chiandussi L, Vaccarino A, Greco F, Muratori F, Cesano L, Indovina D (1963): Effect of drug infusion on the splanchnic circulation. I. Angiotensin infusion in normal and cirrhotic subjects. Proc Soc Exp Biol Med 112: 324–337.

20. Bralet AM, Wepierre J, Bralet J (1973): Distribution of cardiac output and nutritional blood flow in the unanesthetized rat: alterations during experimental renal hypertension. Pfluegers Arch 343: 257–264.

21. Safar ME, Weiss YA, Fontaliran FM, Simon AC, Pauleau NF (1978): Renovascular hypertension: relationship between hepatic blood flow and plasma renin activity. Nephron 20: 119–123.

22. Nowaczynski W, Kuchel O, Genest J (1971): A decreased metabolic clearance rate of aldosterone in benign essential hypertension. J Clin Invest 50: 2184–2191.

23. Kaufmann W, Steiner B, Durr F, Nieth H, Behn C (1967): Aldosteronstoffwechsel bei Nierenarterienstenose. Klin Wochenschr 45: 966–974.

24. Safar ME, London GM (1985): Venous system in essential hypertension. Cli Science 69: 497–504.

25. Svensson CK, Cumella JC, Tronolone M, Middleton E, Lalka D (1985): Effects of hydralazine, nitroglycerin, and food on estimated hepatic blood flow. Clin Pharmacol Ther 37: 464–468.

26. Crossley IR, Bihari D, Gimson AES, Westaby D, Richardson IJ, Williams R (1984): Effect of converting enzyme inhibitor on hepatic blood flow in man. Amer J Med 76 (5B): 62–66.

27. Safar ME, Chau NPh, Levenson JA, Simon ACh, Weiss YA (1978): Pharmacokinetics of intravenous and oral pindolol in hypertensive patients with chronic renal failure. Clin Science and Mol Med 55: 275s–277s.

28. Braillon A, Jiron MI, Valla D, Cales P, Lebreck D (1985): Effect of propranolol on hepatic blood flow in patients with cirrhosis. Clin Pharmac Therapeut 37: 376–380.

29. George CF (1979): Drug kinetics and hepatic blood flow. Clin Pharmacol Cokinet 4: 433–438.

30. Chau NPh, Weiss YA, Safar ME, Lavene DE, Georges DR, Milliez PL (1977): Pindolol availability in hypertensive patients with normal and impaired renal function. Clinical Pharmacol and Therapeut 22: 505–510.

31. Lavene DE, Weiss YA, Safar ME, Loria Y, Agoras N, Georges D, Milliez PL (1977): Pharmacokinetics and hepatic extraction ratio of pindolol in hypertensive patients with normal and impaired renal function. J Clin Pharmacol 17: 501–508.

32. London GM, Safar ME, Weiss YA, Milliez PL (1976): Isoproterenol sensitivity and total body clearance of propranolol in hypertension patients. J Clin Pharmacol 16: 174–182.

33. Shand DG, Evans GH, Nies AS (1971): The almost complete hepatic extraction of propranolol during intravenous administration in the dog. Life Sci 10: 1417–1421.

Part V

Forearm circulation as a model for the study of hypertension

Methods for investigation of the forearm blood flow

BERNARD I. LEVY

The limb circulation is widely used as a model for the study of hypertension and especially for estimation of the hemodynamic modifications induced by the administration of a drug. To understand the circulatory response of a limb, it is necessary to measure the fraction of flow exchanging substances with tissues (nutritive flow) as opposed to flow traversing shunt vessels which are capable of exchanging only heat. The metabolism to perfusion ratio and its distribution within the different tissues of the limb are also important parameters to be estimated. The ideal method must be non-invasive, accurate and reliable, it can be used at frequent intervals and not only at rest but also while the local circulation is varied, as widely as possible, by physical, chemical or nervous influence. Unfortunately, existing methods do not enable all of these measurements to be performed directly. However, considering together results obtained by various methods, most of this information can be obtained.

1. Venous occlusion plethysmography

For measuring the total blood flow, the 'gold standard' method is still the venous occlusion plethysmography. The principles have been described by Brodie and Russel in 1905 [1]: the aim is to arrest the venous blood return completely for a few seconds, without directly interfering with arterial inflow. A continuous record is made of the changes in volume either of the whole limb beyond the level of the venous occlusion, or of a segment of limb between the level of venous occlusion and a distal cuff inflated to a pressure intended to arrest the circulation in all vessels. The initial rate of swelling is the apparent rate of arterial inflow rate (Fig. 1). The assumption is made that this rate is the same as the actual undisturbed rate of arterial inflow immediately before the venous occlusion. Furthermore, the abrupt inflation of the pneumatic collecting cuff must prevent the escape of venous outflow via the deep veins.

There are two main ways to measure the limb swelling after inflation of the

224

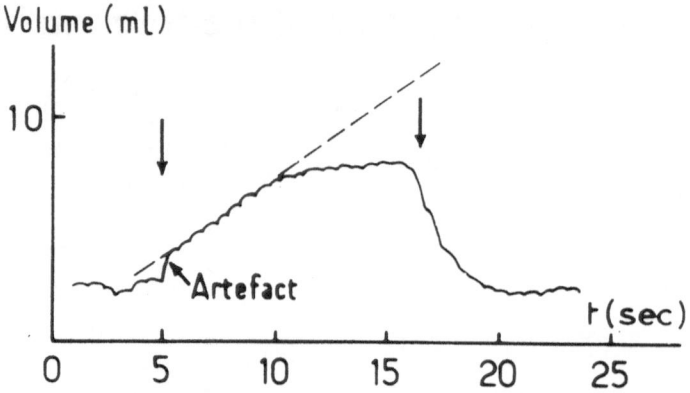

Figure 1. Volume changes of the forearm as measured by venous occlusion plethysmography. Vertical arrows show beginning and end of venous occlusion. Slope of the curve is the apparent blood flow; artifact is due to the displacement of skin during cuff inflation.

collecting pneumatic cuff: water plethysmography and strain gauge plethysmography. Both measure, directly or indirectly, the change in volume following the venous occlusion. The water plethysmograph currently used is shown in Fig. 2. It consists in a horizontal cylinder filled with about 3000 ml of water. A copper coil spiral along the internal wall of the cylinder enables to maintain the water temperature to a constant temperature. A rubber cast of the subject's wrist is applied with collodion bonding to the wrist forming a watertight seal. Volume changes in the plethysmograph are transmitted to a large air-filled compensation tank by a non-distensible water-filled tube. Volume changes are derived from the pressure changes they produce (less than 10 cm H20) within the compensation tank, measured with a high-sensitivity pressure transducer. The instrument is calibrated by introducing known volumes of water into the plethysmograph and measuring the resulting pressure changes.

The water plethysmograph is heavy, difficult to use in unskilled hands, and very sensitive to artefacts due to the subject's movements. To make limb blood flow measurements more convenient, R.J. Whitney introduced in 1953 [2] the mercury-in-rubber strain gauge plethysmography. This method is still widely used today. It is based upon the assumption that the changes in volume of a limb are related to its changes in circumference. The percentage change in volume of a cylinder of a fixed length is, to a close approximation, equal to twice the percentage change in its circumference if only small changes are considered. This approximation also applies for circumferential changes in non-cylindrical objects of non-uniform cross section, if the changes are in uniform proportion at all levels along the axial length. It is thus possible to replace the volume plethysmograph by a strain gauge which can record changes in the circumference of a limb. Two conditions must be assumed: 1) the volume changes of the limb are due to changes

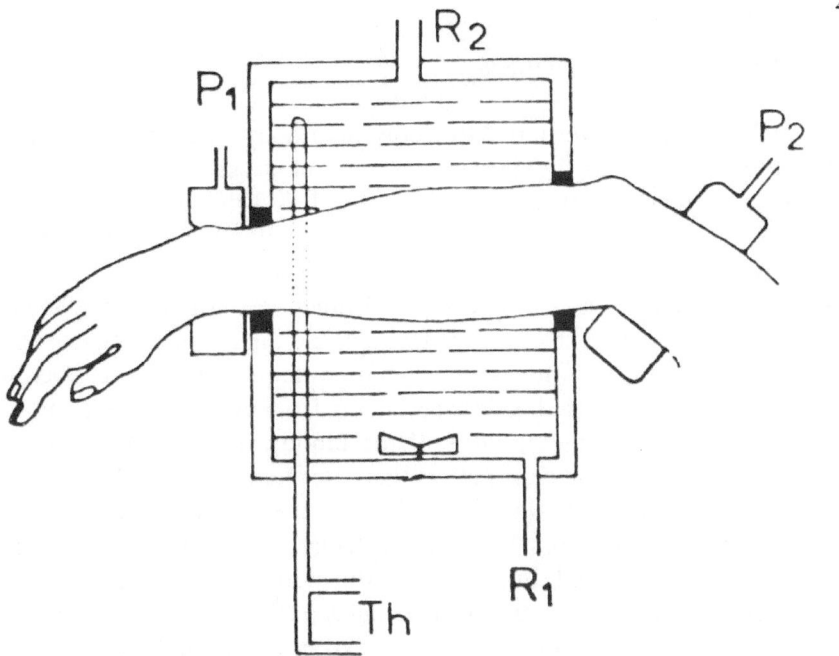

Figure 2. Water plethysmograph: P1 is the wrist cuff, P2 is the collecting venous occlusion cuff, R1 is used for filling the plethysmograph and R2 is connected to the pressure measurement. Th is the thermostatic system.

in radial dimensions without changing axial dimension, 2) the tissues are radially isotropic and the deformation is identical in all transverse directions. Thus, the volume change of a limb segment is assumed to be the integration of the variation of the surface corresponding to successive transverse sections.

The relative variation of the circumference of the forearm after venous occlusion is about 1% to 2%. The mercury-in-rubber strain gauge is a thin mercury-filled silicone tube closed at both ends with copper contacts which assure electrical continuity with the mercury column. The gauge is highly compliant (in the order of 1% extension per 10 g). The resistance of the mercury column varies linearly with the length of the silicone tube; these resistance variations are easily measured with an adjustable Wheastone bridge. Because of the very high compliance of the silicone tube, the pressure exerted on the skin immediately below the gauge is assumed to be negligible.

Blood flow rates measured by venous occlusion plethysmography are expressed as ml. of blood/100 ml. of tissue/minute. Comparison with electro-magnetic flowmetry has shown that the accuracy of the absolute values of flow in human limbs is inevitably in some doubt. Greater confidence attaches to observations of changes in flow in a forearm exposed to a local experimental influence compared with the flow in the opposite untreated limb simultaneously measured [3].

2. Non-plethysmographic methods

Indicator dilution is an alternative to plethysmography. It permits us to measure total limb blood flow but the anatomy of the limb vessels is not favourable for precise measurements by this invasive method. It is difficult to secure mixing of the indicator with the arterial blood, to define the volume of tissue perfused and to obtain a representative sample of the mixed venous blood.

External calorimetry is a simple method much less widely used. It may be utilized for measuring the blood flow through the digits, hands or feet. During steady state, while an extremity is immersed in water at a temperature below that of the skin, the heat released is derived mainly from arriving arterial blood and only slightly from local metabolism. If the blood arrives at the central body temperature and leaves the extremity at the water temperature, the actual blood flow may be calculated. In fact, variations in the arterial and venous blood temperatures introduce errors; blood flow calculated from external calorimetry is thus always underestimated. Furthermore, the method cannot be used to record rapid fluctuations in flow because the thermal capacity of the tissues introduces a major time lag in the response. Conversely, external calorimetry may be useful if integration of the total flow over a long period of time must be measured.

Several other methods are used for measuring local blood flow; these methods 'look' at a small volume of tissue and thus are less used in clinical research.

Heat transfer by the skin partly depends on its blood flow. The principle of local calorimetry consists in heating a small area of skin by an electrical resistance and measuring the induced increase in cutaneous temperature at a given distance from the heat source. Various devices have been proposed: the speed of response is faster than that obtained with calorimetry of the whole part, but the readings are influenced by the blood flow surrounding regions as well as to the skin immediately under the resistance. The calibration of this kind of device is thus very difficult and uncertain [4].

Radioactive substances such as 22 Na, labelled iodoantipyrine or 133 Xe, subcutaneously injected, easily diffuse through the skin and are removed by the local circulation. The rate of removal of these substances is a measure of 'effectiveness of the circulation'. It probably depends mainly on the flow through exchange vessels and it thus reflects 'nutritive' rather than 'total' blood flow. Consequently, it cannot be expressed in volumetric units.

3. Ultrasonic blood flowmetry

Doppler flowmetry is a more recently introduced method and has become of major importance in the measurement of limb blood flow with the development of the range gated apparatus. The method is based upon the frequency change of the emitted ultrasonic wave after its backscattering by moving erythrocytes. $\triangle F$

is a function of the emission frequency (F), the velocity of the red cells (V), and the angle (theta) between the ultrasonic beam and the direction of blood displacement.

$$\triangle F/F = 2\,V \times \cos\,(theta)/C \tag{1}$$

where C is the mean propagation velocity of ultrasounds within tissues (1540 m/ sec). The method was introduced by Satomura [5] and Franklin [6], who used a continuous emission apparatus with one emitting and one receiving transducer. A pulsed range gated instrument transmits repeated short bursts of ultrasounds at a given repetition rate [7, 8]. The transducer is alternatively emitter and receiver. After each burst, the transducer is switched to receive reflected signals until the time of the next emitted burst. Because an electronic gate is opened at an adjustable time after each emission burst, reflected signals are detected and analysed only while the gate is opened. The signals which are detected during a given time interval come from a 'gated' target (the sample volume) that can be moved to cover selected distances from the transducer, and whose width can be altered. The time elapsed between emission and reception and the duration of the gate opening represent depth and thickness of the sample volume along the beam axis respectively. The backscattered Doppler frequencies are usually quantified by means of a zero crosser detector, so that the analogue output of the velocimeter is proportional to the root mean square of the Doppler frequencies detected in the sample volume.

The brachial, ulnar and cubital arteries are easily accessible to the transcutaneous Doppler blood flow measurement [9–12]. With a small gate duration ($0.5\,\mu sec$), vessels walls can be localised and internal diameter measured, from which internal cross-sectional area is calculated with the assumption that the vessel is circular (Fig. 3). When the gate duration is adjusted so that the sample volume exactly encompasses the vessel diameter, the recorded output represents the root mean square of all Doppler frequencies along the vessel diameter. This is taken to be representative of the mean blood velocity (V) over the cross-sectional area. Blood flow rate (BF) is computed as follows:

$$BF = \pi V. \ (d^2/4)$$

where d is the internal diameter.

Using usual single 'pencil' probes, the recorded blood flow velocity signal is uncalibrated because of the unknown angle theta between the ultrasonic beam and the vessel. A double transducer system forming a fixed angle alpha may be used to measure actual blood flow velocity. The probe is designed so that the intersection of the beams occurs in the investigated vessel. To investigate brachial artery, we use a double probe system with an alpha angle fixed at 120°, so that the ultrasonic beams intersect at 12 mm from the skin. The two transducers are

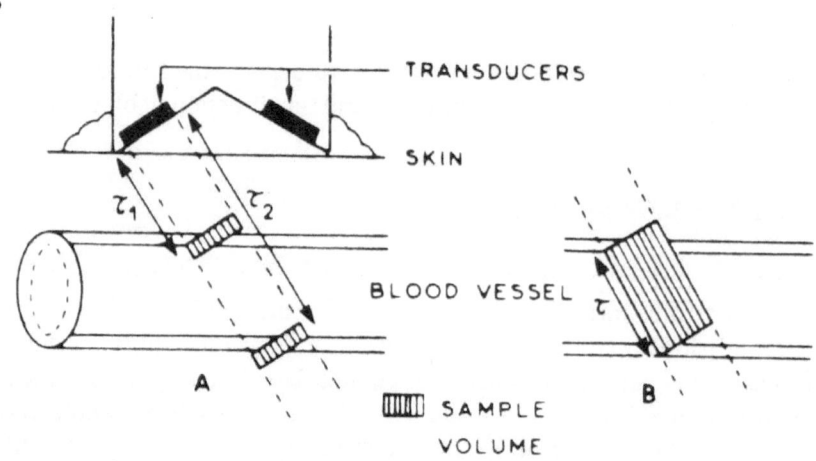

Figure 3. Principle of vessel diameter measurement. A: τ1: delay time for proximal wall, τ2: delay time for distal wall. B: mean cross-sectional velocity measurement, θ = θ2 − τ1.

succesively activated, and a simple calculation provides the longitudinal velocity within the plane defined by the ultrasonic beam and the vessel axis from the apparent velocities measured by each transducer (Fig. 4).

4. Discussion of the validity of plethysmographic and ultrasonic methods

Validity of venous occlusion plethysmography

Three assumptions underlie the technique of venous occlusion plethysmography: 1) the application of the collecting cuff does not affect arterial inflow, 2) the increase in venous pressure due to the blood pooling does not modify the arterial inflow by a direct or reflex effect, 3) the impounded blood causes the hand tissue to swell in proportion to the rate of arterial inflow. The last assumption is quite certainly verified but there is no adequate evidence concerning the two first points. Simultaneous measurements of plethysmographic blood flow and ultrasonic arterial inflow have shown that after inflation of the collecting cuff, there is a significant decrease in arterial inflow. This vasoconstriction induced by the local

Table 1. Brachial artery diameters, blood velocities and blood volume flows (mean + SD) measured at day 1 (D1) and 3 weeks later (D21) in 11 normal subjects.

	D1	D21
diameter (cm)	0.431 + 0.047	0.443 + 0.043
mean blood velocity (cm/sec)	6.1 + 2.6	5.8 + 3.1
blood flow (ml/sec)	56.2 + 36.1	55.6 + 36.7

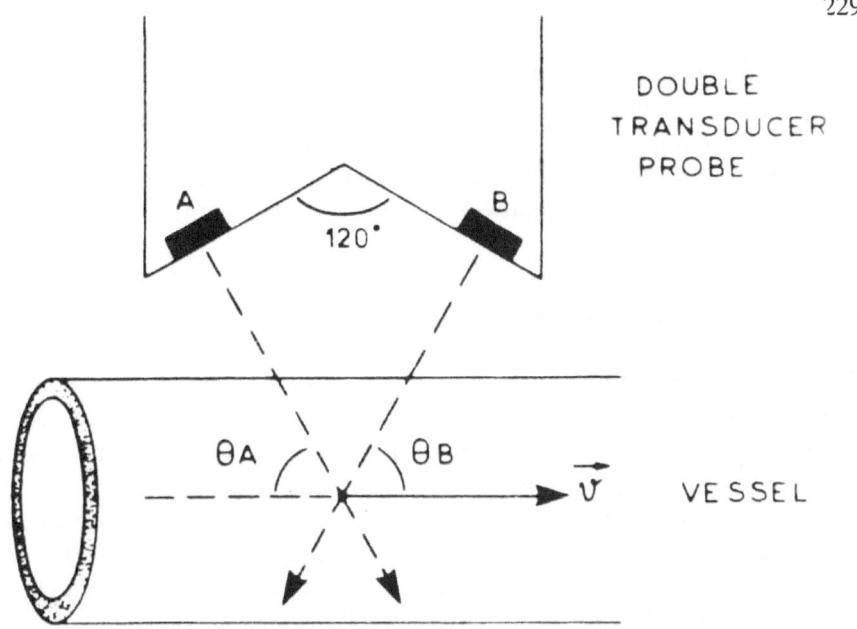

DOUBLE
TRANSDUCER
PROBE

VESSEL

Figure 4. Positioning of the double transducer probe: When Doppler frequencies for transducer A and B are identical, θA and θB = 60°.

venous congestion disappears after exclusion of the hand circulation by inflating a wrist cuff to a suprasystolic pressure [13]. Hence, plethysmographic forearm blood flow estimation in which no wrist cuff is employed is probably unsatisfactory. In the same way, after the release of venous occlusion of the forearm, there is a large brief phase of vasodilatation followed by a longer period of vasoconstriction before blood flow returns to the resting level [14]. In a recent work [15], it has been shown that this probably myogenic vasoconstriction is similar in normotensive and in hypertensive subjects. In contrast the vasodilator component of the response is lower in hypertensive than in normotensive subjects. This difference may be partly attributed to differences in the structure of the vessels in hypertension.

Validity of pulsed Doppler blood flowmetry

The arterial blood velocities in the limbs are relatively low (systolic peak flow lower than 60 cm/sec); this may exclude major errors resulting from saturation of the Doppler frequency measuring system. More problems arise in the determination of the vessel diameter. Several factors may cause errors in this measurement.

First, the step-wise range control of the time delay is responsible for an inaccuracy in the determination of the vessel diameter. If the step-wise range is 0.5 μsec, the location of each vessel wall is known with a maximum error of half a step, that is 0.19 mm. Therefore, with theta equal to 60°, inaccuracy in diameter measurement is $(0.19 \times 2) \sin 60° = 0.34$ mm. The mean diameter of the brachial artery of normal subjects is about 4.5 mm; the relative error is therefore $0.34/4.5 = 8\%$ on diameter, and, hence, of 16% on the cross-sectional area. This value is the maximum error possible with each diameter measurement. Because the absolute error is the same whatever the size of the artery, the relative error will be lower for larger vessels.

The second source of error is the estimation of the angle theta. The problem of measuring theta has been solved by using two transducers making a known angle (120°) with one another. By adjusting the probe so that the Doppler frequency shift, and consequently theta, is the same for both transducers, it can be assumed that theta is half the 120° angle made by the two transducers. It can be calculated that the error introduced by the probe positioning is about 5% by degree [12]. Inaccuracy in probe positioning is therefore the major source of error in the measurement of volume flow. Practically, in skilled hands, the errors in diameter and blood flow measurements are much lower than expected. Table 1 reports the brachial artery diameters, blood velocities and blood flows measured in normal subjects in a double-blind study. Despite a large scattering in individual values, there is no significant difference between these parameters measured at three-week intervals [16].

5. Choice of measuring techniques

Before one can select the best non-invasive flow-measuring technique for a specific application, several questions must be asked [17]: First, under what conditions are the measurements to be made (rest, exercise, tilting, etc ...)? Second, is flow required in a specific vessel, or in the whole limb, or in a specific tissue? Third, is it important to measure pulsatile flow or is mean flow sufficient? Fourth, what is the time response of the blood flow variations to be measured?

In most cases, the method must be chosen between venous occlusion plethysmography, ultrasonic Doppler-shift measurement or calorimetry. Venous occlusion plethysmography measures volume flow expressed as ml/100 ml of tissue/min; calorimetry measures heat loss and is difficult to relate to blood flow. Only the pulsed ultrasonic Doppler method, used with very rigorous methodological precautions, measures the absolute value of volume flow expressed in ml/min and thus seems to be the most useful and accurate method to measure limb blood flow.

References

1. Brodie TG, Russel AE (1905): On the determination of the rate of blood flow through an organ. J Physiol (London), 32: 67–69.

2. Whitney RJ (1953): The measurement of volume changes in human limbs. J Physiol (London), 121: 1–27.
3. Greenfield ADM, Whitney RJ, Mowbray MB (1963): Methods for the investigation of peripheral blood flow. Brit Med Bull, 19: 101–109.
4. Martineaud JP, Seroussi S (1977): Physiologie de la circulation cutanùe. Masson Ed, Paris.
5. Satomura S (1959): A study of the flow patterns in superficial arteries by ultrasonics. J Acoust Soc Jpn, 15: 151–158.
6. Franklin DL, Schlegel W, Rushmer RF (1961): Blood flow measured by Doppler frequency shift of a back scattered ultrasound. Science, 134: 564–577.
7. Baker DW (1970): Pulsed ultrasonic Doppler flow sensing. IEEE Trans Son Ultrason, 17: 170–185.
8. Peronneau P, Hinglais J, Pellet M, Leger F (1970): Vélocimètre sanguin par effet Doppler a ùmission pulsée. Onde Electrique, 50: 3–18.
9. Levy BI, Valladares WR, Ghaem A, Martineaud JP (1979): Comparison of plethysmographic methods with pulsed Doppler blood flowmetry. Am J Physiol 236: H899–903.
10. Levenson JA, Peronneau P, Simon AC, Safar ME (1981): Pulsed Doppler determination of diameter, blood velocity and volume flow of brachial artery in man. Cardiovascular Res, 15: 164–170.
11. Safar ME, Peronneau P, Levenson JA, Toto-Moukoud JA, Simon AC (1981): Pulsed Doppler diameter: diameter, blood flow velocity and volumic flow of the brachial artery in sustained, essential hypertension. Circulation, 16: 220–224.
12. Chauveau M, Levy BI, Dessanges JF, Savin E, Bailliart O, Martineaud JP (1985): Quantitative Doppler blood flow measurement, method and in vivo calibration. Cardiovascular Res, 19: 700–706.
13. Levy BI, Oliva Y, Martineaud JP (1983): Hand arterial blood flow responses to local venous congestion. Am J Physiol, 240: H980–H983.
14. Ireland MA, Davies P, Littler WA (1983): Some aspects of the arterial response to venous occlusion in man. Clin Sci 65: 1–8.
15. Littler WA, Ireland MA (1986): Arterial response to venous occlusion in normotensive and hypertensive subjects. Cardiovasc Res 20: 124–126.
16. Safar ME. Personal communication.
17. Theory and practice of blood flow measurement. JP. Woodcock, Butterworth, 1975.

The contribution of alpha-1 and alpha-2-adrenoceptor mediated vasoconstriction in essential hypertension as assessed by forearm venous occlusion plethysmography

P. BOLLI, W. KIOWSKI and F.R. BÜHLER

Introduction

The contribution of the sympathetic nervous system to essential hypertension has been a point of argument for many years [1–5]. Arguments partly arose because of difficulties in assessing adrenergic activity and measuring its effects on target organs. Interpretation of results obtained from vasoactive substances administered systemically for the investigation of the sympathetic nervous system is hampered by the fact that it elicits a mixture of wanted drug effects and undesired circulatory responses from homeostatic reflex mechanisms. Factors that determine vascular tone can be directly assessed by measuring alterations in regional blood flow following pharmacological interventions. The easy access to the forearm arterial circulation enables to achieve high regional concentrations of vasoactive substances and associated vascular effects without the confounding interference by systemic hemodynamic reflex mechanisms.

Increased sympathetic nervous activity has been implicated in the pathophysiology of essential hypertension [6–9] as reflected by elevated plasma adrenaline concentrations observed in all age groups [10] of patients with essential hypertension [10–13]. This is supported by the relationship of plasma adrenaline to diastolic blood pressure [14], heart rate and to plasma renin activity [15]. Higher plasma adrenaline concentrations were observed not only at rest but also during submaximal exercise [10, 15] and following cold pressor testing [16]. Increased plasma noradrenaline concentrations in some hypertensive patients [9, 17, 18] and the direct relationship of plasma noradrenaline with blood pressure [9, 18, 19] have been taken as evidence for the sympathetic nervous system's contribution to essential hypertension. Others reported that under resting conditions noradrenaline concentrations were not different between normotensives and hypertensives [12, 20, 21] except for some young patients with elevated plasma noradrenaline concentrations [20], particularly those of the high renin type [22]. The short half-life [23] of noradrenaline and its re-uptake in the neuroeffector junction may partly be the reason for the argument whether plasma concentrations of noradrenaline, representing only 10–20% of that released, reflect reliably the degree of sympathetic activity.

Adrenergic mechanisms regulating vascular tone

The sympathetic nervous system regulates vascular tone principally through alpha-adrenoceptor mediated vasoconstriction and beta-adrenoceptor mediated vasodilation (Fig. 1). Noradrenaline released from the sympathetic nerve terminal acts on postjunctional alpha and beta receptors, the sum of its effects determining vascular tone. Noradrenaline regulates its own release through prejunctional alpha-2-adrenoceptors which when stimulated by noradrenaline inhibit its release [24]. Adrenaline is liberated from the adrenal medulla and acts as a circulating neurohormone mainly on postjunctional beta-2-adrenoceptors, the sum of its stimulatory effect being vasodilation. Adrenaline can be taken up by postganglionic nerve endings [25, 26] and released into the synaptic cleft together with noradrenaline as shown in animal experiments [26–28] and in man [29]. Adrenaline enhances noradrenaline release through stimulation of presynaptic beta-adrenoceptors [26, 30–32].

The more recently detected postjunctional alpha-2-adrenoceptors [33–36] appear to be located extrajunctionally and thus represent preferential targets for stimulation by circulating agonists and also for infused substances [37–39]. Alpha adrenoceptors are subdivided according to their different affinities for various agonists and antagonists. Alpha-1-adrenoceptors are particularly sensitive to the agonists phenylephrine [40] and methoxamine [41] and have a high affinity for the antagonist prazosin [42–44] whereas alpha-2-adrenoceptors are particularly sensitive to agonists such as clonidine [40] and BHT 933 [45] and have a high affinity for the antagonist yohimbine [24, 44].

A model for assessing forearm blood flow regulation

All forearm blood flow studies were performed in the morning with the subjects having refrained from smoking and caffeinated beverages for the last 12 hours. They lay down in a quiet air-conditioned room with a constant temperature of 20–22° C. Access to the forearm circulation for infusion of vasoactive substances and for measuring intra-arterial blood pressure was achieved by inserting a small catheter under local anaesthesia into the brachial artery. Thirty minutes later measurements of forearm blood flow under basal conditions and thereafter during pharmacological interventions were performed using venous occlusion plethysmography [46].

Venous occlusion plethysmography [47] measures forearm volume changes after complete arrest of venous return without interfering with arterial flow. Thus

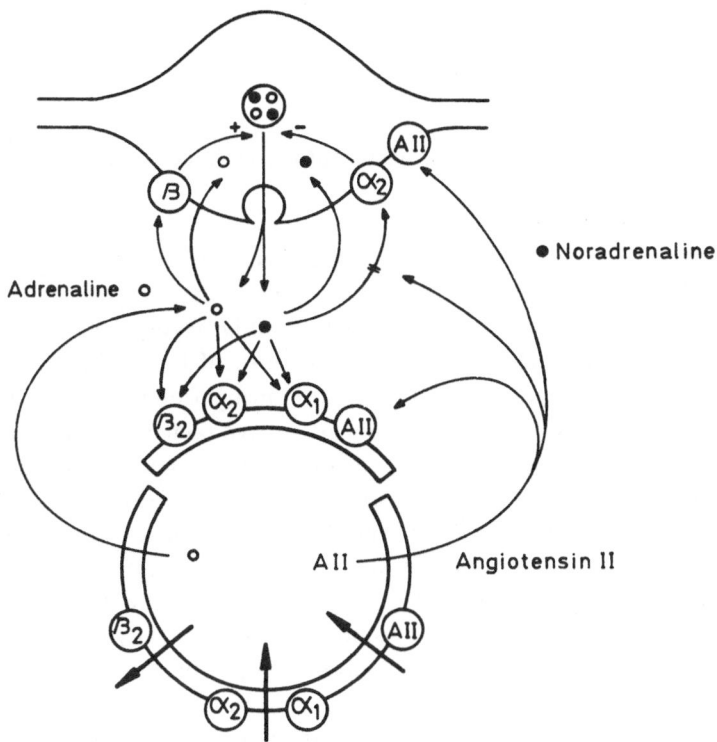

Figure 1. Schematic representation of the neuroeffector junction with adrenergic and angiotensinergic mechanisms regulating vascular tone. Noradrenaline (●) released by exocytosis stimulates postjunctional receptors and regulates its own release through presynaptic alpha-2-adrenoceptors, stimulation of which inhibits noradrenaline release. Adrenaline (O), besides inducing vasodilation through postjunctional beta-2-adrenoceptors, may exert a vasoconstrictor effect through stimulation of postjunctional alpha-2-adrenoceptors and through enhanced noradrenaline release following stimulation of prejunctional beta-adrenoceptors. Adrenaline can be taken up by the sympathetic nerve ending and released again as co-transmitter with noradrenaline.

changes in forearm volume reflect directly arterial blood flow [48, 49]. Forearm volume changes were measured with a mercury-in-silastic strain gauge [50] placed around the proximal third of the forearm, which was slightly elevated above the level of the heart. The strain gauge was coupled to an electronically calibrated plethysmograph (Hokanson EC3) [51]. Venous occlusion was achieved by means of a blood pressure cuff inflated to 40 mm Hg by a rapid cuff inflator (Hokanson EC10) [51] and applied just proximal to the elbow. The hand was excluded from the circulation by inflating a paediatric blood pressure cuff around the wrist to 50 mm Hg above systolic blood pressure for one minute prior to and during the measurement of forearm blood flow. This eliminates the influence of arterio-venous shunts in the hand. Therefore, the measured portion of the forearm represents mainly blood flow in the vascular arterial bed, the skin accounting for about 10% of forearm blood flow.

Enhanced postjunctional alpha-1-adrenoceptor mediated vasoconstriction in essential hypertension

The contribution of increased adrenergic activity in essential hypertension to vascular resistance through postjunctional alpha-1-adrenoceptor mediated vaso-constriction was assessed by measuring the vasodilator response to intra-arterial infusions of a maximal forearm vasodilator dose of the alpha-1-adrenoceptor antagonist prazosin (0.5 μg/min/100 ml tissue) in 24 patients with essential hyper-tension and 16 age- and sex-matched normotensive control subjects [52]. 'Non-specific' (not adrenoceptor mediated) vasodilation was defined by the increase in forearm blood flow to a maximal forearm vasodilator dose of sodium nitro-prusside (0.6 μg/min/100 ml tissue) The greater prazosin induced increase in forearm blood flow in the presence of a comparable response to 'non-specific' vasodilation in both groups unmasked an enhanced postjunctional alpha-1-adre-noceptor mediated vasoconstrictor component in essential hypertension (Fig. 2).

Evidence that enhanced vasoconstriction in essential hypertension is deter-mined by the degree of sympathetic activity is provided by the direct relationship between resting plasma adrenaline concentrations and the increase in forearm blood flow to alpha-1-adrenoceptor blockade with prazosin (Fig. 3). The same could be shown in another study [19] for noradrenaline, where in patients with essential hypertension but not in normotensive subjects the increase in forearm blood flow to alpha-adrenoceptor blockade with phentolamine (0.12 μg/min/ 100 ml tissue) correlated directly with basal plasma noradrenaline concentrations (Fig. 4) as well as with blood pressure (r = 0.73, p<0.01). Therefore, increased adrenergic activity in patients with essential hypertension appears to contribute to their elevated vascular resistance through enhanced alpha-1-adrenoceptor mediated vasoconstriction.

Enhanced postjunctional alpha-2-adrenoceptor mediated vasoconstriction in essential hypertension

Besides the classical postjunctional alpha-1-adrenoceptors there are also post-junctional alpha-2-adrenoceptors functionally participating in the control of vas-cular tone [33–36]. The presence of postjunctional alpha-2-adrenoceptors in the human forearm vasculature was demonstrated by measuring the change in fore-arm blood flow to intra-arterial infusion of the alpha-2-adrenoceptor agonist clonidine and the antagonist yohimbine. Clonidine infused into the forearm of 14 normotensive subjects resulted in a dose-dependent decrease in forearm blood

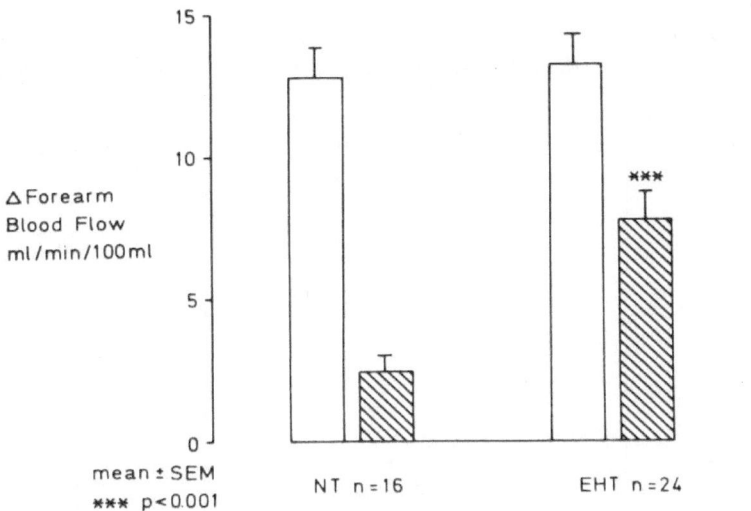

Figure 2. Change in forearm blood flow during intra-arterial infusion of sodium nitroprusside (0.6 μg/min/100 ml tissue; open bars) and the alpha-1-adrenoceptor blocker prazosin (0.5 μg/min/100 ml tissue; hatched bars) in 24 patients with essential hypertension (EHT) and in 16 normotensive subjects (NT). The alpha-1-adrenoceptor blockade-induced increase in forearm blood flow was significantly greater in EHT than in NT.

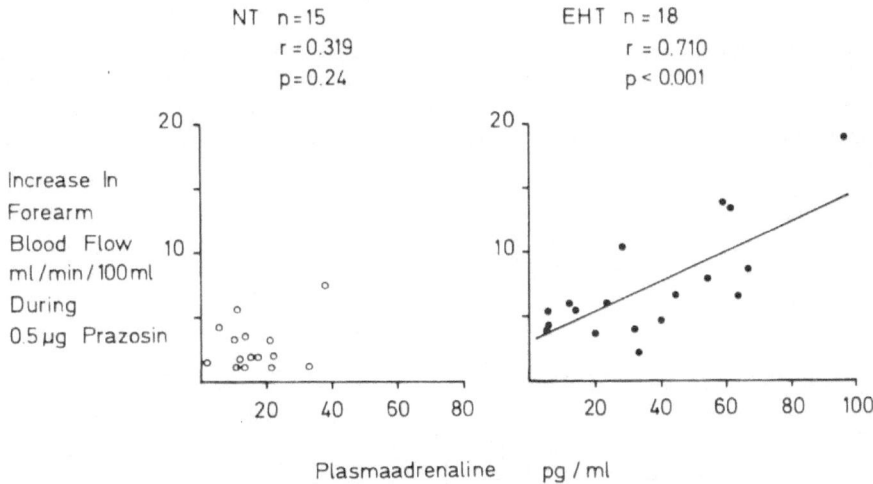

Figure 3. Relationship between basal plasma adrenaline concentration and changes in forearm blood flow induced by postjunctional alpha-1-blockade with prazosin (0.5 μg/min/100 ml tissue) in 20 patients with essential hypertension (EHT; filled circles) and in 16 normotensive subjects (NT; open circles). In EHT prazosin-induced increase in forearm blood flow correlates significantly with plasma adrenaline concentrations.

238

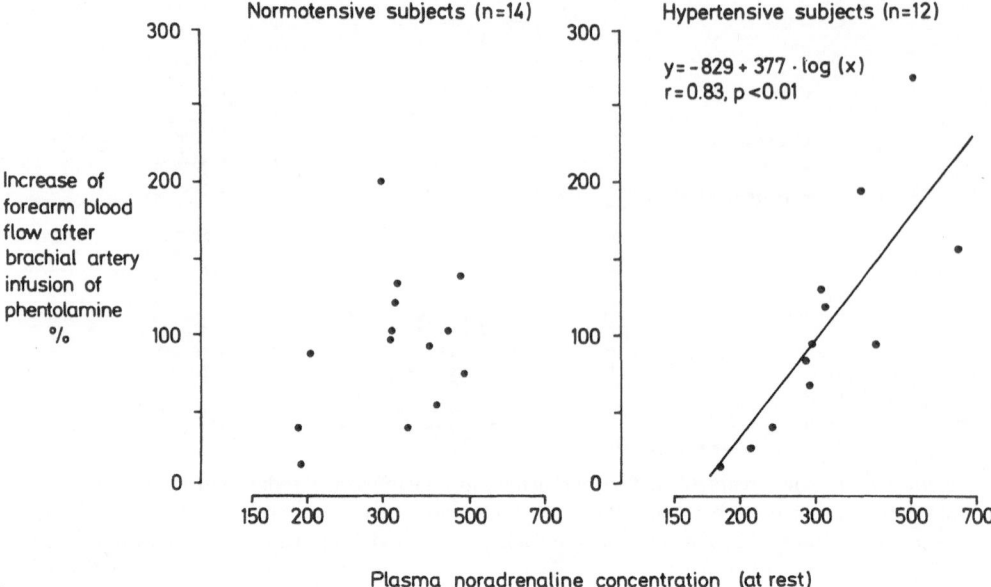

Figure 4. Relationship between basal plasma noradrenaline concentrations and the increase in forearm blood flow during alpha adrenoceptor blockade with intra-arterially infused phentolamine in 12 patients with essential hypertension and 14 normotensive subjects. In hypertensive patients phentolamine-induced increase in forearm blood flow correlates with plasma noradrenaline concentrations (r = 0.62; p<0.05).

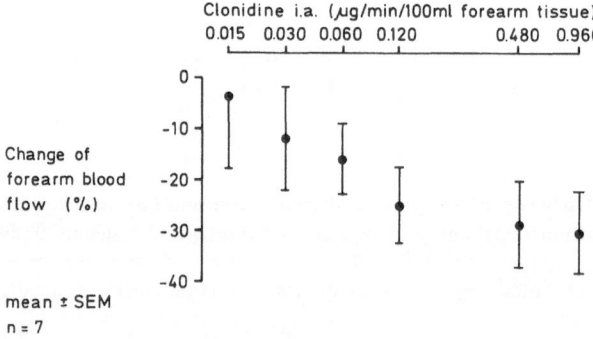

Figure 5. Decrease in forearm blood flow to alpha-2-adrenoceptor stimulation with intra-arterially infused clonidine. The logarithm of the clonidine dose is plotted against the percent change of forearm blood flow observed during the fifth minute of each clonidine infusion. Analysis of variance indicated a significant effect of clonidine on forearm blood flow (p<0.01).

flow (Fig. 5). Concomitant infusion of the alpha-1-adrenoceptor antagonist prazosin (0.5 μg/min/100 ml tissue) did not influence the vasoconstrictor response to clonidine but combined infusions of clonidine with the alpha-adrenoceptor antagonist phentolamine (0.12 μg/min/100 ml tissue) almost abolished the clonidine-induced vasoconstriction [53]. This demonstrates that clonidine-induced postjunctional alpha-2-adrenoceptors mediated vasoconstriction was antagonized by the alpha-2-adrenoceptor blocking component of phentolamine (Fig. 6). This finding could be confirmed [54] by infusion of the more selective alpha-2-adrenoceptor antagonist yohimbine. As shown in Fig. 7 increasing intra-arterial concentrations of yohimbine resulted in a dose-dependent rise in forearm blood flow and decrease in forearm vascular resistance. Therefore, these results together with those of others [55–58] using also different compounds, provide evidence that in man the sympathetic nervous system influences vascular tone not only through postjunctional alpha-1 but also through postjunctional alpha-2-adrenoceptors.

The importance of alpha-2-adrenoceptor mediated vasoconstriction in essential hypertension was assessed by intra-arterial infusions of a maximal forearm vasodilator dose of yohimbine (30 μg/min/100 ml tissue) in patients with essential hypertension and normotensive subjects [59]. Postjunctional alpha-2-adrenoceptor blockade induced a greater increase in forearm blood flow in patients with essential hypertension as compared to normotensive subjects. As the increase in forearm blood flow to non-adrenoceptor mediated vasodilation with sodium nitroprusside was comparable in both groups this difference can be attributed to a greater alpha-2-adrenoceptor mediated vasoconstrictor tone in patients with essential hypertension (Fig. 8). These results are at variance with those found by others [60]; a reason for this could be the different concentrations of yohimbine used. In our studies patients had higher plasma adrenaline concentrations than normotensive subjects (69 ± 31 (S.D.) and 37 ± 13 pg/ml, respectively; $p < 0.05$) reflecting increased sympathetic activity which may have provided a more favourable substrate for demonstrating enhanced alpha-2-adrenoceptor blockade.

Postjunctional alpha-2-adrenoceptor mediated vasoconstriction depends on calcium influx into the vascular smooth muscle cell and can be blocked by calcium antagonists [61]. Calcium influx-dependent vasoconstriction is enhanced in patients with essential hypertension [62, 63] as demonstrated by a greater vasodilator response to calcium entry blockade in hypertensive patients. This tallies with and could be part of the observed enhanced postjunctional alpha-2-adrenoceptor mediated vasoconstriction in essential hypertension.

Adrenaline and postjunctional alpha-2-adrenoceptor mediated vasoconstriction

Postjunctional alpha-2-adrenoceptors have been reported to be located extra-junctionally and thus represent preferential targets for stimulation by circulating

240

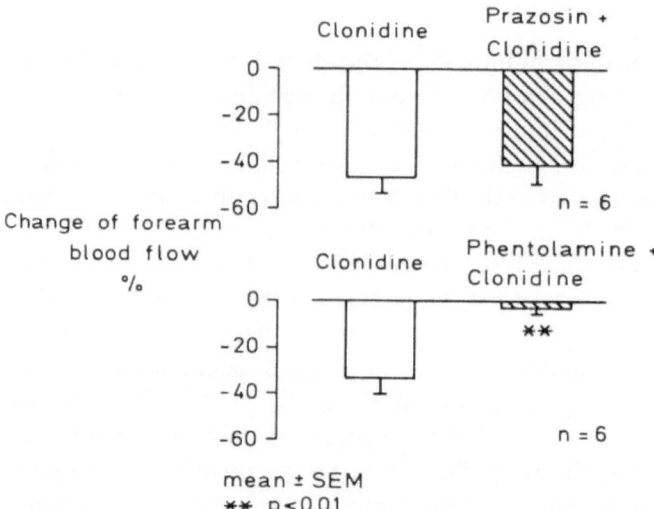

Figure 6. Clonidine effects on forearm blood flow before (open bars) and after pretreatment with prazosin and phentolamine (hatched bars). The percent changes in blood flow following clonidine were similar before and after prazosin (upper panel) whereas the clonidine effect was significantly reduced by pretreatment with phentolamine (lower panel).

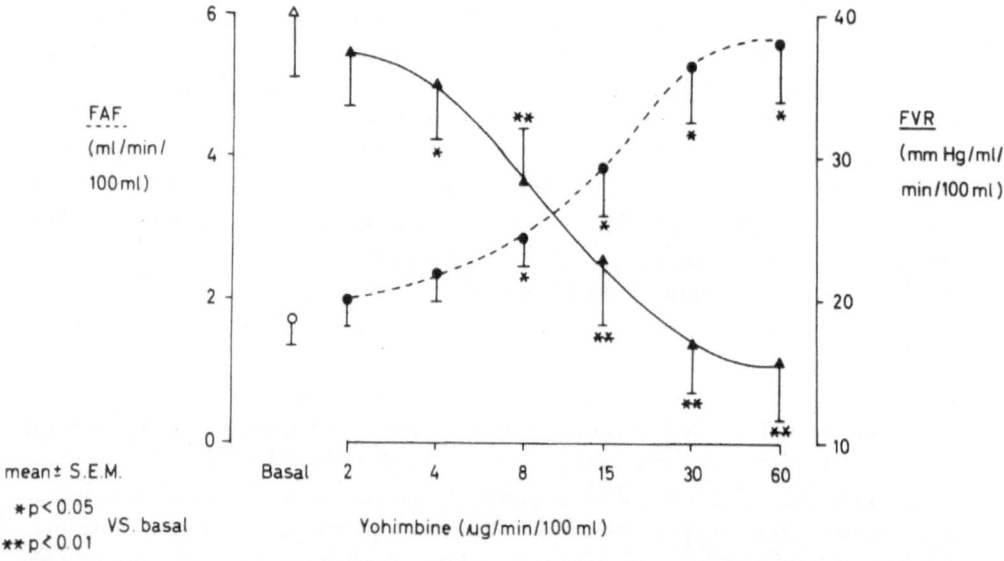

Figure 7. Forearm blood flow (FAF) and forearm vascular resistance (FVR) related to increasing doses of intra-arterially infused yohimbine in 7 normotensive subjects. There was a dose-dependent increase in FAF and decrease in FVR to increasing concentrations of yohimbine. Doses in $\mu g/min/$ 100 ml tissue.

agonists and for infused substances [37–39] raising the question whether adrenaline as a circulating neurohormone could induce vasoconstriction via postjunctional alpha-2-adrenoceptors and thereby contribute to enhanced vascular resistance in essential hypertension. Adrenaline-induced postjunctional alpha-2-adrenoceptor mediated vasoconstriction was shown in the forearm vasculature of 8 normotensive subjects (Fig. 9). Intra-arterial infusion of adrenaline (0.01, 0.02, 0.04, 0.08 μg/min/100 ml tissue) during forearm alpha-1- and beta-adrenoceptor blockade resulted in dose-dependent decreases in forearm blood flow to below basal flow values and this could be blocked by yohimbine. Using the same procedure adrenaline-induced vasoconstriction was greater in patients with essential hypertension (n = 7) than in the normotensive subjects [59]. This is consistent with the findings of Jie *et al.* [60] and reflects greater vascular responses to vasoconstrictor stimuli in hypertensive patients [60, 64–66]. Whether on the basis of this pharmacological evidence adrenaline-induced postjunctional alpha-2-adrenoceptor mediated vasoconstriction may be pathophysiologically important in essential hypertension remains open.

Increased levels of circulating adrenaline could contribute to elevated vascular tone in essential hypertension indirectly through facilitation of noradrenaline release [27, 31, 67] via stimulation of prejunctional beta-adrenoceptors and directly, through stimulation of postjunctional alpha-2-adrenoceptors. Such effects could be more pronounced in the presence of blunted beta-adrenoceptor mediated functions as is known to occur in older subjects and in hypertensive patients [12, 68–73).

The sympatho-adrenal-alpha-2-adrenoceptor mediated vasoconstrictor axis appears to be functionally established, yet under physiological conditions noradrenaline may be primarily responsible for postjunctional alpha-1- and alpha-2-adrenoceptor mediated vascular tone [74]. Under conditions of increased sympatho-adrenal activity [75], e.g. during mental and prolonged physical stress [12, 76, 77], exposure to cold [16], pain and/or anxiety [78], or in patients with pheochromocytoma, this axis may become functionally important potentiating vasoconstriction. As adrenaline's affinity for the prejunctional beta-adrenoceptor is several hundred fold greater than that of noradrenaline [26, 79] high plasma adrenaline concentrations found during stress may induce facilitation of noradrenaline release [80].

The role of prejunctional alpha-2-adrenoceptors?

In vitro and animal experiments demonstrate the presence of an autoinhibitory feedback system for neuronal noradrenaline release at the level of the neuroeffector junction whereby noradrenaline inhibits its own release via stimulation of prejunctionally located alpha-2-adrenoceptors [24]. There is only indirect evidence for the presence of such receptors in man [81]. The existence of such a

242

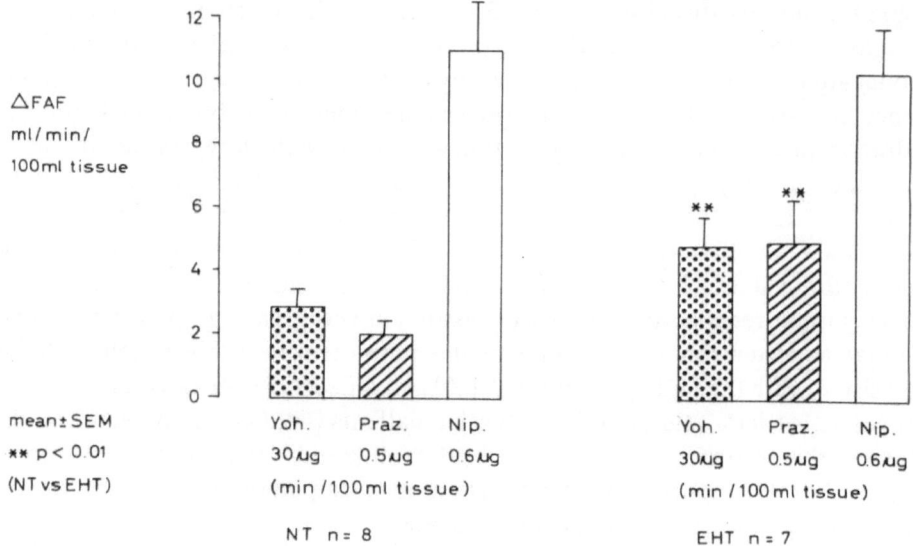

Figure 8. Increase in forearm blood flow ($\triangle$FAF) following postjunctional alpha-2-adrenoceptor blockade with intra-arterially infused yohimbine (Yoh; stippled bars), alpha-1-adrenoceptor blockade with prasozin (Praz; hatched bars) and following 'non-specific' (not adrenoceptor mediated) vasodilation with sodium nitroprusside (Nip; open bars) in 8 normotensive subjects (NT) and 7 patients with essential hypertension (EHT). $\triangle$FAF to Yoh and Praz were greater in EHT than in NT while Nip induced vasodilation was comparable.

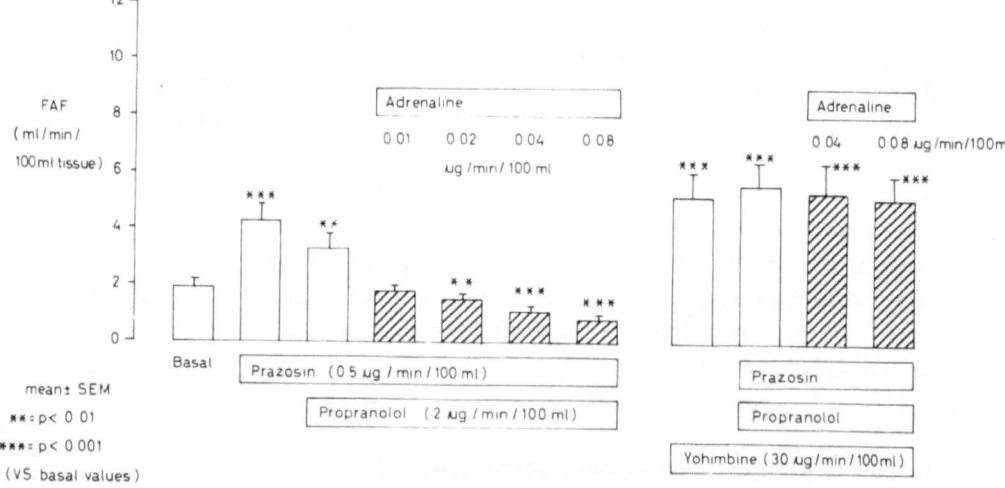

Figure 9. Forearm blood flow (FAF) responses to increasing doses of intra-arterially infused adrenaline (hatched bars) during postjunctional alpha-1-adrenoceptor blockade with prazosin and beta-adrenoceptor blockade with propranolol (left panel) and during additional postjunctional alpha-2-adrenoceptors blockade with yohimbine (right panel) in 8 normotensive subjects. Adrenaline induced a significant decrease in forearm blood flow which was prevented by concomitant alpha-2-adrenoceptors blockade.

negative feedback system was investigated by measuring noradrenaline release from the human forearm under baseline conditions and after infusions into the brachial artery of the alpha-2-adrenoceptors agonist clonidine (0.015, 0.06, 0.48 μg/min/100 ml tissue) in 11 normotensive subjects [82]. Noradrenaline release was estimated as the product of flow and the difference between venous (deep cubital vein) and arterial (brachial artery) noradrenaline concentrations. As shown in Fig. 10 forearm blood flow decreased during infusion of the two larger doses of clonidine as the result of postjunctional alpha-2-adrenoceptor stimulation; but the venous-arterial noradrenaline difference and therefore noradrenaline release remained practically unchanged. There was no reduction in noradrenaline release as would have been expected from prejunctional alpha-2-adrenoceptor stimulation. Therefore, prejunctional alpha-2-adrenoceptors, if at all present in the forearm vasculature, did not become functionally apparent. Demonstration of post- but not prejunctional alpha-2-adrenoceptors in the human forearm could also possibly be due to their different location within the vessel wall and the extrajunctionally located postjunctional alpha-2-adrenoceptors could be more easily accessible to intra-arterially infused clonidine. Alternatively, the forearm vasculature mass may not have been sufficiently big to produce the necessary increase in noradrenaline so as to be detected by current methodology. Nevertheless, this negative finding suggests that results obtained from interference studies with postjunctional alpha-2-adrenoceptors most likely were not confounded by prejunctional alpha-2-adrenoceptor mediated effects.

Alpha-adrenoceptor mediated vasoconstriction and antihypertensive beta-blockade

Since established essential hypertension is characterized by elevated vascular resistance, successful antihypertensive treatment has to be associated with a reduction in vascular resistance. Beta-adrenoceptor blockers interfere with the adrenergic and angiotensinergic vasoconstrictor systems and have been reported to lower vascular resistance [83, 84]. Whether reduction of the enhanced alpha-1-adrenoceptor mediated vasoconstriction forms part of this mechanism was assessed in four male patients (aged 38–55) with essential hypertension whose blood pressure responded to beta-blocker treatment and in four age-matched non-responders [85]. As shown in Fig. 11, starting from a comparable pretreatment pressure, in 'responders' by definition, blood pressure became controlled but remained practically unchanged in 'non-responders' following six weeks treatment with 320 mg propranolol daily. Before treatment, the increase in forearm blood flow to intra-arterial infusion of prazosin (0.5 μg/min/100 ml tissue) was 44% greater in 'responders' than in 'non-responders' confirming enhanced alpha-1-adrenoceptor mediated vasoconstriction. During treatment, in the 'responders' the prazosin-induced increase in forearm blood flow was re-

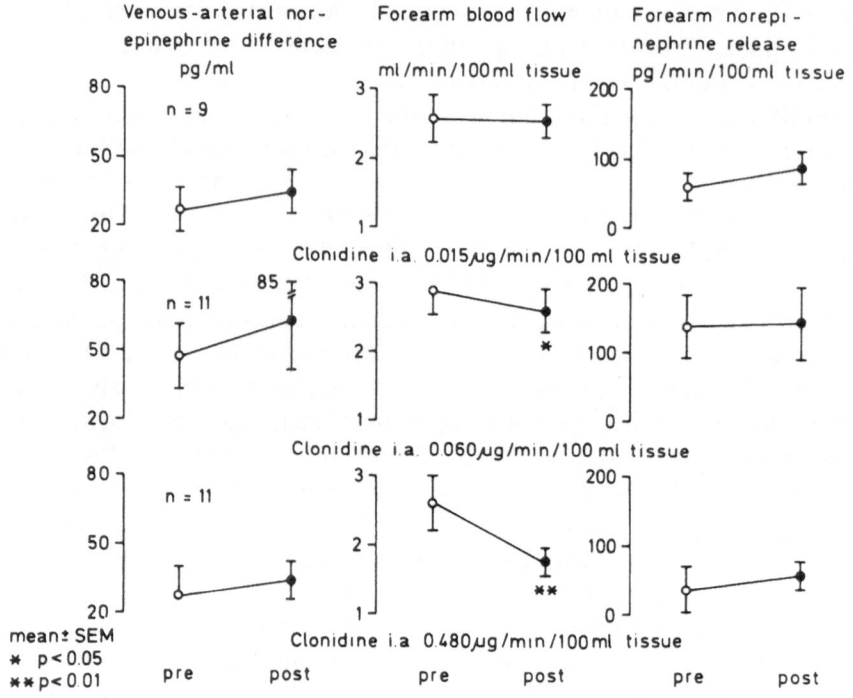

Figure 10. Venous-arterial noradrenaline difference (left panel), forearm blood flow (middle panel) and forearm noradrenaline release (right panel) in 11 normotensive subjects, before and after brachial artery infusion of the alpha-2-adrenoceptor agonist clonidine. There was no decrease in forearm noradrenaline release as would have been expected from prejunctional alpha-2-adrenoceptor stimulation.

duced to that previously found in normotensive subjects. In 'non-responders' the increase in forearm blood flow to alpha-1-blockade remained practically unchanged. The specificity of these differences is supported by the fact that 'non-specific' (not adrenoceptor mediated) vasodilation with sodium nitroprusside was similar in 'responders' and 'non-responders' and was hardly influenced by chronic beta-blockade. Plasma renin activity before and during propranolol treatment was comparable in both groups suggesting a similar effect of beta-blockade on angiotensinergic vasoconstrictor mechanisms. Since responders had a 35% higher mean plasma adrenaline concentration, increased adrenergic activity with enhanced alpha-1-adrenoceptor mediated vasoconstriction as a consequence may be a determinant of antihypertensive beta-blocker response.

Adrenoceptor mediated and calcium influx-dependent vasoconstriction

Various studies demonstrate that increased adrenergic activity contributes to

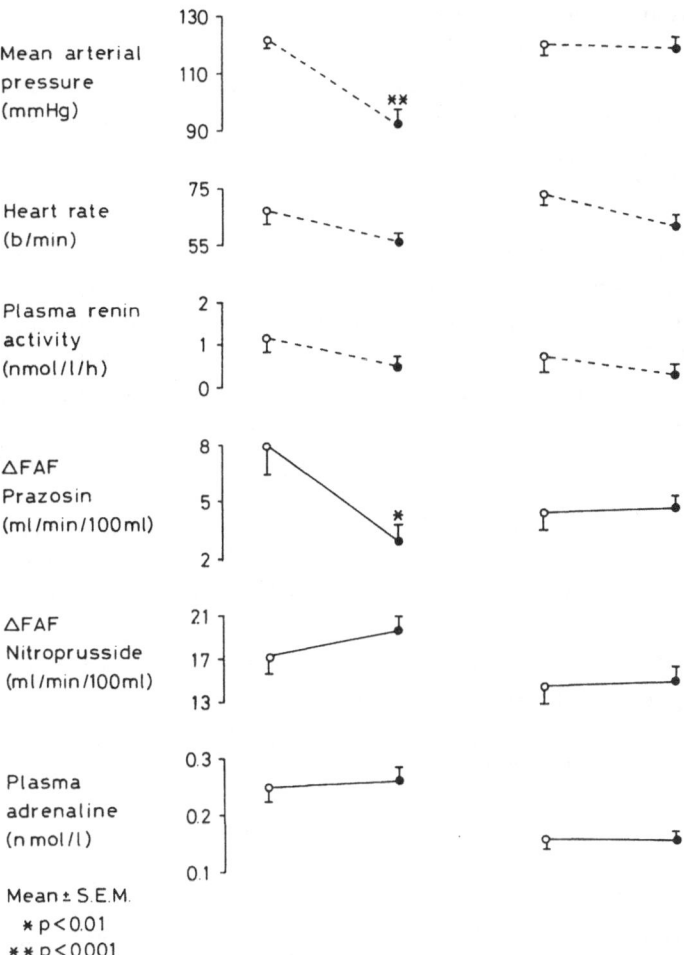

Figure 11. Intra-arterial mean blood pressure, heart rate, plasma renin activity, forearm blood flow to postjunctional alpha-1-adrenoceptor blockade with prazosin (0.5 μg/min/100 ml tissue) and to 'non-specific' vasodilation with sodium nitroprusside (0.6 μg/min/100 ml tissue) and plasma adrenaline concentrations before (●) and after (○) six weeks of propranolol treatment (320 mg/d) in four 'responders' (left panel) and four 'non-responders' (right panel).

vascular resistance in essential hypertension through enhanced alpha-adrenoceptor mediated vasoconstriction. Alpha-adrenoceptor mediated vasoconstriction amounts to about one third of the constrictor component that is generated by calcium influx (Fig. 12). Hyperreactivity of blood vessels to adrenergic stimuli [64–66, 86] on the basis of structural vascular changes [87, 88] can reflect enhanced alpha-adrenoceptor mediated vasoconstriction. Although hyperreactivity becomes obvious with vasoconstrictor responses this does not appear to be a relevant factor influencing vasodilator responses. This is borne out by 'non-specific' vasodilation with sodium nitroprusside or vasodilation following 10 minutes forearm ischaemia which are comparable in hypertensive and normotensive subjects covering a wide dilator range (Fig. 12). Therefore, it seems unlikely that structural vascular changes would account for the difference in alpha-adrenoceptor blockade between hypertensive and normotensive subjects to alpha-adrenoceptor blockade.

Since alpha-2-adrenoceptors via receptor operated calcium channels influence calcium uptake into the vascular smooth muscle cell, enhanced alpha-adrenoceptor mediated vasoconstriction links up with the enhanced calcium influx-dependent vasoconstriction in essential hypertension [62, 63]. It relates to the activity of the adrenergic nervous system [62]. The marked vasorelaxant effect of calcium entry blockade demonstrates its importance for the intracellular free calcium concentration which is the main determinant for vascular smooth muscle contraction [89, 90]. Intracellular free calcium concentration is elevated in patients with essential hypertension [91] reflecting the cellular trigger for enhanced alpha-adrenoceptor mediated and calcium influx-dependent vasoconstriction.

The observation that successful antihypertensive treatment with calcium antagonists or beta-blockers is paralleled by a normalization of platelet intracellular free calcium concentration and the enhanced calcium influx-dependent [92] as well as the enhanced alpha-adrenoceptor mediated vasoconstriction [85] points to a defect in the cellular handling of calcium, perhaps aggravated by adrenergic overactivity. Increasing knowledge of such interactions not only helps to unravel the complex pathophysiology of essential hypertension but also contributes to refine antihypertensive therapy.

Conclusion

The contribution of the adrenergic nervous system to the elevated vascular resistance in essential hypertension has been assessed by forearm venous occlusion plethysmography. In the forearm pharmacological interventions can be done without interference from systemic hemodynamic reflex mechanisms. Post- junctional alpha-1 and alpha-2 adrenoceptor blockade with prazosin and yohimbine, respectively, produced a greater increase in forearm blood flow in patients with essential hypertension as compared to normotensive control subjects. This suggests that an enhanced alpha-adrenoceptor mediated vasoconstriction component contributes to the elevated vascular resistance in essential hypertension. Normalization of the enhanced postjunctional alpha-1-adrenoceptor mediated vasoconstriction parallels the response to antihypertensive beta blockade.

Owing to their extrajunctional localization postjunctional alpha-2-adrenoceptors may be preferential targets for circulating catecholamines, e.g. adrenaline. Adrenaline induced postjunctional alpha-2-adrenoceptor mediated vasoconstriction was demonstrated and this may gain importance as beta adrenoceptor mediated responses decrease as a consequence of age and high blood pressure.

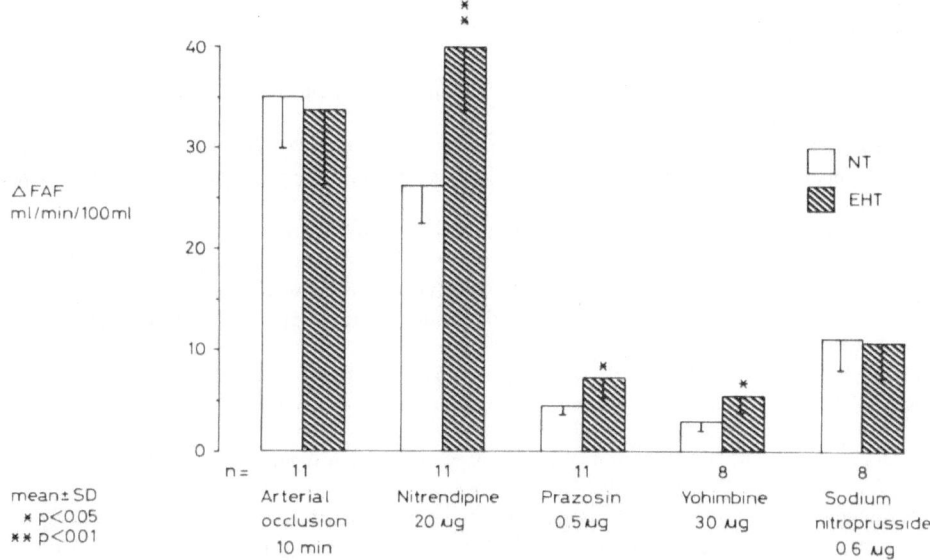

Figure 12. Increase in forearm blood flow ($\triangle$FAF) to calcium entry blockade with nitrendipine, to alpha-1- and alpha-2-blockade with prazosin and yohimbine, respectively, as well as to 'non-specific' (neither adrenoceptor mediated nor calcium influx-dependent) vasodilation after 10 minutes forearm ischaemia (arterial occlusion) and to sodium nitroprusside. Drugs were infused into the brachial artery and doses are given in μg/min/100 ml tissue. Patients with essential hypertension are shown in hatched bars, and age- and sex-matched normotensive control subjects in open bars. The greater increase in forearm blood flow to calcium entry blockade and alpha-1 and alpha-2-adrenoceptor blockade in the presence of comparable values in patients and subjects for 'non-specific' vasodilation indicates enhanced calcium influx-dependent and adrenoceptor mediated vasoconstriction in essential hypertension.

Alpha-1 and alpha-2-adrenoceptor mediated vasoconstriction are comparable and each amount to about one third of calcium influx-dependent vasoconstriction. Calcium influx determines the intracellular calcium and thus the contractile state of smooth muscle cells. As both alpha-adrenoceptor mediated effects had to increase cellular free calcium concentration the enhanced calcium influx-dependent vasoconstriction is in part the consequence of elevated adrenergic activity in essential hypertension.

Acknowledgments

The authors greatly acknowledge the important contributions made by Drs. Wolfgang Amann, Paul Erne, Boa Hua Ji, Lilly Linder, Franco B. Müller and Peter van Brummelen. Last but not least this work and these investigations would not have been possible without the technical and secretarial assistance from Ms. N. Guldimann, Ms. B. Libsig, Ms. R. Mühlethaler and Ms. A. de S. Pinto.

This work was supported by the Swiss National Research Foundation, Grant 3.807.80.

References

1. Alam M, Smirk FH (1938): Blood pressure raising reflexes in health, essential hypertension and renal hypertension. Clin Sci 3: 259–266.
2. Goldenberg M, Pines KL, Baldwin E, Greene DG, Roh CE (1948): The haemodynamic response of man to norepinephrine and epinephrine and its relation to the problem of hypertension. Am J Med 5: 792–806.
3. Pickering GW, Kissin M (1936): The effects of adrenaline and of cold on the blood pressure in human hypertension. Clin Sci 2: 201–207.
4. Fatherree TJ, Hines EA (1938): The blood pressure response to epinephrine administered intravenously to subjects with normal blood pressure and to patients with essential hypertension. Am Heart J 16: 66–71.
5. Doyle AE, Black H (1955): Reactivity to pressor agents in hypertension. Circulation 12: 974–980.
6. DeQuattro V, Miura Y (1973): Neurogenic factors in human hypertension: mechanism or myth. Am J Med 55: 362–378.
7. Julius S, Esler M (1975): Autonomic nervous cardiovascular regulation in borderline hypertension. Am J Cardiol 26: 685–696.
8. Bühler FR (1980): Elevated plasma adrenaline, age-related decrease in beta-adrenoceptor-mediated cardiovascular functions and increase in alpha-receptor mediated vasoconstriction in essential hypertension. In: Central Adrenaline Neurons: Basic Aspects and their Role in Cardiovascular Functions, pp. 305–316, Ed Fuse K, Goldstein M, Hökfelt B and Höfekt T. Pergamon Press, Oxford, New York.
9. DeQuattro V, Can S (1972): Raised plasma catecholamines in some patients with primary hypertension. Lancet i: 806–809.
10. Bühler FR, Kiowski W, van Brummelen P, Amann FW, Bertel O, Landmann R, Lütold BE, Bolli P (1980): Plasma catecholamines and cardiac, renal and peripheral vascular adrenoreceptor-mediated responses in different age groups of normal and hypertensive subjects. Clin Exp Hypertens 2: 409–426.
11. Franco-Morselli R, Elghozi JL, Joly E, Diginilio S, Meyer P (1977): Increased plasma adrenaline concentrations in benign essential hypertension. Br Med J II: 1251–1254.
12. Bertel O, Bühler FR, Kiowski W, Lütold BE (1980): Decreased beta-adrenoreceptor responsiveness as related to age, blood pressure and plasma catecholamines in patients with essential hypertension. Hypertension 2: 130–138.
13. De Champlain J (1981): Use of circulating catecholamines for the detection of autonomic abnormalities in human hypertension. In: Frontiers in Hypertension Research, pp. 306–311. Ed: Laragh JH, Bühler FR, Seldin DW. New York: Springer.
14. Cousineau D, Lapointe L, De Champlain J (1978): Circulating catecholamines and systolic time intervals in normotensive and hypertensive patients with and without left ventricular hypertrophy. Am Heart J 96: 229–234.
15. Bühler FR, Kiowski W, Landmann R, van Brummelen P, Amann FW, Bolli P, Bertel O (1981): Changing role of beta and alpha adrenoceptor-mediated cardiovascular responses in the transition from a high cardiac output into a high peripheral resistance phase in essential hypertension. In: Frontiers in Hypertension Research, pp. 316–426. Ed: Laragh JH, Bühler Fr, Seldin DW. New York: Springer.
16. Bolli P, Amann FW, Hulthén L, Kiowski W, Bühler FR (1981): Elevated plasma adrenaline reflects sympathetic overactivity and enhanced alpha adrenoceptor-mediated vasoconstriction in essential hypertension. Clin Sci 61 (Suppl 7): 161s–164s.
17. Esler MD, Julius S, Zweifler A, Randall O, Gardiner H, DeQuattro V (1977): Mild high-renin essential hypertension. Neurogenic human hypertension? N Engl J Med 296: 405–411.
18. Louis WJ, Doyle AE, Anavekar A (1973): Plasma norepinephrine levels in essential hypertension. N Engl J Med 288: 599–601.

19. Kiowski W, van Brummelen P, Bühler FR (1979): Plasma noradrenaline correlates with alpha-adrenoceptor-mediated vasoconstriction and blood pressure in patients with essential hypertension. Clin Sci 57: 177S–180S.

20. Sever PS, Owikowska B, Birch M, Turnbridge RDG (1977): Plasma noradrenaline in essential hypertension. Lancet I: 1078–1081.

21. Lake CR, Ziegler NG, Coleman MD, Kopin IJ (1977): Age-adjusted plasma norepinephrine levels are similar in normotensive and hypertensive subjects. N Engl J Med 296: 208–209.

22. Kiowski W, Bertel O, Bühler FR (1979): The renin type of essential hypertension and the relationships between catecholamines, renin and age. In: Nervous System and Hypertension, pp. 318–325. Ed: Meyer P, Schmitt H. Paris: Flammarion.

23. Whitby LG, Axelrod J, Weil-Malherbe H (1961): The fate of ^{3}H-norepinephrine in animals. J Pharmacol Exp Therap 132: 193–201.

24. Langer SZ (1977): Presynaptic receptors and their role in the regulation of transmitter release. Sixth Gaddum Memorial Lecture. Br J Pharmaco 60: 481–497.

25. Brown MJ, Macquin I (1981): Is adrenaline the cause of essential hypertension? Lancet II: 1079–1982.

26. Majewski H, MacCulloch MW, Rand MJ, Story DF (1980): Adrenaline activation of prejunctional beta-adrenoceptors in guinea-pig atria. Br J Pharmacol 71: 435–444.

27. Majewski H, Rand MJ, Tung LH (1981): Activation of prejunctional beta-adrenoceptors in rat atria by adrenaline applied exogenously or released as a contransmitter. Br J Pharmacol 73: 669–679.

28. Guimaraes S, Brandao F, Pavia MQ (1978): A study of the adrenoceptor-mediated feedback mechanism by using adrenaline as a false transmitter. Naunyn-Schmiedeberg's Archives of Pharmacol 305: 185–188.

29. Brown MJ, Dollery CT (1984): Adrenaline and hypertension. Clinical and Experimental Hypertension. Part A: Theory and Practice, A6 (1and2): 539–549.

30. Stjärne L, Brundin J (1976): Beta-adrenoceptors facilitating noradrenaline secretion from human vasoconstrictor nerves. Acta Physiol Scand 97: 88–93.

31. Adler-Graschinski E, Langer SZ (1975): Possible role of beta-adrenoceptor in the regulation of noradrenaline release by nerve stimulation through a positive feedback mechanism. Br J Pharmacol 53: 43–50.

32. Rand MJ, McCulloch MW, Story DF (1980): Catecholamine receptors on nerve terminals. In: Adrenergic Activators and Inhibitors. Handbook of Experimental Pharmacology, pp. 224–266, Vol. 54 II. Ed: Szekeres L. Berlin: Springer Verlag.

33. Starke K (1981): Alpha-adrenoceptor subclassification. Rev Physiol Biochem Pharmacol 88: 199–236.

34. Drew GM (1980): Postsynaptic alpha-2 adrenoceptors mediate pressor responses to 2.N-dimethylamino-5,6,dihydroxy-1,2,3,4-tetrahydronaphthalen (M-7). Eur J Pharmacol 65: 85–87.

35. Timmermans PBMWM, Van Zwieten PA (1981): The postsynaptic alpha-2 adrenoceptor. J Auton Pharmacol 1: 171–183.

36. Van Zwieten PA, Van Meel JCA, De Jonge A, Wilffert B, Timmermans PBMWM (1982): Central and peripheral alpha-adrenoceptors. J Cardiovasc Pharmacol 4 (Suppl 1): 19–24.

37. Yamaguchi I, Kopin J (1980): Differential inhibition of alpha-1 and alpha-2 adrenoceptor mediated pressor responses in pithed rats. J Pharmacol Exp Ther 214: 275–281.

38. Langer SZ, Massingham R, Shepperson NB (1980): Presence of postsynaptic alpha-2-adrenoceptors of predominantly extrasynaptic location in the vascular smooth muscle of the dog hind linb. Clin Sci 59: 225s–228s.

39. Wilffert B (1981): Localization of alpha- and beta-adrenoceptors. Naunyn Schmideberg's Arch Pharmacol, Suppl: 316–356.

40. Berthelsen S, Pettinger WA (1977): A functional basis for classification of alpha-adrenergic receptors. Life Sci 21: 595–606.

41. Starke K, Endo T, Taube HD (1975): Relative pre- and postsynaptic potencies of alpha-adrenoceptor agonists in the rabbit pulmonary artery. Naunyn Schmiedeberg's Arch Pharmacol 291: 55–78.
42. Cambridge DM, Davey J, Massingham R (1977): Prazosin, a selective antagonist of post-synaptic alpha-adrenoceptors. Br J Pharmacol 59: 514P–515P.
43. Bentley SM, Drew GM, Whiting SB (1977): Evidence for two distinct types of postsynaptic alpha-adrenoceptors. Br J Pharmacol 61: 116P–117P.
44. Starke K, Docherty JR (1980): Recent development in alpha-adrenoceptor research. J Cardiovasc Pharmacol 2 (Suppl 3): 269–286.
45. Rubin PC, Howden CW, McLean K, Reid JL (1982): Pharmacodynamic studies with a specific alpha 2 adrenoceptor agonist (B-HT 933) in man. J Cardiovasc Pharmacol 4: 527–530.
46. Roddie IC, Wallace WFM (1979): Methods for the assessment of the effects of drugs on the arterial system in man. Br J Clin Pharmacol 7: 317–323.
47. Brodie TG, Russel AE (1905): On the determination of the rate of blood flow through an organ. J Physiol (London) 32: 47–49.
48. Wilkins RW, Bradley SE (1946): Changes in arterial and venous blood pressure and flow distal to a cuff inflated on the human arm. Am J Physiol 147: 260–269.
49. Formel PF, Doyle JT (1957): Rationale of venous occlusion plethysmography. Circ Res 5: 354–356.
50. Greenfield ADM, Whitney RJ, Mowbray JF (1963): Methods for the investigation of peripheral blood flow. Br Med Bull 19: 101–109.
51. Hokanson DE, Summer DS, Strandness DE Jr (1975): An electronically calibrated plethysmograph for direct measurement of limb blood flow. IEEE Trans Biomed Eng BME 22: 25–29.
52. Amann FW, Bolli P, Kiowski W, Bühler FR (1981): Enhanced alpha-adrenoceptor-mediated vasoconstriction in essential hypertension. Hypertension 3 (Suppl 1): 119–123.
53. Kiowski W, Hulthén UL, Ritz R, Bühler FR (1983): Alpha-2-adrenoceptor mediated vasoconstriction in human arterial vessels. Clin Pharmcol Ther 34: 565–569.
54. Bolli P, Erne P, Kiowski W, Ji BH, Amann FW, Bühler FR (1983): Important contribution of the postjunctional alpha-2-adrenoceptor mediated vasoconstrictor response to arteriolar tone in man. J Hypertension 1 (Suppl II): 257–259.
55. Elliott HL, Reid JL (1983): Evidence for postjunctional vascular alpha-2-adrenoceptors in peripheral vascular regulation in man. Clin Sci 65: 237–241.
56. Van Brummelen P, Vermey P, Timmermans PBMWM, van Zwieten PA (1983): Preliminary evidence for a postsynaptic alpha-2-adrenoceptor in the vasculature of the human forearm. Br J Clin Pharmacol 15: 134P–135P.
57. Goldberg MR, Robertson D (1984): Evidence for the existence of vascular alpha-2-adrenergic receptors in humans. Hypertension 6: 551–556.
58. Jie K, van Brummelen P, Vermey P, Timmermans PBMWM, van Zwieten PA (1984): Identification of vascular postsynaptic alpha-1 and alpha-2 adrenoceptors in man. Circ Res 54: 447–452.
59. Bolli P, Erne P, Block LH, Ji BH, Kiowski W, Bühler FR (1984): Adrenaline induces vasoconstriction through postjunctional alpha-2-adrenoceptor stimulation which is enhanced in essential hypertension. J Hypertension 2 (Suppl 3): 115–118.
60. Jie K, van Brummelen P, Vermey P, Timmermans PBMWM, van Zwieten PA (1986): Alpha 1- and alpha 2-adrenoceptor mediated vasoconstriction in the forearm of normotensive and hypertensive subjects. J Cardiovasc Pharmacol 8: 190–196.
61. Timmermans PBMWM, de Jone A, van Meel JCA, Mathy MJ, van Zwieten PA (1983): Influence of nifedipine on functional responses in vivo initiated at alpha-2-adrenoceptors. J Cardiovasc Pharmacol 5: 1–11.
62. Hulthén UL, Bolli P, Amann FW, Kiowski W, Bühler FR (1982): Enhanced vasodilation in essential hypertension by calcium channel blockade with verapamil. Hypertension 4 (Suppl II): 26–31.

63. Robinson BF, Dobbs RJ, Bayley S (1982): Effects of forearm resistance vessels to verapamil and sodium nitroprusside in normotensive and hypertensive man. Clin Sci 63: 33–42.
64. Doyle AE, Fraser JRE, Marshall RJ (1959): Reactivity of forearm vessels to vasoconstrictor substances in hypertensive and normotensive subjects. Clin Sci 18: 441–454.
65. Doyle AE, Fraser JRE (1961): Vascular reactivity in hypertension. Circ Res 9: 775–761.
66. Mendlowitz M (1973): Vascular reactivity in systemic arterial hypertension. Am Heart J 85: 252–259.
67. Stevens MJ, Moulds RFW (1982): The role of facilitatory presynaptic beta-receptors in human digital arteries. Clin Exp Pharmacol Physiol 9: 465–466.
68. Fleisch JH (1980): Age-related changes in the sensitivity of blood vessels to drugs. Pharmacol Ther 8: 477–487.
69. Dillon N, Chung S, Kelly J, O'Malley K (1980): Age and beta-adrenoceptor-mediated function. Clin Pharmacol Ther 27: 769–772.
70. van Brummelen P, Bühler FR, Kiowski W, Amann FW (1981): Age-related decrease in cardiac and peripheral vascular responsiveness to isoproterenol. Clin Sci 60: 571–577.
71. Feldmann RD, Limbird LE, Nadeau J, Robertson D, Wood AJJ (1984): Alterations in leucocyte beta-receptor affinity with aging. N Engl J Med 310: 815–819.
72. Landmann R, van Brummelen P, Amann FW, Bühler FR (1985): Increased beta-adrenoceptor binding capacity is associated with blunted beta-adrenoceptor-mediated cardiovascular responses in essential hypertension. J Cardiovasc Pharmacol 7 (Suppl 6): 168–171.
73. London GM, Safar ME, Weiss YA, Milliez PL (1976): Isoproterenol sensitivity and total body clearance of propranolol in hypertensive patients. J Clin Pharmacol 16: 174–182.
74. Van Brummelen P, Jie K, Vermey P, Timmermans PBMWM, van Zwieten PA (1985): Vascular alpha-adrenoceptors in man: interactions with adrenaline and noradrenaline. Clin Sci 68 (Suppl 10): 151S–153S.
75. Robertson D, Garland AJ, Robertson RM, Nies AS, Shand DG, Oates JA (1979): Comparative assessment of stimuli that release neuronal and adrenomedullary catecholamines in man. Circ 59: 637–643.
76. Perini Ch, Müller FB, Rauchfleisch U, Battegay R, Bühler FR (1986): Hyperadrenergic borderline hypertension is characterized by suppressed aggression. J Cardiovasc Pharmacol 8 (Suppl. 5) 53–56.
77. Bühler FR, Bertel O, Kiowski W (1978): Plasma noradrenaline and adrenaline and beta-adrenoceptor responsiveness in renin subgroups of essential hypertension. Clin Sci Molec Med 55: 57s–60s.
78. Bertel O, Bühler FR, Baitsch G, Ritz R (1982): Plasma adrenaline and noradrenaline in patients with acute myocardial infarction. Chest 82: 64–68.
79. Majewski H, Tung LH, Rand MJ (1982): Adrenaline activation of prejunctional beta-adrenoceptors and hypertension. J Cardiovasc Pharmacol 4: 99–106.
80. Popper CW, Chiueh CC, Kopin IJ (1977): Plasma catecholamine concentrations in unanesthetized rats during sleep, wakefulness, immobilization and after decapitation. J Pharmacol Exp Ther 202: 144–148.
81. Vincent HH, Man in't Veld AJ, Voomsa F, Wenting GJ, Schalekamp MADH (1982): Elevated plasma noradrenaline in response to beta-adrenoceptor stimulation in man. Br J Clin Pharmacol 13: 717–721.
82. Kiowski W, Hulthén UL, Bolli P, Ritz R, Bühler FR (1983): Failure of prejunctional alpha-2 adrenoceptor stimulation to reduce norepinephrine release in normal man. Gen Pharmacol 14: 173
83. Tarazi RZ, Dustan HP (1972): Beta adrenergic blockade in hypertension. Am J Cardiol 29: 633–641.
84. Bühler FR, Burkart F, Lütold BE, Küng M, Marbet G, Pfisterer M (1975): Antihypertensive betablocking action as related to renin and age: a pharmacologic tool to identify pathogenetic mechanisms in essential hypertension. Am J Cardiol 36:653–669.

85. Bolli P, Amann FW, Burkart F, Bühler FR (1982): Role of alpha-adrenoceptor-mediated vasoconstriction for antihypertensive beta-blockade. J Cardiovasc Pharmacol 4 (Suppl 1): S162–S166.
86. Sivertsson R, Olander R (1968): Aspects of the nature of the increased vascular resistance and increased 'reactivity' to noradrenaline in hypertensive subjects. Life Sci 7 (part I): 1291–1297.
87. Folkow B, Grimby G, Thulesius O (1958): Adaptive structural changes of the vascular walls in hypertension and their relation to the control of the peripheral resistance. Acta Physiol Scand 44: 255–272.
88. Conway J (1963): A vascular abnormality in hypertension. A study of blood flow in the forearm. Circulation 27: 520–529.
89. Bolton TB (1979): Mechanisms of action of transmitters and other substances on smooth muscle. Physiol Rev 59: 606–718.
90. Kuriyama H, Yto Y, Suzuki H, Kitamura K, Itoh T (1982): Factors modifying contraction relaxation cycle in vascular smooth muscles. Am J Physiol 243: H641–H662.
91. Erne P, Bolli P, Bürgisser E, Bühler FR (1984): Correlation of platelet calcium with blood pressure. Effect of antihypertensive therapy. N Engl J Med 310: 1084–1088.
92. Bolli P, Erne P, Hulthén UL, Ritz R, Kiowski W, Ji BH, Bühler FR (1984): Parallel reduction of calcium-influx-dependent vasoconstriction and platelet free calcium concentration with calcium entry and beta-adrenoceptor blockade. J Cardiovasc Pharmacol 6: S996–S1001.

Beta-adrenergic receptors and the forearm circulation

P. VAN BRUMMELEN and P.C. CHANG

Introduction

The forearm circulation provides an attractive opportunity to study pathophysiological and pharmacological aspects of various cardiovascular disorders including essential hypertension. In the first place this is due to the fact that in this particular vascular bed blood flow can be measured accurately and repeatedly by non-invasive methods [1]. Among the various possibilities to measure forearm blood flow, venous occlusion plethysmography, using either a mercury-in-silastic or rubber strain gauge or a water-filled reservoir to determine changes in circumference or volume of the forearm respectively, is the technique which has been applied most extensively [1–4]. In addition, cannulation of the brachial artery enables the local infusion of vasoactive drugs and the direct measurement of intra-arterial blood pressure. As long as doses of drugs are infused that exclusively produce local haemodynamic effects, activation of homeostatic cardiovascular reflexes does not occur and responses can be interpreted as direct drug effects on vascular resistance.

Despite its merits there are several limitations to the forearm model. It should be realized that the forearm circulation is not homogeneous since blood is supplied not only to muscle but also to skin and bone. The latter tends to be fairly constant but blood flow to skin is known to vary considerably with changes in temperature and with emotions. Since regional vascular beds may differ in receptor population and in their contribution to total peripheral resistance [5], conclusions drawn from studies in the forearm circulation (or in any other regional vascular bed) cannot be automatically extrapolated to the total circulation. Moreover, with pharmacological interventions only the lower part of dose-response curves can be measured since higher doses of vasoactive drugs will produce pharmacologically active concentrations in the systemic circulation and hence systemic haemodynamic changes. Because these changes will trigger homeostatic reflexes, interpretation of the local haemodynamic effects is made more complex. Finally, the spontaneous variations in forearm blood flow, together with the relatively low basal levels, limit the accuracy with which vaso-constrictor changes can be measured.

In patients with essential hypertension the forearm circulation has been extensively investigated [6]. Studies in patients with borderline hypertension have invariably reported a greater than normal forearm blood flow and hence a normal or only slightly elevated vascular resistance [7–12]. In contrast, patients with sustained hypertension have usually a normal forearm blood flow in spite of the higher perfusion pressure, indicating increased vascular resistance [7, 9, 13, 14]. In this chapter data on the subtypes and functional role of β-adrenoceptors in the forearm circulation are reviewed and their possible relevance for the pathophysiology of essential hypertension will be discussed.

Beta-adrenoceptor subtypes

α- as well as β-adrenoceptors have been identified in the forearm circulation, the former mediating vasoconstriction and the latter mediating vasodilatation when stimulated [5]. Subsequently, β-adrenoceptors have been divided in two subtypes, i.e. β_1 and β_2 [15] and it has been recognized that the catecholamines adrenaline and noradrenaline differ with respect to their affinity for these subtypes: adrenaline has affinity for β_1- as well as for β_2-adrenoceptors whereas noradrenaline has mainly affinity for the β_1-adrenoceptor subtype [15–17]. A functional basis for the β-adrenoceptor subdivision could therefore be that β_1-adrenoceptors are innervated receptors sensitive to the neurotransmitter noradrenaline, whereas β_2-adrenoceptors are not innervated and sensitive to the circulating hormone adrenaline [18]. The β-adrenoceptors of the forearm vasculature, especially those of the muscle blood vessels, are mainly of the β_2-subtype [5, 19].

Studies in the hindlimb circulation of dogs [20–23] and cats [24–25] suggest the presence of a noradrenaline sensitive β-adrenoceptor mediating vasodilatation in skeletal muscle blood vessels. This β-adrenoceptor seems to be sensitive to circulating noradrenaline [20, 21, 25] as well as to neuronally released noradrenaline [22–24] and, in order to reveal its presence, β-adrenoceptor blockade is required. Recently, Vatner et al. [23] demonstrated that these β-adrenoceptors belong to the β_1-subtype, which is not surprising in face of their sensitivity to noradrenaline. The presence of a vasodilating β_1-adrenoceptor in the human forearm remains to be demonstrated.

Apart from the above-mentioned β_2- and β_1-adrenoceptors on vascular smooth muscle, it is conceivable that presynaptic β-adrenoceptors located on adrenergic nerve terminals also play a role in the regulation of vascular resistance via their influence on neurotransmitter release [26, 27]. Indeed, *in vitro* experiments with isolated superfused strips of human blood vessels have shown facilitation of noradrenaline release upon β-adrenoceptor stimulation [28]. Subsequently evidence has been presented that these receptors are of the β_2-subtype [29]. Results of *in vivo* studies in man are in accordance with a presynaptic β_2- adrenoceptor facilitating noradrenaline release upon nerve stimulation [30, 31]. However, the presence and importance of this mechanism in the forearm vascular bed remains to be established.

In summary, the postjunctional β_2-adrenoceptor mediating vasodilatation is the prevailing β-adrenoceptor in the vasculature of the human forearm, but contributions of a vasodilating β_1-adrenoceptor and of a presynaptic β_2-adrenoceptor to the regulation of vascular resistance cannot be dismissed.

β-adrenoceptor mediated vasodilatation

The contribution of β-adrenoceptor mediated vasodilatation to basal vascular tone in the forearm (or leg) circulation has been investigated by measuring the change in blood flow in response to local intra-arterial infusion of beta-blockers [32–35]. Although in one study [33] a slight decrease in basal blood flow was found during intra-arterial infusion of the non-selective beta-blocker propranolol, this was not confirmed by others [32, 33, 35]. Also the local infusion of the β_1-selective beta-blocker atenolol had no influence on resting forearm blood flow [35]. Thus, blockade of β-adrenoceptors in the forearm seems to have little influence on blood flow in basal conditions.

This indicates that under these circumstances β_2-adrenoceptor stimulation by circulating adrenaline and possibly also β_1-adrenoceptor stimulation by neuronally released noradrenaline are relatively unimportant determinants of vascular resistance. Surprisingly, also the exercise-induced increase in muscle blood flow is not influenced by the local infusion of propranolol or atenolol [34, 35]. It seems therefore that vasoactive metabolites released in working muscles [36] have more significance than stimulation of β-adrenoceptors for the vasodilatation in skeletal muscle during exercise.

The effects of local infusion of beta-blockers with intrinsic sympathomimetic activity (ISA) warrant special mention. These drugs are partial agonists and from experimental studies there is evidence for a direct vasodilatory effect [37–39]. We have studied the local haemodynamic effect of pindolol, a non-selective beta-blocker with relatively strong ISA [40], in the forearm circulation of healthy volunteers [41]. Different from non-selective and selective beta-blockers without ISA, pindolol produced a dose-dependent vasodilatation upon infusion in the brachial artery (Fig. 1). This effect was due to stimulation of vascular β_2-adrenoceptors because it could be prevented by stimultaneous infusion of propanolol (Fig. 1). Whether the vasodilating effect of pindolol (and of similar partial agonists) contributes to the blood pressure lowering effect remains to be established, but it could well be of relevance for the divergent systemic haemodynamic pattern observed during treatment of hypertensive patients with these drugs [42, 43].

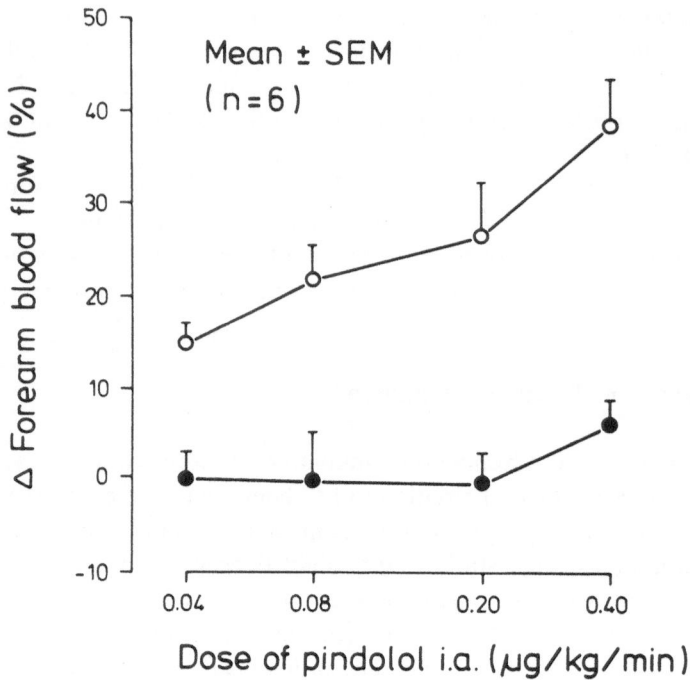

Figure 1. Percentage change in forearm blood flow during cumulative dose infusion of pindolol into the brachial artery of healthy volunteers. Pindolol was given in the presence of saline (open circles) and with a concomitant infusion of propranolol 1 μg/kg/min (closed circles). Each dose was given for 3 minutes and forearm blood flow was measured by plethysmography (for details see ref. 41).

Stimulation of vascular β-adrenoceptors by local infusion of adrenaline [44–46] or isoprenaline [44, 47, 48] produces considerable vasodilatation in the forearm circulation. For adrenaline α-adrenoceptor blockade is required to reveal its full vasodilatory potency [46]. Evidence from experimental studies [49, 50] suggests that β-adrenoceptor mediated vasodilatation diminishes with increasing age. We have studied the age dependency of β-adrenoceptor mediated vasodilatation in healthy subjects [48]. Intra-brachial infusions of isoproterenol, in doses that did not produce systemic haemodynamic effects, produced a significantly greater vasodilatation in subjects younger than 25 years than in subjects older than 50 years of age [48]. This age-related decrease in vascular responses to β-adrenoceptor agonists is paralleled by a diminished heart rate response to exercise [51] and to β-adrenoceptor stimulation by isoproterenol [51–53]. The mechanism underlying decreased β-adrenoceptor responsiveness in the eldery has not been fully clarified. A diminished cyclic AMP content of vascular smooth muscle has been reported [50] suggesting a defect in the second messenger system of the β-adrenoceptor at higher age. This notion is supported by the finding of diminished cyclic AMP production upon isoproterenol stimulation in lymphocytes of older individuals [54]. However, the latter finding could not be confirmed by others [55]. Thus there is suggestive evidence for diminished cardiovascular responses to β-adrenoceptor stimulation with age but the mechanism remains as yet speculative.

Forearm blood flow in hypertension

As mentioned before, patients with borderline hypertension have an increased forearm blood flow when compared to normotensive controls [7–12]. There are several arguments in favor of a role for β-adrenoceptor mediated vasodilatation in this respect. For instance, circulating levels of adrenaline are elevated in patients with mild to moderate essential hypertension [51, 56], and in young normotensive individuals plasma adrenaline concentrations were directly related to forearm blood flow [48]. More direct evidence stems from a study of Levenson and coworkers [12] who studied the haemodynamic effect of β_1-selective and non-selective β-blockade in a group of borderline hypertensives. Both beta-blockers diminished cardiac output but brachial blood flow was normalised only after non-selective beta-blockade [12]. So far there is no experimental support for a noradrenaline sensitive vasodilating β-adrenoceptor in the forearm. In fact the findings of Levenson and coworkers [12] argue against this possibility in borderline hypertensives.

There is evidence that not only age but also hypertension is accompanied by diminished β-adrenoceptor mediated responses [51, 56]. It should be realised, however, that this has been more clearly demonstrated for cardiac responses [51] than for peripheral vascular responses [56]. Moreover, the fact that β-adrenoceptor blockade has no influence on forearm blood flow is difficult to reconcile with an important role for β-adrenoceptor mediated vasodilatation in this vascular bed. Therefore a contribution of blunted β-adrenoceptor responsiveness to the increased vascular resistance in long-standing hypertension remains as yet speculative.

References

1. Roddie IC, Wallace WFM (1979): Methods for the assesment of the effects of drugs on the arterial system in man. British Journal of Clinical Pharmacology 7: 317–323.
2. Brodie TG, Russel AE (1905): On the determination of the rate of blood- flow through an organ. Journal of Physiology (London) 32: 47–49.
3. Whitney RJ (1953): The measurement of volume changes in human limbs. Journal of Physiology (London) 121: 1–27.
4. Greenfield ADM, Whitney RJ, Mowbray JF (1963): Methods for the investigation of peripheral blood flow. British Medical Bulletin 19: 101–109.
5. Shepherd JT, Vanhoutte PM (1979): The human cardiovascular system. Facts and concepts. New York: Raven Press.

6. Conway J (1984): Hemodynamic aspects of essential hypertension in humans. Physiological Reviews 64: 617–648.
7. Abramson DI, Fierst SM (1942): Resting blood flow and peripheral vascular response in hypertensive subjects. American Heart Journal 23: 84–98.
8. Brod J, Fencl V, Hejl Z, Jirka J (1962): General and regional haemodynamic pattern underlying essential hypertension. Clinical Science 23: 339–349.
9. Conway J (1963): A vascular abnormality in hypertension. A study of blood flow in the forearm. Circulation 27: 520–529.
10. Amery A, Bossaert H, Verstraete M (1969): Muscle blood flow in normal and hypertensive subjects. Influence of age, exercise and body position. American Heart Journal 78: 211–216.
11. Temmar MM, Safar ME, Levenson JA, Totomoukouo JM, Simon ACh (1981): Regional blood flow in borderline and sustained essential hypertension. Clinical Science 60: 653–658.
12. Levenson J, Simon AC, Safar ME, Bouthier JD, London GM (1985): Elevation of brachial arterial blood velocity and volumic flow mediated by peripheral β-adrenoceptors in patients with borderline hypertension. Circulation 71: 663–668.
13. Pickering GW (1936): The peripheral resistance in persistent arterial hypertension. Clinical Science 2: 209–235.
14. Folkow B, Grimby G, Thulesius O (1959): Adaptive structural changes of the vascular walls in hypertension and their relation to the control of the peripheral resistance. Acta Physiologica Scandinavica. 44: 255–272.
15. Lands AM, Arnold A, McAuliff JP, Luduena FP, Brown TG (1967): Differentiation of receptor systems activated by sympathomimetic amines. Nature (London) 214: 597–598.
16. Hjemdahl P, Belfrage E, Daleskog M (1979): Vascular and metabolic effects of circulating epinephine and norepinephrine. Journal of Clinical Investigation 64: 1221–1228.
17. Weiner N (1980): Norepinephrine, epinephrine and the sympathomimetic amines. In: the Pharmacological Basis of Therapeutics (6th ed), edited by A. Goodman, L.S. Goodman, and A. Gilman. New York: Macmillan, 138–175.
18. Ariens EJ, Simonis AM (1983): Physiological and pharmacological aspects of adrenergic receptor classification. Biochemical Pharmacology 32: 1539–1545.
19. Nickerson M (1973): Adrenergic receptors. Circulation Research 32 and 33, supplement 1: 53–59.
20. Glick G, Epstein SE, Wechsler AS, Braunwald E (1967): Physiological differences between the effects of neuronally released and bloodborne norepinephrine on beta adrenergic receptors in the arterial bed of the dog. Circulation Research 21: 217–227.
21. Brungardt JM, Swan KG, Reynolds DG (1974): Adrenergic mechanisms in canine hind limb circulation. Cardiovascular Research 8: 423–429.
22. Saeed M, Sommer O, Holtz J, Bassenge E (1982): α-Adrenergic blockade by phentolamine causes β-adrenergic vasodilation by increased cathecholamine release due to presynaptic α-blockade. Journal of Cardiovascular Pharmacology 4: 44–52.
23. Vatner SF, Knight DR, Hintze TH (1985): Norepinephrine – induced β₁-adrenergic peripheral vasodilation in conscious dogs. American Journal of Physiology 249: H 49–H 56.
24. Lundvall J, Järhult J (1976): Beta adrenergic dilator component of sympathetic vascular responce in skeletal muscle. Influence on the microcirculation and on transcapillary exchange. Acta Physiologica Scandinavica 96: 180–192.
25. Lundvall J, Hillman J (1978): Noradrenaline evoked beta adrenergic delatation of precipillary sphincters in skeletal muscle. Acta Physiologica Scandinavica 102: 126–128.
26. Langer SZ (1977): Presynaptic receptors and their role in the regulation of transmitter release. British Journal of Pharmacology 60: 481–497.
27. Starke K (1977): Regulation of noradrenaline release by presynaptic receptor systems. Revues of Physiology, Biochemistry and Pharmacology 77: 1–124.
28. Stjärne L, Brundin J (1975): Dual adrenoceptor-mediated control of noradrenaline secretion from human vasoconstrictor nerves: facilitation by β-receptors and inhibition by α-receptors. Acta Physiologica Scandinavica 94: 139–141.

29. Stjärne L, Brundin J (1976): β_2-adrenoceptors facilitating noradrenaline secretion from human vasoconstrictor nerves. Acta Physiologica Scandinavica 97: 88–93.
30. Vincent HH, Man in 't Veld AJ, Boomsma F, Wenting GJ, Schalekamp MADH (1982): Elevated plasma noradrenaline in response to β-adrenoceptor stimulation in man. British Journal of Clinical Pharmacology 13: 717–721.
31. Vincent HH, Boomsma F, Man in 't Veld AJ, Derkx FHM, Wenting GJ, Schalekamp MADH (1984): Effects of selective and nonselective β-agonists on plasma potassium and norepinephrine. Journal of Cardiovascular Pharmacology 6: 107–114.
32. Brick I, Glover WE, Hutchison KJ, Roddie IC (1966): Effect of propanolol on peripheral vessels in man. American Journal of Cardiology 18: 329–332.
33. Johnsson G (1967): The effects of intra-arterially administered propranolol and H 56/28 on blood flow in the forearm – a comparative study of two β-adrenergic receptor antagonists. Acta Pharmacologica and Toxicologica 25: 63–74.
34. Juhlin-Dannfelt A, Aström H (1979): Influence of β-adrenoceptor blockade on leg blood flow and lactate release in man. Scandinavican Journal of Clinical and Laboratory Investigation 39: 179–183.
35. Hartling OJ, Noer I, Svendsen TL, Clausen JP, Trap Jensen J (1980): Selective and non-selective β-adrenoceptor blockade in the human forearm. Clinical Science 58: 279–286.
36. Mellander S, Johansson B (1968): Control of resistance, exchange and capacitance functions in the peripheral circulation. Pharmacological Reviews 20: 117–196.
37. Thulesius O, Gjöres JE, Berlin E (1982): Vasodilating properties of β-adrenoceptor blockers with intrinsic sympathomimetic activity. British Journal of Clinical Pharmacology 13 (suppl 2) 229 S–230 S.
38. Clark BJ, Bertholet A (1983): Effects of pindolol on vascular smooth muscle. General Pharmacology 14: 117–119.
39. Syberts EJ, Baum T, Pula KK, Nelson S, Eynon E, Sabin C (1982): Studies on the mechanism of the acute antihypertensive and vasodilator actions of several β-adrenoceptors antagonists. Journal of Cardiovascular Pharmacology 4: 749–758.
40. Frishman WH (1983): Pindolol: a new β-adrenoceptor antagonist with partial agonist activity. New England Journal of Medicine 308: 940–944.
41. Chang PC, van Brummelen P, Vermey P (1985): Acute vasodilator action of pindolol in humans. Hypertension 7: 146–150.
42. Man in 't Veld AJ, Schalekamp MADH (1983): Effect of 10 different β-adrenoceptor antagonists on haemodynamics, plasma renin activity and plasma norepinephrine in hypertension: the key role of vascular resistance changes in relation to partial agonist activity. Journal of Cardiovascular Pharmacology 5 (suppl 1): S30–S45.
43. v.d. Meiracker A, Man in 't Veld AJ, Ritsema van Eck H, Wenting GJ, Schalekamp MADH (1984): Direct 24-hour haemodynamic monitoring after starting β-blocker therapy: studies with pindolol in hypertension. Journal of Hypertension 2 (suppl 3): 581–583.
44. Barcroft H, Konzett H (1949). On the action of noradrenaline, adrenaline and isopropyl noradrenaline on the arterial blood pressure, heart rate and muscle blood flow in man. Journal of Physiology (London) 110: 194–204.
45. Whelan RF (1952): Vasodilatation in human skeletal muscle during adrenaline infusions. Journal of Physiology (London) 118: 575–587.
46. Whelan RF, de la Lande IS (1963): Action of adrenaline on limb blood vessels. British Medical Bulletin 19: 125–131.
47. Allwood MJ, Cobbold AF, Ginsburg J (1963): Peripheral vascular effects of noradrenaline, isopropylnoradrenaline and dopamine. British Medical Bulletin 19: 32–36.
48. van Brummelen P, Bühler FR, Kiowski W, Amann FW (1981): Age-related decrease in cardiac and peripheral vascular responsiveness to isoprenaline: studies in normal subjects. Clinical Science 60: 571–577.

49. Fleisch JH, Maling HM, Brodie BB (1970): β-Receptor activity in aorta: variations with age and species. Circulation Research 26: 151–162.
50. Ericsson EE, Lundholm L (1975): Adrenergic β-receptor activity and cyclic AMP metabolism in vascular smooth muscle: variations with age. Mechanisms of Aging and Development 4, 1–16.
51. Bertel O, Bühler FR, Kiowski W, Lütold BE (1980): Decreased β-adrenoceptor responsiveness as related to age, blood pressure and plasma catecholamines in patients with essential hypertension. Hypertension 2: 130–139.
52. London GM, Safar ME, Weiss YA, Milliez PL (1976): Isoproterenol sensitivity and total body clearance of propranolol in hypertensive patients. Journal of Clinical Pharmacology 16: 174–182.
53. Vestal RE, Wood AJJ, Shand DG (1979): Reduced β-adrenoceptor sensitivity in the elderly. Clinical Pharmacology and Therapeutics 26: 181–186.
54. Dillon N, Chung S, Kelly J, O'Malley K (1980): Age and beta adrenoceptor-mediated function. Clinical Pharmacology and Therapeutics 27: 769–772.
55. Kraft CA, Castleden CM (1981): The effect of aging on β-adrenoceptor stimulated cyclic AMP formation in human lymphocytes. Clinical Science 10: 587–589.
56. Franco-Morselli R, Elghozi JL, Joly E, Diginilio S, Meyer P (1977): Increased plasma adrenaline concentrations in benign essential hypertension. British Medical Journal 2: 1251–1254.
57. Bühler FR, Kiowki W, Landmann R, van Brummelen P, Amann W, Bolli P, Bertel O (1981): Changing role of beta- and alpha-adrenoceptor-mediated cardiovascular responses in the transition form high cardiac output into a peripheral resistance phase in essential hypertension. In: Frontiers in Hypertension Research edited by J.H. Laragh, F.R. Bühler and O.W. Seldin, pp. 316–324, Springer New York.

Converting enzyme inhibitors and hypertensive large arteries

ALAIN SIMON and JAIME LEVENSON

Because increased peripheral resistance is hemodynamically admitted as the primary cause of blood pressure elevation in essential hypertension [1], any antihypertensive drug might theoretically decrease peripheral resistance. This is the case of angiotensin converting enzyme (ACE) inhibitors which have been demonstrated to lower blood pressure through a fall in total peripheral resistance [2–3]. However, increasing attention must be also given to the action of drugs on the large arteries the distensibility of which is a major determination of the cardiac afterload [4] and of the arterial cyclic stress [4], two factors which strongly contribute in long-term to the occurrence of cardiovascular damage [5]. Moreover, since the large arteries of hypertensive patients are the site of various abnormalities including an increase in arterial calibre [6], an increase in pulse-wave velocity [6, 7] and a diminution of arterial compliance [8, 9], it must be a primary objective of antihypertensive treatment to reverse these arterial changes. The reason is that correction of these alterations in hypertensive large arteries might help to improve prophylaxis against the atherosclerotic complications of the disease. Thus the response of the large arteries to antihypertensive treatment represents a line of pharmacological research that should be followed up in the coming years. In this respect, the effects of two angiotensin converting enzyme (ACE) inhibitors (captopril and enalapril) have been studied on large arteries of essential hypertensive patients. These investigations concerned the whole arterial tree (aorta and peripheral arteries) evaluated by means of systemic arterial compliance [8], and also the large arteries of the forearm studied by means of pulsed Doppler velocimetry of the brachial artery [10].

I. Methodological approach

At present two methods are available for investigating the effects of ACE inhibitors on the large arteries in hypertension in man: the first, general in character, is based on the evaluation of systemic arterial compliance [8]. The second method, involving the arterial circulation of the forearm, has recourse to pulsed Doppler velocimetry of the brachial artery (see Part III).

1) Systemic arterial compliance

Systemic arterial compliance is an index representing the volumic distensibility of the aorta and the large peripheral arteries; it thus expresses the capacity to increase the arterial volume per unit of arterial pressure increase [11]. The most reliable evaluation of arterial compliance is based on analysis of the exponential diastolic pressure decay of the intrabrachial arterial pressure by using a simple model of arterial circulation [8]; in this way arterial compliance can be measured from 2 parameters [8]: a) the slope of the exponential decay of the intrabrachial diastolic pressure; b) the total peripheral resistance, which it is standard to calculate as the ratio of the mean brachial arterial pressure to the cardiac output.

2) Arterial circulation in the forearm

To facilitate analysis of the effects of hypertension on the large arteries a non-invasive technique based on pulsed Doppler velocimetry has been used for direct exploration of the brachial artery and its branches, the site where blood pressure is measured in human beings. The pulsed Doppler velocimeter used in clinical investigation of the arterial circulation of the forearm has been widely described and validated and allows the diameter of the brachial artery and the velocity of the circulating column of blood inside the artery to be measured transcutaneously [9, 10]. Besides measuring the diameter of the artery and its flow rate, the pulsed Doppler apparatus permits forearm arterial compliance to be evaluated [9, 12] by means of two methods.

The first one is based on the analysis of simultaneous recordings of the brachial artery pressure and flow according to a first-order model of the arterial circulation of the forearm during diastole [9]. Forearm arterial compliance is calculated as the ratio between the time constant of the diastolic pressure decay computorized according to the equations of the arterial model and the forearm vascular resistance calculated as the ratio between mean flow and pressure in the brachial artery [9]. The main limitation of this method is that it requires a punction of the brachial artery for the recording of the diastolic pressure wave.

The second method of evaluation of forearm arterial compliance [12] is completely non-invasive, can be applied to the long-term study of ambulatory patients, and is derived from the analysis of the brachial artery blood velocity contour recorded by pulsed Doppler. This contour exhibited a systolic flow followed by a constant plateau during diastole (Fig. 1). Brachial artery blood velocity can thus be represented as the sum of two components: a constant

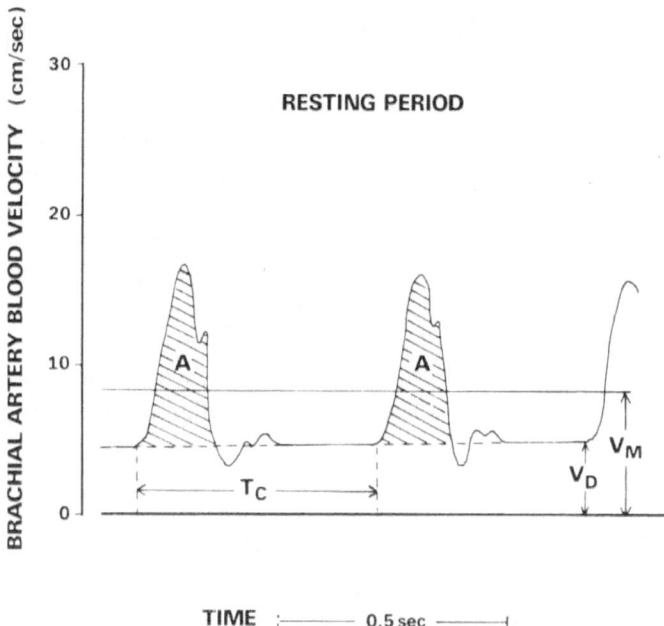

Figure 1. Typical brachial artery blood velocity contour. A, the hatched area, represents the integral of the part of the systolic blood velocity located above the extrapolation (dotted line) of diastolic velocity. Modified from Simon *et al.* [16].

velocity which is the extrapolation of the diastolic velocity (V_d) through the entire cardiac cycle, and a phasic velocity (V_s) which is the additional systolic velocity superimposed on the constant velocity. The amount of flow consequent on the distension of the large arteries, (vol), is equal to the integral of phasic velocity (hatched area of Fig. 1) multiplied by the brachial artery cross-sectional area [5], and is easily deduced from measurements of mean velocity (V_m) and diastolic velocity (V_d) and cardiac time T_c, using the formula vol = $(V_m - V_d) T_c \cdot S$. This (vol) rapidly introduced into the forearm arterial system corresponds, according to the waterhammer formula [16], to an increase in pressure equal to the pulse pressure (PP). The forearm arterial compliance (FAC), which represents the ratio of any change in arterial volume to corresponding change in arterial pressure of the forearm [10], can be calculated as the ratio of vol to PP, as follows: FAC = $(V_m - V_d) T_c \cdot S/PP$. The values of forearm arterial compliance obtained with the two methods were expressed in 10^{-4} ml/mm Hg and were found strongly correlated between them with a slope of regression not significantly different from unit and an y-axis intercept not statistically different from zero [12].

3) Pharmacological procedures

These arterial methodologies were applied to test the effects of ACE inhibitors

264

on hypertensive large arteries. For this purpose, two drugs (captopril and enal-april) were administered in uncomplicated essential hypertensive patients (I or II WHO) without any treatment at least one month before. Captopril was given in two different conditions [13]: (i) an acute experiment after a single dose of 100 mg in 7 patients, and (ii) a short-term treatment of five days (300 ± 20 mg per day) ± SEM in 5 other patients. Enalapril was randomly assigned at the end of a 4-week placebo period to 14 patients during 3 to 6 months of double-blind treatment with propranolol, and the mean dose obtained at the end of the third month of active treatment was 25 ± 5 mg per day [12, 14]. Group data were expressed as mean ± standard error of mean (SEM) and the comparison of the value of arterial parameters before and after drug was made by using the paired-t-test [15]. Differences in means and correlations were considered significant if the p value was less than 0.05.

II. Effects of ACE inhibitors on large arteries in hypertension

1) Systemic arterial compliance

Acute and short-term administration of captopril increased significantly systemic arterial compliance in essential hypertensive patients and concomitantly de-creased total peripheral resistance [13, 16] (Table 1). These results are in agree-ment with the increase in arterial compliance found in normal mildly sodium-depleted subjects after acute enalapril [17], and demonstrate that arterial effects of acute ACE inhibition are not only restricted to the arterioles but also concern the large arteries. Moreover, the comparison between acute and short-term arterial effects of captopril leads to two observations [16] (Fig. 2): (i) systemic arterial compliance is increased to the same extent in acute and short-term administration, but the decrease in total peripheral resistance is more pro-nounced after short-term than after acute captopril, suggesting that effects of

Table 1. Acute effects of captopril on systemic and forearm vascular resistance and arterial compliance in patients with essential hypertension. Data are shown as means ± SEM. * p<0.05. B = before, A = after captopril.

	Arterial Compliance (ml/mm Hg)		Vascular Resistance dynes · sec · cm^{-5}	
	Baseline	Captopril	Baseline	Captopril
Systemic Arteries	1.59 ± 0.06	1.95 ± 0.07*	1388 ± 66	1306 ± 72*
Forearm Arteries	(92 ± 7) 10^{-4}	(120 ± 10) 10^{-4}*	(208 ± 40) 10^3	(156 ± 36) 10^3*

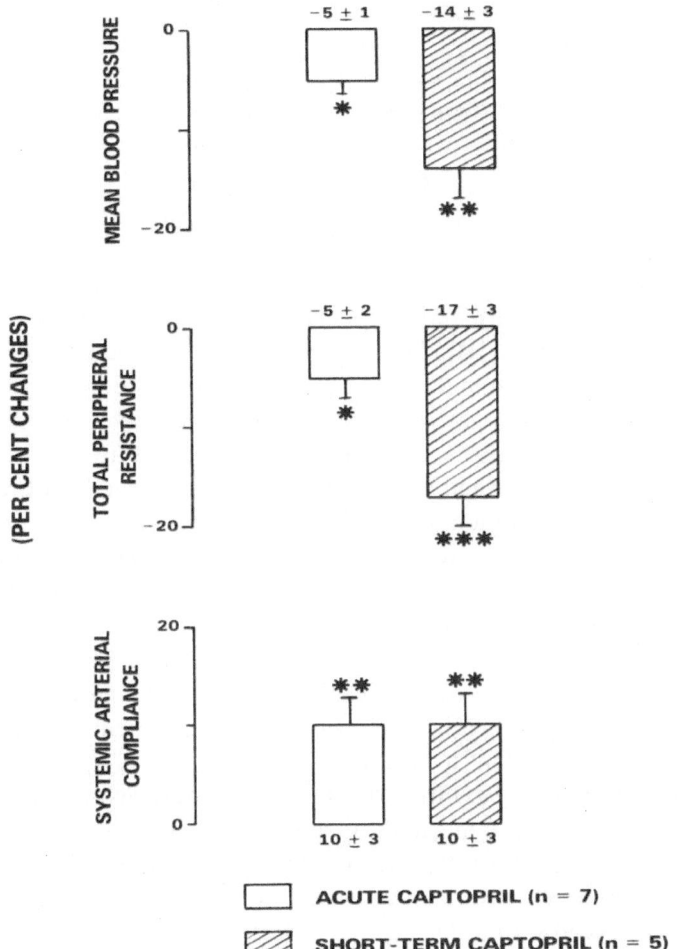

Figure 2. Percent change from baseline in mean blood pressure, total peripheral resistance, and systemic arterial compliance after acute and short-term administration of captopril in patients with essential hypertension. Data are shown as mean ± SEM. * p<0.05, * * p<0.01, * * * p<0.001. From Simon *et al.* [13] with permission.

ACE inhibition appear earlier on the large arteries than on the arterioles in essential hypertension; (ii) the decrease in total peripheral resistance is almost parallel with the decrease in blood pressure after acute and short-term captopril, but the increase in arterial compliance is not influenced by the degree of pressure fall, demonstrating that the improvement in arterial distensibility after captopril is not exclusively a mechanical consequence of pressure fall on the arterial stretch but may also signify a direct action of the drug on the arterial smooth muscle.

2) Forearm large arteries

Acute captopril increased significantly the diameter of the brachial artery [18]. The same arterial dilation was also obtained on long-term ACE inhibition, at 3 and 6 months of treatment with enalapril given alone [12, 14] (Fig. 3). However, the arterial dilation of captopril and enalapril can be counterbalanced by the blood pressure fall consecutive to the administration of these drugs in hypertension [11]. Indeed, a decrease in systemic pressure inside the lumen of large arteries, must mechanically and passively decrease their caliber because of a lesser stretch of their walls [11]. These opposite effects of active dilation of large arteries by ACE inhibition and passive arterial contraction induced by pressure fall are illustrated in the negative correlation between change in brachial artery diameter and change in mean blood pressure observed after acute captopril, indicating that dilation of the brachial artery is counterbalanced by the magnitude of pressure fall inside its lumen, so that the greater arterial dilation corresponds to the lesser reduction in pressure [13]. This observation finally demonstrates that ACE inhibitors may act directly on the large arteries independently of their action of lowering blood pressure.

Acute captopril increased arterial compliance and decreased simultaneously vascular resistance of the forearm (Table 1). Similar increase in arterial compliance of the forearm was also found on chronic treatment with enalapril [16] (Fig. 3). Thus it is important to consider how converting enzyme inhibition may increase arterial compliance. First, the increase in arterial compliance with ACE inhibitors may be a simple mechanical consequence of the pressure reduction, resulting in less distension of the arterial walls [11]. Second, arterial compliance may increase consecutively to a reduction in the smooth muscle tone of the brachial artery because of a decrease in angiotensin II concentration in plasma and/or in the walls of large arteries owing to inhibition of converting enzyme by enalapril. This hypothesis is supported by experimental studies in spontaneously hypertensive rats, showing that renin concentration was elevated in the walls of large arteries [18], and that this elevation responded to negative feedback inhibition, as suggested by the increase in renin activity in arterial tissue after inhibition of angiotensin II synthesis by captopril [19]. A further consideration in this respect is that both captopril and enalapril inhibit angiotensin-converting enzyme in large arteries to a greater extent than in other tissues of spontaneously hypertensive rats [20].

III. Consequences of arterial effects of ACE inhibitors on the function of large arteries

The large arteries serve two clear functions in the circulation, the conducting and the buffering function [4], and they also contain inside their walls the barorecep-

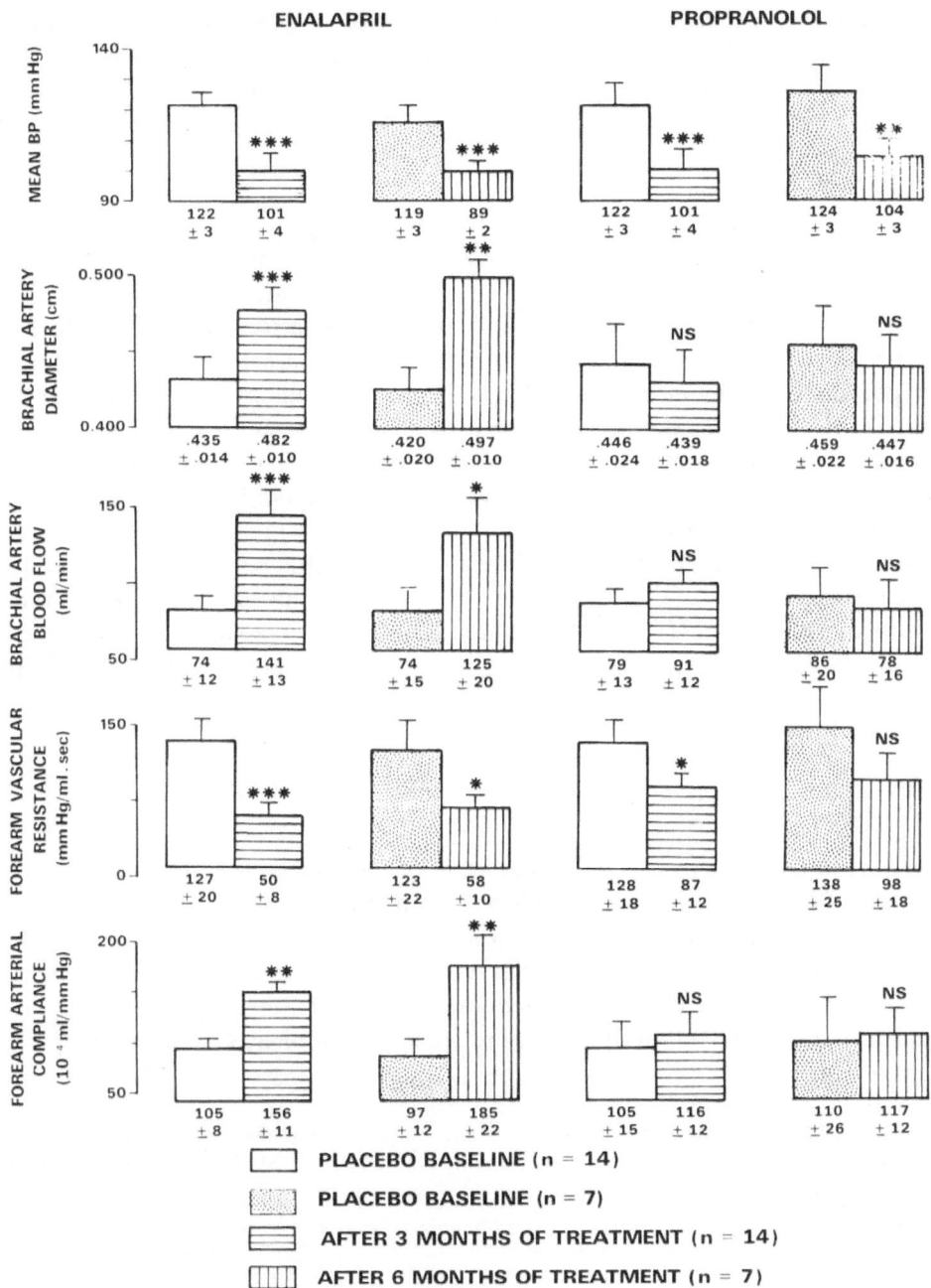

Figure 3. Changes in mean blood pressure (BP) and forearm arterial variables from placebo (baseline) to 3 and 6 months of treatment with enalapril or propranolol (n = number of patients). Data expressed as means ± 1 SEM. Asterisks indicate significant difference: one, p<0.05, two, p<0.01, three, p<0.001. From Simon *et al.* [16] with permission.

tors which participate to the baroreflex control of pressure and heart rate. Important modifications of these arterial functions may be expected from the effects of ACE inhibitors on large arteries in hypertension.

1) Buffering function

The buffering function of large arteries which consists in dampening the pulsatility of arterial pressure is altered in hypertension, as attested by the decreased arterial compliance [8, 9]; it ensues an increase in the arterial pulsatility which is reflected by an increased amplitude of pulse pressure [4]. Such an arterial hyperpulsatility, by causing a cyclic stress to the walls of large arteries, may induce in long-term the degradation of the bio-elastomeres constituting their walls [5]. In this respect, it is important to observe that acute and short-time angiotensin converting enzyme inhibition by captopril significantly reduced pulse pressure, the simplest index of pulsatility of arterial pressure (Table 2). The increase in arterial compliance induced by captopril is responsible for the decrease in pulse pressure as demonstrate by the observation of correlation between these two parameters (Fig. 4). Similar results were observed in chronic treatment with enalapril which significantly decreased pulse pressure at 3 and 6 months of treatment [16].

2) Conducting function

A second consequence of ACE inhibition of large arteries concerns their conducting function. Assuming that blood flow in a large artery equals the product between its section and the cross-sectional blood velocity inside its lumen [10], the dilation of large arteries obtained with ACE inhibition participates in the increase in arterial flow. This can be observed for the brachial artery with acute captopril [13] and chronic enalapril [16, 14] where brachial dilation acts concomitantly with

Table 2. Effects of acute and short-term captopril on mean blood pressure and pulse pressure in essential hypertensive patients; data are shown as mean ± 1 SEM. * $p<0.05$, ** $p<0.01$, *** $p<0.001$.

	Acute Captopril (n = 7)		Short-term Captopril (n = 5)	
	Before	After	Before	After
Mean Blood Pressure (mm Hg)	113 ± 4	106 ± 4**	139 ± 3	112 ± 4***
Pulse pressure (mm Hg)	80 ± 3	73 ± 3**	85 ± 6	71 ± 4*

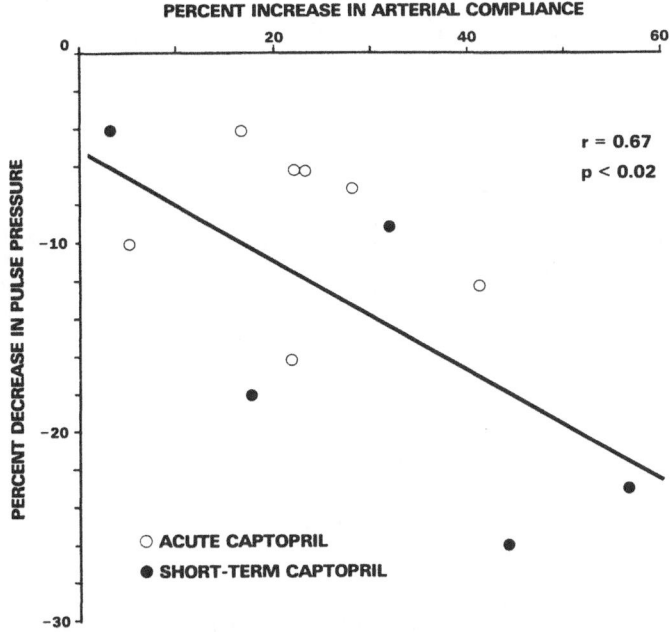

Figure 4. Correlation between percent increase in arterial compliance and percent decrease in pulse pressure after acute and short-term administration of captopril in essential hypertensive patients.

the increased blood velocity to increase strongly arterial flow (Fig. 3). However, the interest to increase arterial flow in the forearm must be questioned because blood flow in skeletal muscle and skin of mild to moderate hypertensive patients has been found to be within the normal range prior to treatment [10]. Moreover, the increase in flow in the forearm circulation by angiotensin converting enzyme inhibitors must be considered as a local effect which cannot be extrapolated to the systemic circulation; it does raise the question of whether this type of drugs affects other regional circulations in a similar or contrary way.

3) Baroreceptors stimulation

The dilation of the large arteries which accompanies ACE inhibition may modify the stimulation of baroreceptors, induced by the decrease in systemic pressure, because the baroreceptors located inside the walls of large arteries are stimulated not by arterial pressure itself but by the tension applied to the arterial walls [21]. The arterial wall tension can be simply evaluated by the law of Laplace $T = P \times R/h$ where T is the tangential tension of the artery, R and P the arterial radius and pressure en h the arterial thickness [22]. It ensues that change in tension (delta T) of large arteries depends not only on change in pressure (delta P) inside

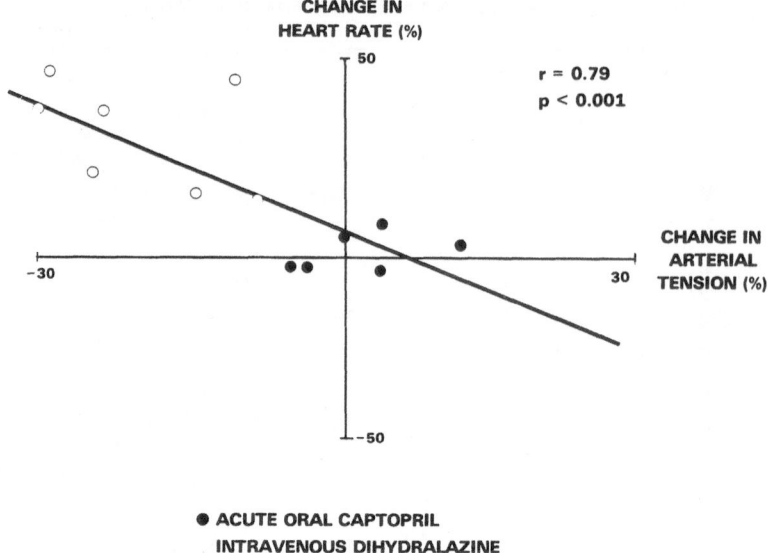

Figure 5. Correlation between change in brachial artery tension and change in heart rate after captopril and dihydralazine administration in essential hypertensive patients. From Simon *et al.* [16] with permission.

the lumen, but also on change in arterial radius (delta R) according to the formula delta T = P × delta R + R × delta P, on the condition that the wall thickness is assumed to be constant, which is a convenient hypothesis at least in acute conditions. The pulsed Doppler measurement of brachial artery radius before and after acute captopril has permitted to show with the latter formula that variation in tangential tension of the brachial artery was insignificant (1 ± 1 mm Hg/cm) because the arterial dilation counterbalances the decrease in systolic pressure and maintains the arterial tension normal [14, 16]. Such an effect may be extrapolated at the site of baroreceptors after captopril and suggests that unchanged tension of baroreceptors may participate in the lack of baroreflex tachycardia despite the reduction in arterial pressure. In contrast, the concomitant decrease in brachial artery caliber and pressure previously described with acute administration of a classical vasodilating drug, such as dihydralazine induces a strong reduction in arterial tension which stimulates the baroreceptors and produces a reflex tachycardia [23]. An additional argument in favour of the role of tension of large arteries on baroreflex response is given in the observation of a correlation between the change in brachial artery tension and the change in heart rate after acute captopril and intravenous dihydralazine administration in essential hypertensive patients [16] (Fig. 5). Lastly, the dilation of large arteries may also play a role on the baroreceptor sensitivity by increasing arterial compliance; baroreceptor sensitivity has indeed been demonstrated to increase in parallel with elevation of systemic arterial compliance after acute administration of enalapril in normal subjects [17], and it is well known that baroreflex sensitivity is closely related to arterial compliance [24]. Probably, the greater distensibility of large arteries after ACE inhibition increases the stimulation of baroreceptors inside their walls for a lower level of pressure in addition to other mechanisms relating ACE inhibition and sympathetic nervous activity.

IV. Conclusion

In conclusion, ACE inhibition induces acute and chronic dilation and increased compliance of hypertensive large arteries. Such an effect is not exclusively dependent on pressure fall which accompanies these drugs; it expresses also a direct response of the walls of large arteries to converting enzyme inhibition. These large artery modifications have several consequences on the arterial function. They dampen the baroreceptor stimulation induced by the systemic pressure fall and might so explain partly the lack of reflex tachycardia observed with these drugs. The response of large arteries to converting enzyme inhibitors produce also an improvement of their conducting and buffering function. This latter effect by reducing the arterial pulsatility might be at long term advantageous for the prevention of degenerative arterial disease, which continues to affect many hypertensive patients treated with classical antihypertensive drugs [25].

References

1. Folkow B (1982): Physiological aspects of primary hypertension. Physiol Reviews, 62: 347–503.
2. Tarazi RC, Bravo EL, Fouad FM, Corvik P, Cody JP (1980): Hemodynamic and volume changes associated with captopril. Hypertension, 2: 576–584.
3. Fouad FM, Tarazi RC, Bravo EL, Textor SO (1982): Antihypertensive effects of MK 421: Hemodynamic and humoral correlates. Clin Pharma Ther 31: 227–233.
4. O'Rourke MF (1982): Arterial function in health and disease (1982): Churchill Livingstone, Edinburgh-London-Melbourne-New York, pp. 196–252.
5. Gent AN. Fracture of elastomeres. In: Fracture H, Liebowith (ed), Academic Press, New York.
6. Simon A, Levenson J, Bouthier J, Safar M, Avolio AP (1985): Evidence of early degenerative changes in large arteries in human essential hypertension. Hypertension 7: 675–680.
7. Gribbin B, Pickering TG, Sleight P (1979): Arterial distensibility in normal and hypertensive man. Clin Science 56: 413–417.
8. Simon ACh, Safar ME, Levenson JA, London GM, Levy BI, Chau NP (1979): An evaluation of large arteries compliance in man. Am J Physiol 237 [5] H: 550–554.
9. Simon ACh, Laurent S, Levenson JA, Bouthier JE, Safar ME (1983): Estimation of forearm arterial compliance in normal and hypertensive men from simultaneous pressure and flow measurements in the brachial artery, using a pulsed Doppler device a first-order arterial model during diastole. Cardiovasc Res, 17: 331–338.
10. Levenson JA, Peronneau P, Simon ACh, Safar ME (1981): Pulsed Doppler: determination of diameter blood velocity and volume flow of brachial artery in man. Cardio Vasc Res 15: 164–170.

11. Hallock P, Benson IC (1937): Studies on the elastic properties of human elastic aorta. J Clin Invest, 16: 595–602.
12. Simon ACh, Levenson JA, Bouthier JD, Safar ME (1985): Effects of chronic administration of Enalapril and Propranolol on the large arteries in essential hypertension. J Cardiovasc Pharmacol 7: 856–861.
13. Simon ACh, Levenson JA, Bouthier JE, Safar ME (1984): Captopril induced changes in large arteries in essential hypertension. Amer J Med, 76 (5B): 71–75.
14. Simon ACh, Levenson JA, Bouthier JE & al (1984): Comparison of oral MK 421 and propranolol in mild and moderate essential hypertension and their effects on arterial and venous vessels of the forearm. Amer J Cardiol 53: 781–785.
15. Draper N, Smith H (1966): Applied regression analysis. New York, John Wiley: pp. 4–33.
16. Simon ACh, Levenson JA, Bouthier J, Maarek B, Safar ME (1985): Effects of acute and chronic angiotensin-converting enzyme inhibition on large arteries in human hypertension. J Cardiovasc Pharmacol 7: S45–S51.
17. Ibsen H, Egan B, Osterziel K, Vander H, Julius S (1983): Reflex hemodynamic adjustments and baroreflex sensitivity during converting enzyme inhibition with MK 421 in normal humans. Hypertension, 5: 184–191.
18. Swales JD (1979): Arterial wall or plasma renin in hypertension. Clin Sci 56: 593–303.
19. Assad MM, Antonaccio MJ (1982): Vascular wall renin in spontaneously hypertensive rats. Potential relevance to hypertension. Maintenance and antihypertensive effects of captopril. Hypertension 4: 487–493.
20. Cohen ML, Kurz KD (1982): Angiotensin converting enzyme inhibition in tissues from spontaneously hypertensive rats after treatment with captopril or MK 421. J Pharmacol Exper Ther 220: 63–69.
21. Milnor WR (1982): Hemodynamics. Williams and Wilkins, Baltimore.
22. Rushmer RK (1970): Cardiovascular Dynamics. Philadelphia, W.B. Saunders, pp. 163–167.
23. Safar ME, Simon ACh, Levenson JA, Cazor SL (1983): Hemodynamic effects of diltiazem in hypertension. Circul Res (Sup I) 52: 169–173.
24. Randal US, Elser MD, Bulloch GF & al (1976): Relationship of age and blood pressure to baroreflex sensitivity and arterial compliance in man. Clin Sci 51: 357–360.
25. Freis ED (1982): The veterans' trial and sequelae. Brit J Clin Pharm 13: 67–72.

Calcium entry blockers and the forearm arterial bed

BRIAN F. ROBINSON

The smooth muscle cells in the walls of blood vessels are endowed with several mechanisms by which the concentration of calcium in the cytosol can be raised and contraction initiated [1, 2]. One important system is that of the voltage-dependent calcium channels in the plasma membrane. Voltage-dependent channels, as their name implies, open to permit the influx of calcium when the membrane is depolarised either spontaneously or in response to a stimulus; some channels with similar characteristics are, however, thought to be linked to α_2-adrenoceptors and may thus be directly activated by noradrenaline. The influx of calcium through channels of the voltage-dependent type is inhibited by calcium entry blockers such as verapamil, diltiazem and compounds of the dihydro-pyridine group including nifedipine and nitrendipine.

The importance of the voltage-dependent calcium channels in triggering contraction varies greatly between differing types of vessel [3]. Some vascular responses appear wholly dependent on this system. The phasic activity of rat portal vein and the contraction of veins or arterial strips depolarised by exposure to high concentrations of potassium are mediated entirely by this system of activation. Contractions arising in this way are completely inhibited by relatively low concentrations of verapamil or nifedipine. Other mechanisms of activation exist, however, and are of major importance in certain types of contraction. The contraction of a hand vein induced by noradrenaline provides a good example of a response that depends almost entirely on these other mechanisms. Activation is initiated by the interaction of the agonist with specific receptors in the surface membrane; this leads to the release of calcium from the endoplasmic reticulum and it is possible that there is also calcium entry through membrane channels that are solely operated through receptors and have quite different characteristics to the voltage-dependent channels. The existence of such receptor-operated channels is, however, uncertain. Contractions induced through the receptor-operated system are less easily inhibited by verapamil than similar contractions induced by depolarisation and they are completely resistant to nifedipine [4]. They are, however, selectively inhibited by sodium nitroprusside and glyceryl trinitrate. It should be noted, however, that agonists such as noradrenaline are not limited to acting through the receptor-operated system but can also activate the voltage-dependent system directly through their ability to depolarise the membrane.

It thus appears that the two main activation systems for vascular smooth muscle can be differentially inhibited by calcium entry blockers and sodium nitroprusside respectively. Examination of the comparative effects of these two types of dilator on a particular vessel or vascular bed may therefore provide some insight into the activation mechanisms responsible for the maintenance of vascular tone.

In relation to the development of primary hypertension, the behaviour of the resistance vessels is clearly of major importance. There is evidence to suggest that the maintenance of tone in the resistance vessels involves contributions from both activation systems. In the forearm, which provides the only vascular bed easily available for study in man, the resistance vessels are sensitive to relatively low concentrations of calcium entry blockers and also sodium nitroprusside; neither class of dilator, however, is able to induce complete relaxation when given by itself [5]. This suggests that the contraction of the smooth muscle in the vessel walls is in part dependent on the entry of calcium through voltage-dependent channels, but also involves activation of the receptor-operated mechanism. It is to be expected that other resistance vessels will show a similar pattern although the relative contribution from the two activation systems may well differ. In the skin, for example, sympathetically mediated constriction dominates and intrinsic tone is relatively weak; this is likely to result in greater activity of the receptor-operated system than in the forearm with a corresponding reduction in voltage-dependent activity.

Responsiveness of forearm resistance vessels to calcium entry blocking agents in normal subjects and patients with hypertension

The responsiveness of the forearm arterial bed to dilator agents can conveniently be assessed by infusing drugs into the brachial artery while measuring the resultant change in forearm flow by venous occlusion plethysmography using mercury-in-silastic gauges. Local administration of drugs has the advantage that systemic circulatory effects can be avoided and the interpretation of flow changes is not confused by simultaneous changes in arterial pressure. This approach has been used in my own laboratory and it has also been extensively employed by Professor F. Bühler and Dr P. Bolli in Basel. The summary that follows is based on work carried out by both groups.

The dilator response of the forearm vascular bed to local infusion of verapamil is increased in patients with hypertension when compared to normal subjects (Fig. 1). At all dose rates the increase in flow induced by verapamil is greater in patients than in controls and the difference in response persists when the dose is increased to produce a maximal response [5, 6]. The increase in responsiveness is

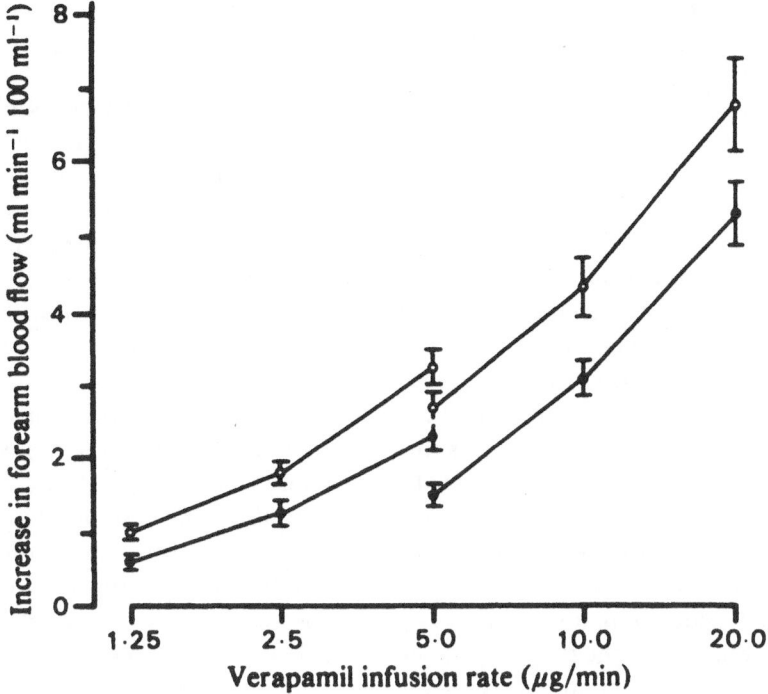

Figure 1. Increase in forearm blood flow in response to infusion of verapamil into the brachial artery. At every dose, the response in 20 patients with hypertension (open circles) is greater than that in 23 normotensive controls (closed circles); values shown are mean ± SEM. Reproduced with permission from Clinical Science [6].

not specific to verapamil and has also been demonstrated with nicardipine [7].

There are two possible explanations for the increased sensitivity of hypertensive resistance vessels to the dilator action of calcium entry blocking agents. It could result from a functional change in the smooth muscle cells. It could, however, arise as a direct consequence of structural change in the arterioles in which case no functional disorder of the smooth muscle need be inferred. Folkow has pointed out that the increase in wall thickness that is known to accompany raised arterial pressure must be expected to augment both constrictor and dilator responses: the inner part of the thickened wall encroaches on the lumen and the effect on resistance of any change in contraction of the smooth muscle will necessarily be increased [8].

If the enhanced response to calcium entry blockers in patients with hypertension was entirely dependent on altered vascular geometry, a similar increase in response should be seen with other dilators. In considering the importance of the structural factor it is therefore important to observe the response to a dilator which has a different mechanism of action to that of the calcium entry blockers.

Sodium nitroprusside is a suitable drug for this purpose. Its exact mechanism of action remains uncertain, but it is clear that it induces relaxation by inhibiting mechanisms of contraction other than those affected by calcium entry blockers.

At doses just above threshold, the dilator response of the forearm vascular bed to local infusion of sodium nitroprusside is similar in patients to that in normal subjects [6]; at higher doses the response in patients may even be depressed (Fig. 2). This finding makes it very unlikely that the increased response to verapamil is the result of structural changes in the vessels since if this was so, the response to nitroprusside should be similarly increased.

The relation between the response to verapamil and that to nitroprusside is most clearly seen when responses to the two drugs are compared in individual subjects (Fig. 3). In normal subjects, the increases in blood flow induced by verapamil and nitroprusside vary widely, but there is a close correlation between responses to the two drugs. This is interpreted as showing that the non-specific factors that influence the magnitude of the response to any infused drug (arm size, resting blood flow, distribution of infused drug) affect the response to the two dilators equally. In about two thirds of the patients with hypertension, the response to verapamil is considerably in excess of that expected from the response to nitroprusside. In many of these patients, the response to verapamil is abso-lutely increased and the response to nitroprusside is within the normal range. In a few, however, the response to verapamil appears normal and it is the response to nitroprusside that is reduced; it cannot be excluded that some patients show a true reduction in responsiveness to this drug. It seems likely, however, that in most patients the primary abnormality is enhancement of the response to verapamil rather than depression of the response to nitroprusside since, as will be seen, induced alterations in the functional state of the vessel always cause changes in the response to verapamil rather than in that to nitroprusside. It thus seems reasonable to conclude that the hypertensive resistance vessel exhibits a real increase in its responsiveness to verapamil and that this reflects an underlying functional change in the vascular smooth muscle.

Nature of the functional change in the resistance vessels of patients with hypertension

The most likely explanation of the enhanced dilator response to verapamil in the hypertensive resistance vessel is an increase in the contribution of the voltage-dependent system for calcium entry to the maintenance of smooth muscle tone. There are, however, two other possibilities that need to be considered.

One concerns the possibility of a functional rather than a mechanical effect of medial thickening. In small arteries, sympathetic nerve terminals are confined to the outer aspect of the media [9] and there is presumably a similar distribution of innervation in the arterioles. In patients with hypertension, the smooth muscle

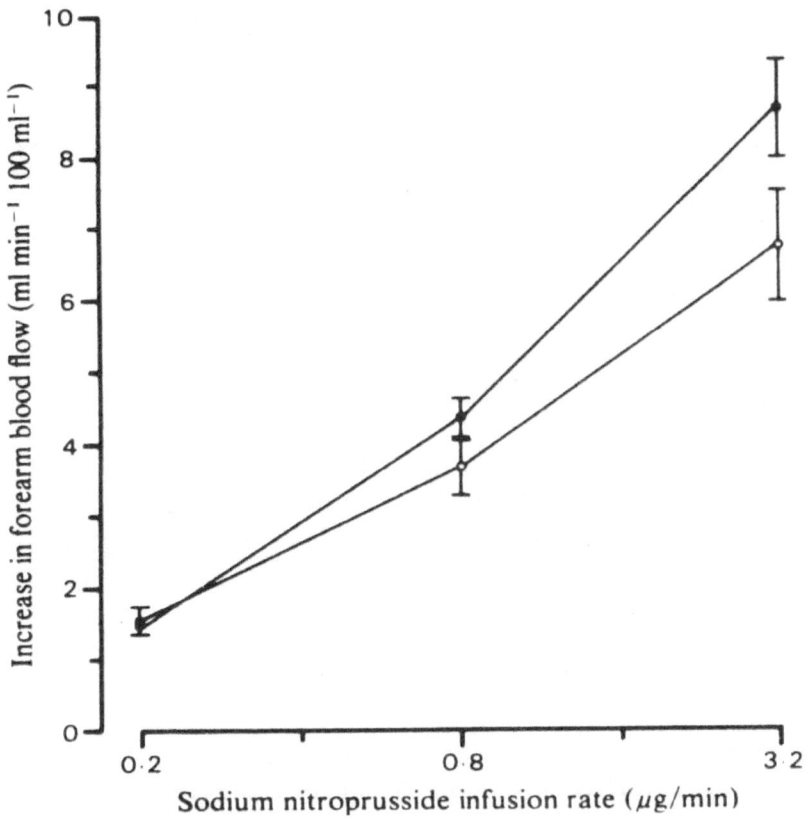

Figure 2. Increase in forearm blood flow in response to infusion of sodium nitroprusside into the brachial artery. Response in the 20 patients with hypertension (open circles) is similar to that in the 23 normotensive controls (closed circles) at the lower doses, but tends to be reduced at the highest dose (P = 0.06). Reproduced with permission from Clinical Science [6].

layer is thickened and the inner cells will, in consequence, be further from the source of noradrenaline release. It is at least possible that this would make them more dependent on the voltage-dependent mechanism for their activation and less dependent on the receptor-operated mechanism with a resultant change in sensitivity to dilator agents. This would imply that the functional change in the vessels was an indirect consequence of structural adaptation and did not result from a fundamental change in the cells themselves.

The second possibility relates to impaired removal of calcium from the cell: if calcium efflux were depressed, this would augment the effect of any change in calcium influx on the concentration of the ion in the cytosol and this might lead to an exaggerated dilator response to calcium entry blocking agents. The extrusion of calcium from vascular smooth muscle cells is thought to be dominated by the activity of the ATP-dependent calcium pump [10]. There is conflicting evidence as to the functional state of this system in primary hypertension. Studies of inside-

278

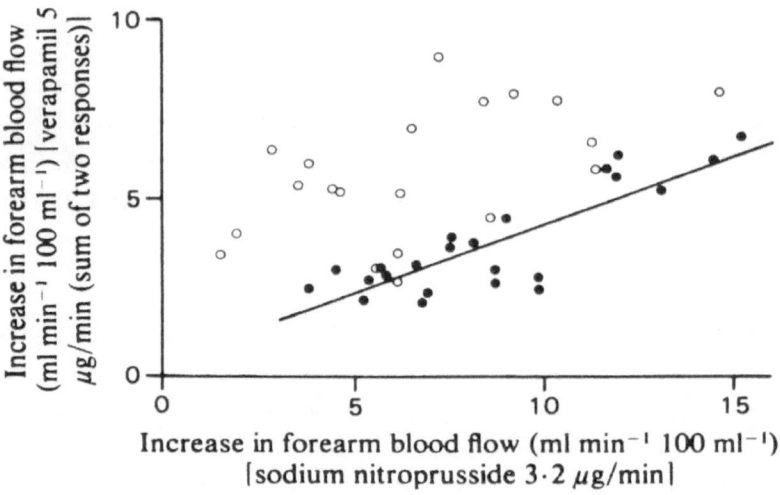

Figure 3. Response of forearm blood flow to verapamil (sum of duplicate responses to 5 μg/min) related to response to sodium nitroprusside (3.2 μg/min). In normal subjects (closed circles), there is a close correlation between responses to the two drugs (r = 0.85; P<0.001). In most patients with hypertension (open circles), the response to verapamil is enhanced relative to that to nitroprusside. Reproduced with permission from Clinical Science [6].

out membrane vesicles derived from mesenteric arteries of the spontaneously hypertensive rat (SHR) have shown ATP-dependent calcium uptake to be reduced [11]. This has been thought to reflect impaired function of the ATP-dependent calcium pump, but the same change would be observed if the vesicles were abnormally permeable to calcium so that the ion leaked away more rapidly than usual. Calcium fluxes in both lymphocytes and platelets of the SHR have been measured by methods which enable influx and efflux to be studied separately. In these experiments, calcium influx was found to be raised but there was no significant change in calcium pumping ability [12]; these findings suggest that the reduced calcium accumulation by the inside-out vesicles may indeed result from increased leakage rather than decreased pumping. No comparable studies have been carried out in man, but evidence is accumulating which indicates that the Ca^{2+}-dependent ATPase of platelet plasma membrane is in some way abnormal in patients with primary hypertension. The specific activity of the Ca^{2+}-dependent ATPase is increased, but the enzyme is functionally abnormal in that it is less easily inhibited by La^{3+} [13] and less easily stimulated by calmodulin [14] than that from normal subjects. It thus appears that there is an increase in the total amount of enzyme in the membrane, but that it may be less effective in pumping calcium. The net effect of these changes on the extrusion of calcium from the platelet is uncertain and the implication for calcium pump function in the cells of the vascular smooth muscle quite unknown. Nevertheless, these studies indicate that there are abnormalities of the Ca^{2+}-dependent ATPase of the platelet plasma membrane in patients with hypertension, and the possibility that impaired ATP dependent calcium pumping contributes to the observed alteration in responsiveness of the resistance vessels cannot be excluded.

Whatever the underlying cause of the functional change in the hypertensive resistance vessel, the degree of abnormality bears a direct relation to the severity of the hypertension [15]: responsiveness to verapamil is significantly correlated with mean arterial pressure over a wide range from normal to severe hypertension (Fig. 4). This relationship does not, of course, imply that there is a causal correlation between the functional change in the vessels and the rise in arterial pressure. It is even possible that the functional change is a consequence of the elevated pressure but this seems unlikely.

Effect of local infusion of ouabain and calcium on vascular responsiveness

The leucocytes of patients with hypertension show an increase in intracellular sodium and this results from reduced activity of the sodium pump [16]. The dilator response to local infusion of low concentrations of potassium is mediated by stimulation of the sodium pump; the response to potassium is significantly reduced in the forearm vascular bed of patients with hypertension [17] and this suggests that sodium pump activity is reduced in the resistance vessels in a manner analogous to that in the leucocytes. It seemed possible that the enhanced response to verapamil observed in patients with hypertension might depend in some way on the reduction in sodium pump activity. We therefore investigated the effect of an acute depression of sodium pump activity in normal subjects produced by local infusion of ouabain [18]. The drug was infused into the brachial artery at a rate calculated to produce a plasma concentration about 100 times greater than those that are achieved during systemic administration and have been shown to cause acute depression of sodium pump activity. During the infusion of ouabain, there was an increase in forearm vascular resistance and the dilator response to local infusion of K^+ was reduced by 33%, confirming that significant inhibition of the sodium pump had been achieved. The dilator response to verapamil was, however, unchanged and there was no significant change in the response to nitroprusside. This study showed that the enhanced response to verapamil is not a consequence of the impaired activity of the sodium pump.

Modest changes in plasma calcium concentration cause changes in the response of the resistance vessels to verapamil. In normal subjects, infusion of calcium into the brachial artery at a rate sufficient to increase the concentration in venous blood leaving the arm by about 0.5 mmol/l caused a small fall in forearm blood flow with a proportionately larger fall in the response to verapamil [19]. This is interpreted as showing inactivation of voltage-dependent calcium channels by the increased extracellular calcium concentration. When the infusion of calcium was

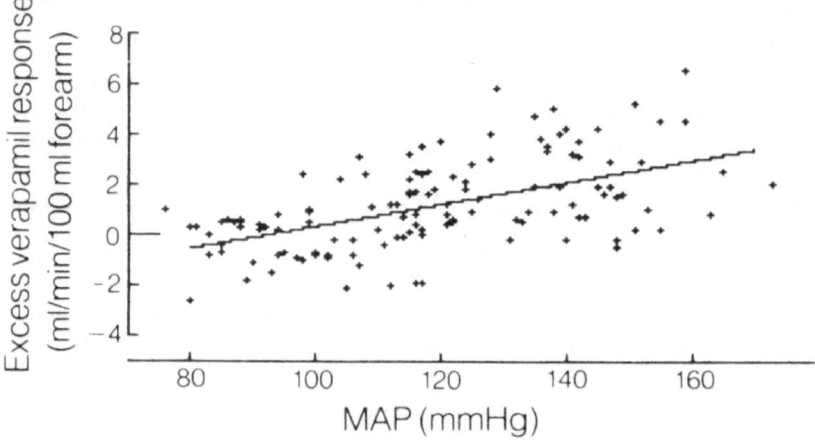

Figure 4. Relative responsiveness of forearm resistance vessels to verapamil related to mean arterial pressure in 127 men. The 'excess verapamil response' is the amount by which the sum of the responses to two infusions of verapamil at $5\,\mu$g/min exceeds that predicted for the observed response to nitroprusside from the regression line in normal subjects (Fig. 3). There is a highly significant relation between response to verapamil and arterial pressure ($r = 0.55$; $P<0.001$). Reproduced with permission from J. Hypertension [15].

discontinued, resting flow returned to the control level, but in most subjects response to verapamil increased so that in a series of 11 normal men, the control level was, on average, exceeded by 34% (Fig. 5). The mechanism of this rebound is unknown. In parallel studies in which response to nitroprusside was examined, no significant change was seen either during or after infusion of calcium. In patients with primary hypertension, infusion of calcium depressed the response to verapamil to a similar extent to that seen in normal subjects [20]. In a subsequent study of 13 men with primary hypertension in whom the response to verapamil was examined after calcium was discontinued, the pattern was found to differ from that in normal subjects in that there was no increase in the dilator effect of verapamil when the plasma calcium concentration fell back to normal (Fig. 5). These observations indicate that responsiveness to verapamil is influenced by changes in plasma calcium concentration and they suggest that there may be differences in the regulation of voltage-dependent calcium channels between patients with hypertension and normal subjects. Increased activity of the calcium channels in patients might thus result from a defect in regulatory mechanisms rather than an increase in the number of channels.

Effect of treatment

Treatment of hypertension with a diuretic, two different β-adrenoceptor blockers and a calcium entry blocker has in all cases been shown to diminish the respon-

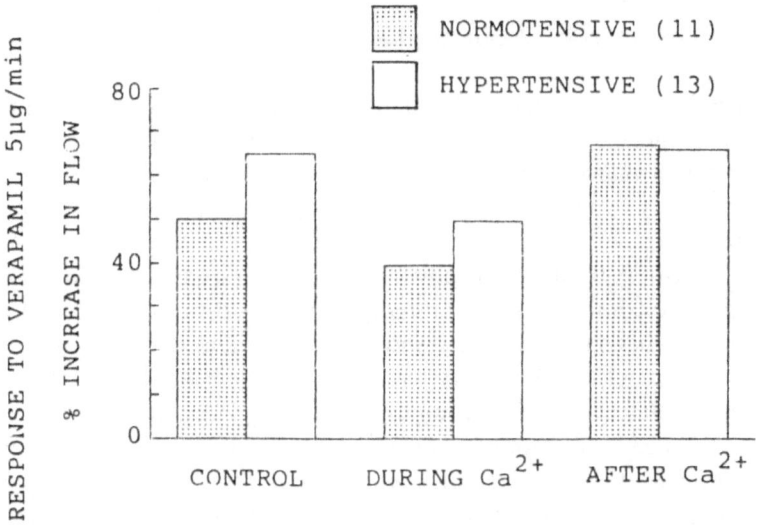

Figure 5. Response to paired infusions of verapamil, 5 μg/min, expressed as percentage increase over control flow, in 11 men with normal arterial pressure and 13 men with mild to moderate hypertension. Before infusion of calcium, response to verapamil tends, as expected, to be lower in normal subjects than in the patients. During infusion of calcium at 10 μmol/min, response to verapamil is depressed in both groups. When calcium is discontinued, response to verapamil rebounds above control level in normal subjects, but not in the patients. Both groups now show very similar responsiveness. The results suggest that the regulation of calcium channels by extra cellular calcium may differ from normal in patients with hypertension.

siveness of the forearm vascular bed to local infusion of a calcium entry blocker.

In all of 16 patients with primary hypertension, treatment with chlorthalidone 50 mg daily for one month caused a decrease in the relative responsiveness of the forearm resistance vessels to verapamil [21]. The effect on responsiveness was proportionately greater than the effect on arterial pressure, suggesting that the change in sensitivity to verapamil was not merely secondary to the change in pressure. A similar, though slightly less consistent reduction in responsiveness to verapamil was observed during treatment with atenolol [21] and reduced responsiveness to nitrendipine has been observed during treatment with acebutolol [22]. A similar reduction in responsiveness to local nitrendipine was observed during oral treatment with the same drug [22].

It is not surprising that systemic treatment with a calcium entry blocking agent reduces the local response to the same drug. It is, however, of considerable interest that treatment with such diverse agents as diuretics and β-adrenoceptor blockers should have the same effect. The reduced responsiveness to calcium entry blockers might reflect no more than an indirect effect of both types of antihypertensive such as, for example, an increase in sympathetic activity at α-adrenoceptors. It is possible, however, that normalisation of the functional disorder in the resistance vessels represents a mechanism through which both types of drug act to reduce arterial pressure.

Relation between forearm vascular bed and the circulation as a whole

The forearm resistance vessels make up no more than a small fraction of the total peripheral resistance and the relevance of the abnormalities found in the forearm bed to the performance of the general circulation may well be questioned. In studies with many drugs, however, the forearm bed has given results that appeared representative of the circulation as a whole. Patients with hypertension have been reported to show proportionately larger reductions in pressure in response to acute administration of nifedipine than is the case in normal subjects [23, 24]. This has been interpreted as showing a generalised increase in sensitivity to calcium entry blockade similar to that observed experimentally in the forearm. The validity of relating the fall in pressure induced by drugs to the initial pressure has, however, been questioned and it is difficult to interpret the results of systemic administration of drugs since reflex effects may limit the fall in pressure. It is therefore difficult to demonstrate a generalised increase in sensitivity to the dilator action of calcium entry blocking agents.

Even if the increased responsiveness to verapamil were confined to the vessels of skeletal muscle, it might still be of considerable importance in the genesis and maintenance of hypertension. Skeletal muscle accounts in total for a substantial fraction of the peripheral vascular bed and since flow in muscle can vary more widely in response to changes in pressure than is the case in organs such as the kidney and brain, the muscle bed may play an important role in circulatory control, serving as a safety valve to accommodate transient increases in cardiac output. Any alteration in the responses of the resistance vessels in the muscular bed might thus be of critical importance to the behaviour of the circulation as a whole, and a sustained increase in resistance in this bed alone might serve to initiate the hypertensive process.

References

1. Carafoli E (1984): How calcium crosses plasma membranes including the sarcolemma. In: Opie LH (ed) Calcium antagonists and cardiovascular disease. New York, Raven Press, pp. 29–41.
2. Triggle DJ (1985): Calcium ions and respiratory smooth muscle function. Br J Clin Pharmacol 20: 213s–219s.
3. Robinson BF, Collier JG, Dobbs RJ (1979): Comparative dilator effect of verapamil and sodium nitroprusside in forearm arterial bed and dorsal hand veins in man: functional differences between vascular smooth muscle in arterioles and veins. Cardiovasc Res 13: 16–21.
4. Robinson BF, Dobbs RJ, Kelsey CR (1980): Effects of nifedipine on resistance vessels, arteries and veins in man. Br J Clin Pharmacol 10: 433–438.
5. Hulthén UL, Bolli P, Amann FW, Kiowski W, Bühler FR (1982): Enhanced vasodilatation in essential hypertension by calcium channel blockade with verapamil. Hypertension, 4 suppl II: 26–31.
6. Robinson BF, Dobbs RJ, Bayley S (1982): Response of forearm resistance vessels to verapamil and sodium nitroprusside in normotensive and hypertensive men: evidence for a functional

abnormality of vascular smooth muscle in primary hypertension. Clin Sci 63: 33–42.

7. Bühler FR, Bolli P, Hulthén UL (1984): Calcium influx-dependent vasoconstrictor mechanisms in essential hypertension. In: Opie LH (ed) Calcium antagonists and cardiovascular disease. New York, Raven Press, pp. 313–322.

8. Folkow B (1978): Cardiovascular structural adaptation: its role in the initiation and maintenance of primary hypertension. Clin Sci Mol Med 55 (suppl 4): 3s–22s.

9. Keatinge WR (1979): Blood-vessels. Br Med Bull 35: 249–254.

10. Brading AF, Lategan TW (1985): Na-Ca exchange in vascular smooth muscle. J Hypertension 3: 109–116.

11. Kwan CY, Belbeck L, Daniel EE (1980): Abnormal biochemistry of vascular smooth muscle plasma membrane isolated from hypertensive rats. Mol Pharmacol 17: 137–140.

12. Bruschi G, Bruschi ME, Orlandini G, Cavatorta A, Borghetti A, Ferrandi M, Bianchi G (1985): Why is Ca_i^{2+} increased in blood cells in primary hypertension?: J. Hypertension 3 (suppl 3): s45–s47.

13. Graham JM, Robinson BF, Wilson RBJ (1985): (Ca^{2+} + Mg^{2+})-ATPase activity of a platelet membrane fraction from normal subjects and patients with hypertension (Abstract). J Hypertension 3: 664.

14. Resink TJ, Tkachuk VA, Erne P, Bühler FR (1986): Platelet membrane calmodulin-stimulated calcium-adenosine triphosphatase: altered activity in essential hypertension. Hypertension 8: 159–166.

15. Robinson BF (1984): Altered calcium handling as a cause of primary hypertension. J Hypertension 2: 453–460.

16. Hilton PJ (1986): Cellular sodium transport in essential hypertension. N Engl J Med 314: 222–229.

17. Phillips RJW, Robinson BF (1984): The dilator response to K^+ is reduced in the forearm resistance vessels of men with primary hypertension. Clin Sci 66: 237–239.

18. Robinson BF, Phillips RJW, Wilson PN, Chiodini PL (1983): Effect of local infusion of ouabain on human forearm vascular resistance and on response to potassium, verapamil and sodium nitroprusside. J Hypertension 1: 165–169.

19. Robinson BF, Phillips RJW (1984): Effect of small increments in plasma calcium concentration on the responsiveness of forearm resistance vessels to verapamil in normal subjects. Clin Sci 67: 613–618.

20. Robinson BF, Benjamin N, Phillips RJW (1984): Small increments in plasma calcium concentration reduce the responsiveness of forearm resistance vessels to verapamil in men with primary hypertension. J Hypertension 2 (suppl 3): 507–509.

21. Robinson BF, Dobbs RJ, Phillips RJW (1983): Effect of treatment with chlorthalidone and atenolol on response to dilator agents in the forearm resistance vessels of men with primary hypertension. Br J Clin Pharmacol 16: 327–332.

22. Bolli P, Erne P, Hulthén UL, Ritz R, Kiowski W, Ji BH, Bühler FR (1984): Parallel reduction of calcium-influx-dependent vasoconstriction and platelet-free calcium concentration with calcium entry and β-adrenoceptor blockade. J Cardiovasc Pharmacol 6: S996–S1001.

23. MacGregor GA, Markandu ND, Rotellar C, Smith SJ, Sagnella GA (1983): The acute response to nifedipine is related to pre-treatment blood pressure. Postgrad Med J 59 (suppl 2): 91–94.

24. Lederballe Pedersen O, Christensen NJ, Rämsch KD (1980): Comparison of acute effects of nifedipine in normotensive and hypertensive man. J Cardiovasc Pharmacol 2: 357–366.

Cations and the forearm circulation in hypertensive humans

A. TAKESHITA and T. IMAIZUMI

1. Introduction

Epidemiological studies suggest that excess salt intake contributes to the prevalence of essential hypertension in humans [1]. For the past 15 years, there has been a considerable interest in the effects of excess salt intake on blood pressure and vascular resistance in humans [2–13]. Several important features as to the relationship between excess salt intake and blood pressure in humans have been delineated in these studies. First, it has been clearly shown that effects of dietary salt loading on blood pressure and vascular resistance vary considerably among subjects. Dietary salt loading may produce a marked increase in blood pressure in some but may not alter blood pressure in others [4–6, 11, 13]. Generally speaking, hypertensive patients are more sensitive to dietary salt loading than normotensive subjects [5, 7, 8, 10, 11]. However, it has also been shown that there is a considerable variation in responses to salt loading even among hypertensive patients [4, 6, 13]. The findings of variable responses to salt loading in humans are consistent with the findings in experimental animals [14–18]. Excess salt intake increases blood pressure and vascular resistance in rats with genetic hypertension but does not alter them in normotensive control rats [14–18].

Second, it has been shown that a reduced natriuretic capacity is a characteristic common to salt-sensitive humans [4,5] and rats [19]. An impaired renal ability to excrete sodium leads to a greater retention of body fluid during excess salt intake. It has been shown that increases in body weight and cardiac output during excess salt intake are greater in patients with essential hypertension whose blood pressure rises in response to salt loading (salt-sensitive) than in those whose blood pressure does not rise (salt-nonsensitive) [4, 13].

Third, there seem to be differences in control of vascular resistance during dietary salt loading between salt-sensitive and salt-nonsensitive humans. In salt-nonsensitive subjects, vascular resistance decreases during salt loading [2, 5, 8, 20]. In these men, the decrease in vascular resistance compensates the increase in cardiac output and thus blood pressure does not rise. In contrast, such compensatory decrease in vascular resistance does not occur in salt-sensitive patients with essential hypertension, which leads to the rise in blood pressure [10, 11, 13]. Thus, an abnormal control of vascular resistance in addition to a greater volume retention may contribute to the salt-induced elevation of blood pressure in salt-sensitive patients with essential hypertension.

In this chapter, we will focus on control of forearm vascular resistance during excess salt intake in humans. In particular, the following two subjects will be discussed: 1) the difference between the effects of acute increase in sodium concentration in blood and those of dietary salt loading on control of forearm vascular resistance and 2) the difference in control of forearm vascular resistance between salt-sensitive and non-sensitive humans. In addition, we will discuss 3) the effect of excess salt intake on forearm venous distensibility and 4) the effect of potassium and diuretics on control of forearm vascular resistance.

2. Excess salt intake and control of forearm vascular resistance

a) Effects of the local increase in sodium and those of dietary salt loading on control of forearm vascular resistance

Studies in experimental animals suggest that excess sodium may facilitate sympathetic neurotransmission and the release of endogenous norepinephrine from nerve endings [17, 18, 23]. Excess sodium may also increase vascular smooth muscle tone or vascular reactivity to humoral vasoactive substances through an effect on transmembrane cation gradients [24], calcium movement [25] or contractile proteins [25]. In addition, excess sodium may increase responses to vasoconstrictor stimuli by increasing salt and water content and the wall-to-lumen ratio of resistance vessels [21, 22].

On the other hand, dietary salt loading and associated water retention reduce production of angiotensin and aldosterone and may stimulate the release of atrial natriuretic peptide from the atria [26]. Dietary salt loading also decreases plasma norepinephrine in normotensive subjects [3, 8, 9]. These hormonal adjustments to excess salt intake may decrease vascular smooth muscle tone or vascular reactivity to vasoactive substances.

It has been suggested that effects of excess salt intake on blood pressure and vascular resistance in humans may depend on the balance between the effects which increase vascular resistance and the opposing hormonal and hemodynamic adjustments [2, 10, 14]. Investigators at the University of Iowa have examined the effects of acute changes in sodium concentration in blood and those of dietary excess salt intake on control of forearm vascular resistance in normotensive young men [2, 10, 27].

Heistad, Abboud and Ballard examined the effects of three different sodium solutions on vascular reactivity in normotensive subjects [27]. Solutions, which contained normal (145 mEq/L), high (193 mEq/L) or no sodium were infused into the brachial artery. Sodium contents of the venous effluents were paralleled with the sodium concentration of the infused solutions. Osmolarity was maintained at the normal level (305 mOsm/L) in each solution. During infusion of each solution, forearm vascular responses to intra-arterial injections of norepinephrine and angiotensin and to lower body negative pressure were examined. Lower body negative pressure pools blood in the lower extremities and causes reflex neurogenic vasoconstriction in the forearm. Forearm blood flow was measured by a plethysmograph. The magnitudes of the decreases in forearm blood flow in response to norepinephrine, angiotensin and lower body negative pressure were directly correlated with the concentration of sodium in the infused solution [29]. Thus, the acute increase in the local sodium concentration augments vascular responses to neurohumoral vasoconstrictor stimuli in the forearm in normotensive young men.

Abboud and his colleagues examined the effects of changes in chronic dietary salt intake on control of forearm vascular resistance in normotensive subjects [2]. Subjects were given three different salt diets; low (10 mEq/day), moderate (210 mEq/day) and high (410 mEq/day). Each diet was given for a month and potassium content was constant (100 mEq/day). Metabolic and hormonal examinations revealed parallel decreases in plasma renin and aldosterone with sodium intake. Inulin space and exchangeable sodium tended to increase during high salt intake. Central venous pressure increased in every subject during high salt intake. These results were consistent with increased blood volume during high salt intake.

However, mean blood pressure did not change and surprisingly, resting forearm blood flow increased but did not decrease during high salt intake. Inulin clearance, which reflects glomerular filtration and possibly renal blood flow, also increased during high salt intake. Thus, in normotensive subjects, dietary salt loading decreased forearm vascular resistance and possibly renal vascular resistance. The decrease in vascular resistance during dietary salt loading is the opposite to what might be expected from the direct or local effects of excess sodium which are to increase vascular resistance [27].

They also examined forearm vascular responses to intra-arterial injections of norepinephrine and to lower body negative pressure after a month of low and high salt intake. Responses to norepinephrine were augmented but those to lower body negative pressure were not altered during high salt intake as compared to those during low salt intake. Thus, the acute increase in sodium in blood augmented forearm vascular responses to lower body negative pressure [27] whereas chronic dietary salt loading did not augment reflex forearm vasoconstriction despite the fact that vascular reactivity to norepinephrine was augmented [2].

These results suggest that compensatory adjustments had occurred during dietary salt loading and prevented increases in vascular resistance and reflex neural vasoconstriction in normotensive subjects. Several mechanisms might be involved in compensatory adjustments. First, volume expansion and the increase in atrial pressure during dietary salt loading might have stimulated cardiac receptor reflex and produced reflex forearm vasodilatation [28]. Second, humoral vasoconstrictor substances in blood, such as norepinephrine, angiotensin and vasopressin, were likely to be decreased during dietary salt loading and volume expansion. The release of vasodilating atrial natriuretic peptide from the atria also might be increased during excess salt intake and volume expansion [26]. Such decreases in vasoconstrictor humoral substances and possible increases in vasodilator substance might have contributed to vasodilatation. Third, it is known that these vasoacting substances modify reflex neural vasoconstriction by acting at various levels of the reflex arc [29–31].

In summary, an acute increase in sodium concentration in blood augments vascular reactivity to vasoconstrictor stimuli. However, chronic dietary salt loading causes neurohumoral adjustments which modify the direct or local effect of excess sodium. In normotensive subjects, dietary salt loading does not alter blood pressure and causes forearm vasodilatation because of such neurohumoral adjustments. It may be possible that abnormalities in neurohumoral adjustments may lead to the increase in blood pressure and vascular resistance during dietary salt loading in hypertensive patients.

b) Control of forearm vascular resistance during dietary salt loading in normotensive subjects and patients with essential hypertension

As discussed in the previous section, the study by Abboud and coworkers has shown that 410 mEq/day salt diet for a month did not alter blood pressure and caused forearm vasodilatation in normotensive subjects [2]. Mark and coworkers from the same institution later examined the effects of 10 and 410 mEq/day salt diet for a month on blood pressure and control of forearm vascular resistance in patients with borderline hypertension [10]. In contrast to the results in normotensive subjects, high salt diet increased blood pressure and forearm vascular resistance in patients with borderline hypertension [10] (Fig. 1). We also examined the effects of low (70 mEq/day) and high (345 mEq/day) salt diet for a week on blood pressure and forearm vascular resistance in patients with essential hypertension [13]. Salt loading increased forearm vascular resistance in patients with essential hypertension whose mean blood pressure rose by more than 10% as compared with that during low salt diet (salt-sensitive). Forearm vascular resistance did not change in patients with essential hypertension whose blood pressure did not rise with salt loading (salt-nonsensitive) (Fig. 2). Thus, it appears that forearm vascular responses to dietary salt loading differ between normotensive subjects whose blood pressure does not rise during salt loading and patients with borderline or essential hypertension who respond to salt loading by increasing blood pressure. It should also be mentioned that forearm vascular response to dietary

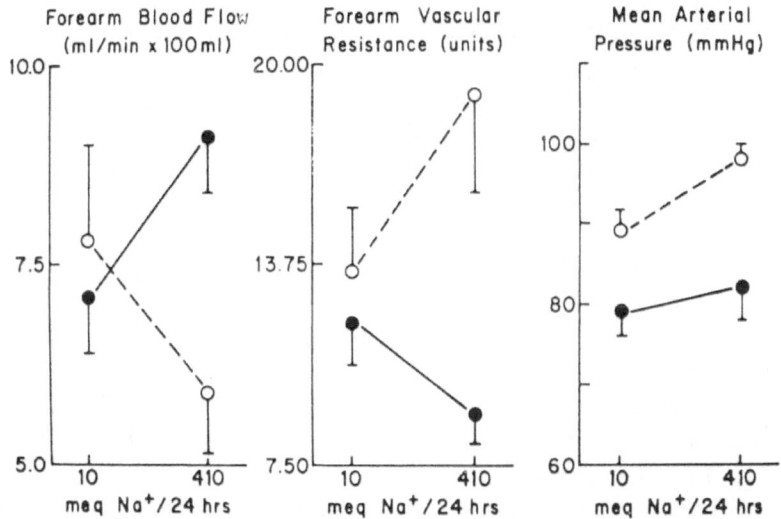

Figure 1. Forearm blood flow, forearm vascular resistance and mean arterial pressure in borderline hypertensive (n = 6, broken lines) and normotensive (n = 6, solid lines) men during low (10 mEq/day) and high (410 mEq/day) salt diets. (taken from reference [10])

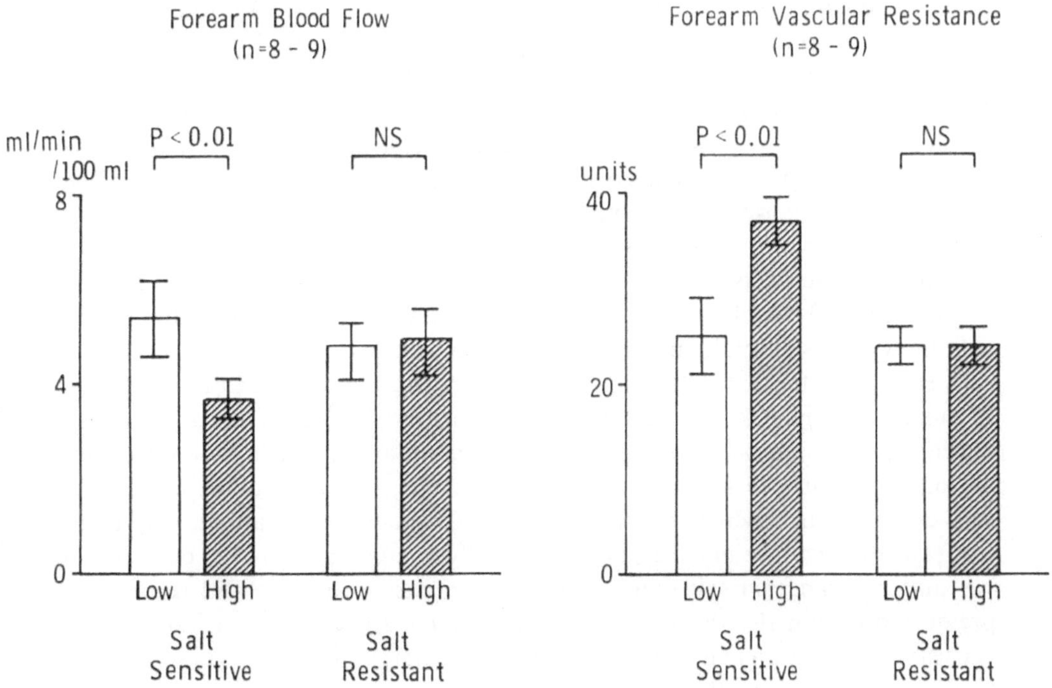

Forearm Blood Flow (n=8 - 9)

ml/min /100 ml

P < 0.01   NS

8

4

0

Low   High   Low   High

Salt Sensitive   Salt Resistant

Forearm Vascular Resistance (n=8 - 9)

units

P < 0.01   NS

40

20

0

Low   High   Low   High

Salt Sensitive   Salt Resistant

Figure 2. Forearm blood flow and forearm vascular resistance in salt-sensitive (n = 8) and salt-nonsensitive (n = 9) patients with essential hypertension during low (70 mEq/day, open bars) and high (345 mEq/day, shaded bars) salt diet.

salt loading in salt-nonsensitive patients with essential hypertension differed from those in normotensive subjects. Forearm vascular resistance decreased during dietary salt loading in normotensive subjects [2] whereas it did not change in salt-nonsensitive patients with essential hypertension [13].

These findings on forearm circulation are consistent with the results of the studies which examined total peripheral vascular resistance during low and high salt intake [5, 8, 11]. In patients with borderline hypertension who responded to salt loading by increasing blood pressure, cardiac output increased during dietary salt loading but total peripheral vascular resistance did not adequately fall [5, 11]. However, in normotensive subjects whose blood pressure did not increase during salt loading, the increase in cardiac output was adequately compensated by the fall of total peripheral vascular resistance [5, 8, 11]. Similar differences have been found between salt-sensitive and salt-nonsensitive patients with essential hypertension [4]. In salt-sensitive patients with essential hypertension, dietary salt loading increased cardiac output but total peripheral vascular resistance did not change [4]. On the other hand, salt loading did not significantly alter cardiac output or total peripheral vascular resistance in salt-nonsensitive patients with essential hypertension [4].

Salt-sensitive patients with borderline or essential hypertension had greater increases in cardiac output during salt loading as compared with those in normotensive subjects or salt-nonsensitive patients with essential hypertension [4, 5]. However, a greater increase in cardiac output by itself did not fully explain the salt-induced elevation of blood pressure in these patients. The magnitudes of the rise in blood pressure during salt loading in patients with borderline hypertension did not correlate with the changes in cardiac output but did correlate with the changes in total peripheral vascular resistance [5]. It is interesting to note that extremely high salt intakes of 800 to 1500 mEq/day increased blood pressure in normotensive subjects, but this increase resulted entirely from higher cardiac output and total peripheral vascular resistance tended to decrease even with the extremely high salt intake in normotensive subjects [8].

In summary, these results suggest that there are abnormalities in control of vascular resistance during dietary salt loading in salt-sensitive patients with borderline or essential hypertension. It appears that the rise in blood pressure during salt loading in salt-sensitive patients results from inadequate compensatory decreases in vascular resistance during the increase in cardiac output. In contrast, the increase in cardiac output is fully compensated by the decrease in vascular resistance in salt-nonsensitive normotensive subjects and thus blood pressure does not rise during dietary salt loading. In the forearm, salt loading causes vasodilatation in normotensive subjects whereas it produces vasoconstriction in salt-sensitive patients with borderline or essential hypertension.

c) Possible mechanisms for altered control of vascular resistance in salt-sensitive patients with essential hypertension

What might be the mechanisms by which control of vascular resistance during dietary salt loading is altered in salt-sensitive patients with borderline or essential hypertension? We will consider three possible mechanisms: 1) total body auto-regulation, 2) neurogenic mechanisms and 3) structural vascular changes.

It has been considered that increased cardiac output might lead to the increase in vascular resistance by the mechanism of autoregulation [32]. This view is consistent with the findings that salt-sensitive patients with borderline or essential hypertension have greater increases in cardiac output during salt loading as compared with those in normotensive subjects or salt-nonsensitive patients with essential hypertension [4, 5]. However, we consider it unlikely that the mechanism of autoregulation totally accounts for the salt-induced vasoconstriction. First, dietary salt loading increased blood flow and decreased vascular resistance in the forearm in normotensive subjects [2], suggesting that autoregulation did not occur. Second, Onesti and coworkers have shown that volume expansion caused blood pressure elevation in anephric patients with a history of hypertension prior to nephrectomy whereas it did not increase blood pressure in anephric patients with no previous history of hypertension [33].

Studies in Dahl rats [17, 18] and rats with DOCA-salt hypertension [23] have suggested that increased neurogenic mechanisms may be involved in the salt-induced vasoconstriction. The possibility that neurogenic mechanisms may contribute to altered control of vascular resistance during dietary salt loading in humans has been studied by Mark and coworkers [10]. They examined forearm vascular responses to lower body negative pressure and intra-arterial injections of norepinephrine in patients with borderline hypertension after a month of low (10 mEq/day) and high (410 mEq/day) salt diet [10]. In normotensive subjects, salt loading tended to decrease forearm vasoconstrictive responses to lower body negative pressure [2], whereas in patients with borderline hypertension it increased reflex vasoconstrictive responses to lower body negative pressure (Fig. 3). The increase in reflex vasoconstrictive responses to lower body negative pressure in patients with borderline hypertension might reflect facilitated neurogenic vasoconstriction or increased responsiveness to the adrenergic neurotransmitter norepinephrine. To evaluate these alternatives, they examined the ratio of vasoconstrictive responses to lower body negative pressure to responses to norepinephrine. Dietary salt loading tended to decrease this ratio in normotensive subjects whereas it increased the ratio in patients with borderline hypertension (Fig. 3). These results suggest that dietary salt loading facilitated neurogenic vasoconstriction in patients with borderline hypertension but not in normotensive subjects. These results are consistent with the results of studies which examined plasma norepinephrine during dietary salt loading [3–5, 8, 9]. Dietary salt loading decreased plasma norepinephrine in normotensive subjects [3, 8, 9] whereas in

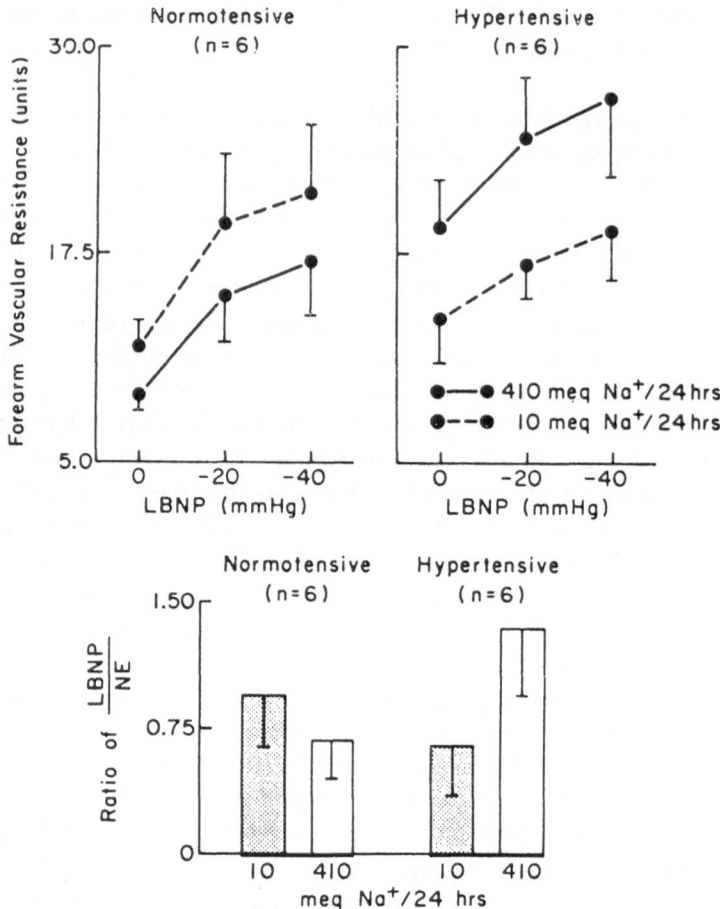

Figure 3. Effect of salt intake on neurogenic vasoconstriction. Top panel, responses to lower body negative pressure (LBNP) at −20 and −40 mm Hg during low (10 mEq/day) and high (410 mEq/day) salt diet. Bottom panel, effect of low and high salt intake on the ratio of responses to LBNP divided by responses to norepinephrine (NE). The ratio was calculated by dividing the sum of increases in forearm vascular resistance with the two levels of LBNP by the sum of increases in resistance with the two doses of NE (taken from reference [10]).

salt-sensitive patients with essential hypertension expected decreases in plasma norepinephrine during salt loading did not occur [3–5].

We examined the possibility that salt loading may produce structural changes of the forearm resistance vessels by increasing the wall-to-lumen ratio in patients with essential hypertension [13]. It has been shown that dietary salt loading causes structural changes in resistance vessels in spontaneously hypertensive rats [34]. To determine whether there were structural vascular changes of the forearm resistance vessels during salt loading, we examined maximal vasodilator capacity of the forearm resistance vessels after 7 days of low (70 mEq/day) and high (345 mEq/day) salt diets. Maximal vasodilator capacity was assessed by measuring minimal forearm vascular resistance during peak reactive hyperemia following 10 minutes of arterial occlusion. It was previously shown that increasing metabolic vasodilator stimulus by combining handgrip exercise and 10 minutes of arterial occlusion did not lower minimal vascular resistance more than that following 10 minutes of arterial occlusion alone [20, 35]. These results suggest that there was maximal vasodilatation during peak reactive hyperemia after 10 minutes of arterial occlusion [20, 35]. Dietary salt loading increased forearm vascular resistance and decreased maximal vasodilator capacity in salt-sensitive patients with essential hypertension but did not alter them in salt-nonsensitive patients (Fig. 4). These results are consistent with the view that, in hypertensive patients who responded to salt loading with a greater rise of blood pressure, salt loading produced structural changes of the forearm resistance vessels and structural changes contributed to the salt-induced increase in forearm vascular resistance [13].

In summary, dietary salt loading causes vasoconstriction in salt-sensitive hypertensive patients. It has been suggested that facilitated neurogenic vasoconstriction and/or structural vascular changes may contribute to salt-induced forearm vasoconstriction in salt-sensitive hypertensive patients. There is obviously much to be learned about the mechanisms which contribute to altered control of vascular resistance during salt loading in salt-sensitive humans.

3. Excess salt intake and forearm venous distensibility

Fujita and coworkers have shown that salt-sensitive hypertensive patients had a greater increase in cardiac output during salt loading than did salt-nonsensitive hypertensive patients [4]. A greater increase in cardiac output was attributed to greater volume retention resulting from reduced natriuretic response to salt loading [4]. We considered the possibility that salt loading might produce changes in veins as well as arteries in salt-sensitive patients with essential hypertension [12]. If salt loading produces changes in veins and decreases venous distensibility, such changes might contribute to redistribution of venous blood from peripheral to cardiopulmonary circulation and thus to the increase in cardiac output.

The venous pressure-volume relationship was determined in the forearm with a water-filled plethysmograph in patients with essential hypertension after 7 days of low (70 mEq/day) and high (345 mEq/day) salt diet [12]. Patients were arbitrarily divided into two groups, salt-sensitive and salt-nonsensitive, based on their blood pressure responses to salt loading. While on the low salt diet, venous pressure-volume curves were not different between salt-sensitive and nonsensitive patients. High salt intake shifted the curve toward the pressure axis for salt-sensitive patients (Fig. 5), whereas it did not alter the curve for salt-nonsensitive

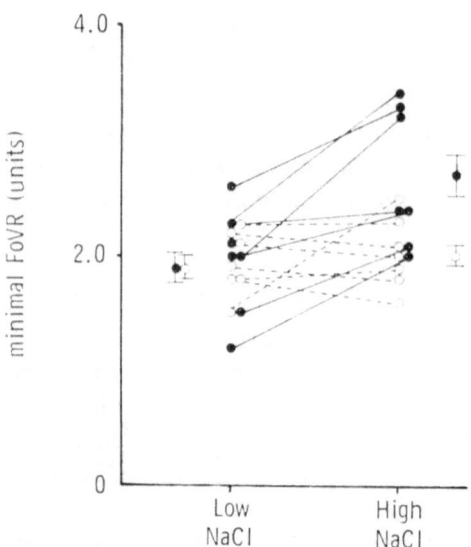

Figure 4. Minimal forearm vascular resistance during peak reactive hyperemia after 10 minutes of arterial occlusion in salt-sensitive (closed circles) and salt-nonsensitive (open circles) patients with essential hypertension during low (70 mEq/day) and high (345 mmEq/day) salt diet (taken from reference [13]).

VENOUS DISTENSIBILITY IN SALT-NONSENSITIVE PATIENTS

(n=8)

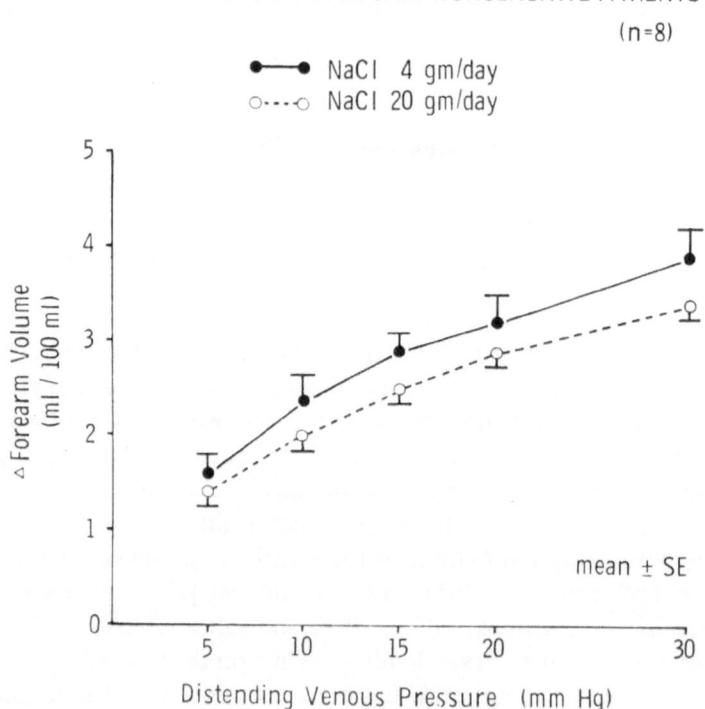

Figure 5. Venous pressure-volume curves in salt-sensitive patients with essential hypertension during low and high salt diet.

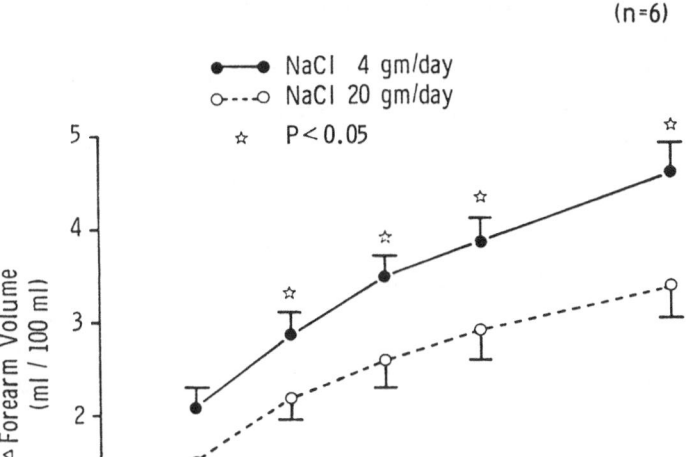

Figure 6. Venous pressure-volume curves in salt-sensitive patients with essential hypertension during low and high salt diet.

patients (Fig. 6). These results suggest that salt loading decreased venous distensibility in salt-sensitive patients but not in salt-nonsensitive patients. The mechanisms for salt-induced decreases in venous distensibility in salt-sensitive hypertensive patients are unknown but it was considered that adrenergic mechanisms were unlikely to be involved since phentolamine did not alter the venous pressure-volume curve in these patients. It is possible that dietary salt loading produced structural changes in veins as it did in arteries [13] in salt-sensitive patients with essential hypertension, which resulted in decreased venous distensibility. These changes in veins may contribute to salt-induced hypertension by causing an increase in cardiac output.

4. Potassium, diuretics and forearm circulation

In contrast to the vasoconstricting effect of sodium, potassium has been known to have a vasodilator effect [36, 37]. An infusion of potassium into the brachial artery causes vasodilatation of forearm resistance vessels [38, 39]. Overbeck and coworkers [38] and Phillip and Robinson [39] compared vasodilator response to intra-arterially infused potassium in the forearm between normotensive subjects and patients with essential hypertension. It was found that vasodilator response to potassium was reduced in patients with essential hypertension as compared with that in normotensive subjects [38, 39]. Potassium-induced vasodilation is thought to result from stimulation of the Na^+–K^+ pump since it is inhibited by prior administration of ouabain [40]. Thus, the observation of a reduced dilator response to potassium in patients with essential hypertension has been considered to suggest that the activity of the Na^+–K^+ pump in the resistance vessels is impaired in patients with essential hypertension [38, 39]. However, this is not conclusive since a recent study has shown that vasoconstrictive response of forearm resistance vessels to ouabain is increased in patients with essential hypertension, suggesting that the activity of the Na^+–K^+ pump may be increased in hypertensive patients [41].

It is also known that dietary high potassium chloride intake has an antihypertensive effect [37]. In particular, potassium chloride supplementation attenuates the hypertensive effects of high salt intake [5, 36, 37]. It has been suggested that, in addition to the direct vasodilator effect of potassium, other mechanisms also may be involved in this antihypertensive effect of dietary potassium chloride supplementation [5, 36, 42]. Dietary potassium chloride supplementation increases natriuresis [5, 36] and thus reduces sodium retention during salt loading. Dietary potassium chloride supplementation also reduced plasma norepinephrine, suggesting that it may decrease sympathetic nervous activity [5, 36]. However, the effects of dietary high potassium chloride intake on control of vascular resistance, such as that in the forearm, have not been studied in humans.

The antihypertensive effects of diuretics result not only from volume depletion but also from the decrease in vascular resistance [43]. The long-term antihypertensive effects of diuretics may be related to its effect on vascular resistance since the antihypertensive effects of diuretics are not correlated with their natriuretic potentials [44]. There are several studies which have examined the effects of diuretics on forearm circulation [45–48]. Diuretics may dilate resistance vessels with no change in the diameter of large vessels in the forearm in patients with essential hypertension [45]. However, the mechanisms by which diuretics decrease vascular resistance are not clear. It has been shown that diuretics may reduce the vasoconstrictive responses of forearm resistance vessels to norepinephrine in normotensive subjects [46]. Recently, Robinson and coworkers have shown that the vasodilator response of forearm resistance vessels to verapamil is augmented more in patients with essential hypertension than in normotensive subjects [47], and that the treatment with chlorthalidone for a month normalizes the vasodilator response to verapamil but not to sodium nitroprusside [48]. What these results might indicate is still not clear.

5. Conclusion

Studies of forearm circulation have contributed importantly to understanding vascular responses to dietary salt loading in humans. Dietary salt loading increases forearm vascular resistance in salt-sensitive patients with borderline or essential hypertension whereas it decreases forearm vascular resistance in salt-nonsensitive normotensive subjects. Dietary salt loading also decreases forearm venous distensibility in salt-sensitive patients with essential hypertension. It has been suggested that facilitated neurogenic mechanisms and/or structural vascular changes may contribute to altered control of vascular resistance and venous capacitance in salt-sensitive patients with borderline or essential hypertension. However, there is much to be learned about the salt-sensitivity in humans. Further studies need to be done to clarify the mechanisms by which salt sensitivity is determined in humans.

6. Acknowledgement

We appreciate secretarial assistance of Tomoko Hirokawa.

References

1. Freis ED (1976): Salt, volume and the prevention of hypertension. Circulation 53: 589–596.
2. Abboud FM (1974): Effets of sodium, angiotensin, and steroids on vascular reactivity in man. Fed Proc 33: 143–149.
3. Campese VM, Romoff MS, Levitan D, Saglikes Y, Friedler RM, Massry SG (1982): Abnormal relationship between sodium intake and sympathetic nervous activity in salt-sensitive patients with essential hypertension. Kidney Int 21: 371–378.
4. Fujita T, Henry WL, Bartter FC, Lake CR, Delea CS (1980): Factors influencing blood pressure in salt-sensitive patients with hypertension. Am J Med 69: 334–344.
5. Fujita T, Node , Ando K (1984): Sodium susceptibility and potassium effects in young patients with borderline hypertension. Circulation 69: 468–476.
6. Kawasaki T, Delea CS, Bartter FC, Smith H (1978): The effect of high-sodium and low-sodium intakes on blood pressure and other related variables in human subjects with idiopathic hypertension. Am J Med 64: 193–198.
7. Kirkendall WM, Connor WE, Abboud FM, Rastogi SP, Anderson TA, Fry M (1976): The effect of dietary chloride on blood pressure, body fluids, electrolytes, renal function, and serum lipids of normotensive man. J Lab Clin Med 87: 418–434.
8. Luft FC, Rankin LI, Bloch R, Weyman AE, Willis LR, Murray RH, Grim CE, Weinberger MH (1979): Cardiovascular and humoral responses to extremes of sodium intake in normal black and white men. Circulation 60: 697–706.
9. Luft FC, Rankin LI, Henry DP et al. (1979): Plasma and urinary norepinephrine values at extremes of sodium intake in normal man. Hypertension 1: 261–266.
10. Mark AL, Lawton WJ, Abboud FM, Fitz AE, Connor WE, Heistad DD (1975): Effects of high and low sodium intake on arterial pressure and forearm vascular resistance in borderline hypertension. Circ Res 36–37 (suppl): I-194–I-198.

298

11. Sullivan JM, Ratts TE, Taylor JC, Kraus DH, Barton BR, Patrick DR, Read SW (1980): Hemodynamic effects of dietary sodium in man. A preliminary report. Hypertension 2: 506–514.
12. Takeshita A, Ashihara T, Yamamoto K, Imaizumi T, Hoka S, Ito N, Nakamura M (1984): Venous responses to salt loading in hypertensive subjects. Circulation 69: 50–56.
13. Takeshita A, Imaizumi T, Ashihara T, Nakamura M (1982): Characteristics of responses to salt loading and deprivation in hypertensive subjects. Circ Res 51: 457–464.
14. Dahl LK, Heine M, Tassinari L (1962): Effects of chronic salt ingestion. Evidence that genetic factors play an important role in susceptibility to experimental hypertension. J Exp Med 115: 1173–1190.
15. Mark AL, Gordon FJ, Takeshita A (1981): Sodium, vascular resistance and genetic hypertension. In: Hypertension, ed. by Brenmer BM and Steun JH, Churchill Livingstone, p. 21–38.
16. Takeshita A, Imaizumi T, Ashihara T, Nakamura M (1982): Adrenergic mechanisms do not contribute to salt-induced vasoconstriction in stroke-prone spontaneously hypertensive rat. Hypertension 4: 288–293.
17. Takeshita A, Mark AL (1978): Neurogenic contribution to hindquarters vasoconstriction during high sodium intake in Dahl strain of genetically hypertensive rats. Circ Res 43 (suppl I): I-86–I-91.
18. Takeshita A, Mark AL, Brody M (1979): Prevention of salt-induced hypertension in the Dahl strain by 6-hydroxydopamine. Am J Physiol 236: H48–H52.
19. Tobian L, Lange J, Azar S, Iwai J, Koop D, Coffee K, Johnson MA (1978): Reduction of natriuretic capacity and renin release in isolated blood perfused kidneys of Dahl hypertension-prone rats. Circ Res 43 (suppl I): I-92–I-98.
20. Takeshita A, Mark AL (1980): Decreased vasodilator capacity of forearm resistance vessels in borderline hypertension. Hypertension 2: 610–615.
21. Folkow B (1971): Haemodynamic consequences of the adaptive structural changes of the resistance vessels in hypertension. Clin Sci 41: 1–12.
22. Tobian L Jr, Binion JT (1952): Tissue cations and water in arterial hypertension. Circulation 5: 754–758.
23. deChamplain J, Krakoff LR, Axelrod J (1968): Relationship between sodium intake and nor-epinephrine storage during the development of experimental hypertension. Circ Res 23: 479–491.
24. Bohr DF, Seidel C, Sobieski J (1969): Possible role of sodium-calcium pumps in tension development of vascular smooth muscle. Microvasc Res 1: 335–343.
25. Hollander W, Shibata N (1968): Mode of action of sodium on the contractile proteins of the arteries. J Clin Invest 47: 47a.
26. Needleman P, Adams SP, Cole BR, Currie MG, Geller DM, Michener ML, Saper CG, Schwartz D, Standert DG (1985): Atriopeptins as cardiac hormones. Hypertension 7: 469–482.
27. Heistad DD, Abboud FM, Ballard DR (1971): Relationship between plasma sodium concentration and vascular reactivity in man. J Clin Invest 50: 2022–2032.
28. Zoller RP, Mark AL, Abboud FM, Schmid PG, Heistad DD (1972): The role of low pressure baroreceptors in reflex vasoconstrictor responses in man. J Clin Invest 51: 2967–2972.
29. Guo GB, Abboud FM (1984): Angiotensin II attenuates baroreflex control of heart rate and sympathetic activity. Am J Physiol 246: H80–H89.
30. Imaizumi T, Takeshita A, Higuchi S, Higashi H, Nakamura M (1986): Effects of atrial extract and synthetic atrial natriuretic peptide on arterial baroreflex control of lumbar sympathetic nerve activity. Jap Circ J 50: 1135–1136.
31. Undersser KP, Hasser EM, Haywood JR, Johnson AK, Bishop VS (1985): Interactions of vasopressin with the area postrema in arterial baroreflex function in conscious rabbits. Circ Res 56: 410–417.
32. Coleman TG, Granger HJ, Guyton AC (1971): Whole body circulatory autoregulation and hypertension. Circ Res 28/29 (suppl II): II-76–II-87.
33. Onesti G, Kim KE, Greco JA, Del Guerico ET, Fernandes M, Schwartz C (1975): Blood pressure regulation in end-stage renal disease and anephric man. Circ Res 36 (suppl I): I-145–I-152.

34. Limas C, Westrum B, Limas CJ, Cohn JN (1980): Effect of salt on the vascular lesions of spontaneously hypertensive rats. Hypertension 2: 477–489.
35. Takeshita A, Imaizumi T, Ashihara T, Yamamoto K, Hoka S, Nakamura M (1982): Limited maximal vasodilator capacity of forearm resistance vessels in normotensive young men with a familial predisposition to hypertension. Circ Res 50: 671–677.
36. Fujita T, Ando K (1984): Hemodynamic and endocrine changes associated with potassium supplementation in sodium-loaded hypertensives. Hypertension 6: 184–192.
37. Meneely GR, Ball COT, Youmans JB (1957): Chronic sodium chloride toxicity: Protective effect of added potassium chloride. Ann Intern Med 47: 263–273.
38. Overbeck HW, Derifield RS, Pamnani MB, Sozen T (1974): Attenuated vasodilator responses to K^+ in essential hypertensive men. J Clin Invest 53: 678–686.
39. Phillips PJW, Robinson BF (1984): The dilator response to K^+ ions reduced in the forearm resistance vessels of men with primary hypertension. Clin Sci 66: 237–239.
40. Chen WT, Brace RA, Scott JB, Anderson DK, Haddy FJ (1972): The mechanism of the vasodilator action of potassium. Proc Soc Exp Biol Med 140: 820–824.
41. Hulthén UL, Bolli P, Kiowski W, Bühler FR (1984): Forearm vasoconstrictor response to ouabain: studies in patients with mild and moderate hypertension. J Cardiovasc Pharmacol 6 (suppl): S75–S81.
42. Young DB, McCaa RE, Pan YJ, Guyton AC (1976): The natriuretic and hypotensive effects of potassium. Circ Res 38 (suppl II): II-84–II-89.
43. Lund-Johansen P (1970): Hemodynamic changes in long-term diuretic therapy of essential hypertension. Acta Med Scand 187: 509–518.
44. Matterson BJ, Oster JR, Michael UF, Bolton SM, Burton ZC, Stambaugh JE, Morledge J (1978): Dose-response to chlorothiazide in patients with mild hypertension. Efficacy of a lower dose. Clin Pharmacol Ther 22: 519–527.
45. Bouthier JA, Safar ME, Levenson JA, Simon A: Hemodynamic effects of a diuretic-like substance on the forearm circulation of men with essential hypertension (personal communication).
46. Khalil FA, Eckstein JW, Horsley AW, Keasling HH (1961): Effects of chlorothazide on forearm vascular responses to norepinephrine. J Appl Physiol 16: 549–552.
47. Robinson BF, Dobbs RJ, Bayley S (1982): Response of forearm resistance vessels to verapamil and sodium nitroprusside in normotensive and hypertensive men: evidence for a functional abnormality of vascular smooth muscle in primary hypertension. Clin Sci 63: 33–42.
48. Robinson BF, Dobbs RJ, Phillips RJW (1983): Effects of treatment with chlorthalidone and atenolol on response to dilator agents in the forearm resistance vessels of men with primary hypertension. Br J Clin Pharmac 16: 327–332.

Conclusion

Homeostatic mechanisms and structural modifications of the cardiovascular system in essential hypertension

M.E. SAFAR

The understanding of hypertension is largely dependent on the methodology which may be used to investigate the disease. This methodology is different in animal and in man.

In animal hypertension, the sequence of events occurring in the course of the disease may be described extensively [1–3]. In several examples, the initiating factors of the disease are well known. The general concept is that a drastic change in a given causative factor leads with time to major modifications of the cardiovascular system with a resulting elevation in blood pressure and complex interactions between the heart, the small vessels, the kidney and the autonomic nervous system.

In hypertension in man, long-term longitudinal studies are almost impossible to perform. Initiating factors are largely unknown. The general assumption is that, with cross-sectional studies, somewhat significant (but never drastic) changes in any given parameter may be observed as in the renin-angiotensin, the prostaglandin systems, the autonomic nervous system, the cation pumps ... However, in hypertensive humans, with the exception of the elevated blood pressure, most of the important functions of the body, such as the maintenance of blood flow and sodium balance, the capillary exchange and the nutritional needs of tissues, appear to be largely maintained. Thus, the basic problem in clinical hypertension is as follows: how may homeostasis (or autoregulation as a synonym) be preserved in hypertensive humans?

The purpose of this review is to discuss the problem of homeostasis in hypertension, but only on the basis of clinical investigation. First, an example of homeostasis will be presented, principally taking into account the control of cardiac output. Second, the concept of vascular resistance will be analysed and applied to the general understanding of hypertension. On the basis of hemodynamic data introduced into models of the cardiovascular system, the structural and the functional components of vascular resistance will be described and discussed. Then, the structural modifications of vascular resistance (and more generally of the cardiovascular system) will be studied in hypertension and assessed on the basis of clinical data. The present review is restricted to the problem of men with uncomplicated sustained essential hypertension.

Homeostasis of cardiac output in essential hypertension

Basic knowledge about cardiac output in essential hypertension results both from cross-sectional and longitudinal studies.

Cross-sectional studies

In patients with sustained essential hypertension, all reports in the literature point to normal values of cardiac output and cardiac index in supine, upright and sitting positions with a gaussian distribution of the parameters [4–6]. The reduction of cardiac output with age occurs in similar fashion as in normal subjects [4–5]. However, several dissimilarities may be observed when hypertensives are compared with healthy controls. First, heart rate is slightly elevated while there is a tendency towards lower values of stroke volume [4–6]. Second, regional blood flows remain largely within the normal range, although renal blood flow is reduced in patients with severe hypertension and decreases with age more than in the normal population [7–8]. Third, cardiac output is positively correlated to oxygen consumption both at rest and during exercise, but with a shallower slope than in controls [5]: at any given value of oxygen consumption, cardiac output is lower in hypertensives than in normal subjects. Finally, studies of hemodynamic correlates in large populations of subjects indicate that cardiac output, measured in steady-state conditions, is poorly correlated with heart rate but strongly and positively correlated with intravascular volume [9–11].

The hemodynamic situation is quite different from that of age- and sex-matched patients with borderline hypertension. In this particular population, cardiac output, when measured in supine position, is increased in 30 to 60% of the patients [6–12]. The decrease with age seems to be more rapid than in normal subjects. The elevated cardiac output is related to an increase in heart rate, to an increase in stroke volume or both [4–6, 12]. In addition to the increased cardiac output, patients with borderline hypertension exhibit several other hemodynamic abnormalities. First, regional blood flows are modified, with an increase in muscle blood flow and normal values of hepatic and renal blood flows, a situation which is often observed in normal subjects submitted to beta-stimulation [8]. Second, although cardiac output is elevated at rest in the supine position, it remains constantly within the normal range in upright and sitting position and also during exercise [4–6, 12]. Finally, study of hemodynamic correlates in large populations of subjects clearly indicate that cardiac output, measured in steady-state conditions is strongly and positively correlated with heart rate while no significant correlation is observed with intravascular volume [9–11].

Since the gaussian distribution of blood pressure implies that the definition of hypertension is arbitrary [13], it may be difficult using cross-sectional studies to demonstrate the fundamental differences in cardiac output regulation observed in patients with sustained essential hypertension, in normal subjects and in patients with borderline hypertension. For that reason, mathematical methods [9–11] for the evaluation of clinical data have been developed to illustrate the changes in cardiac output control observed in patients with elevated blood pressure. In order to avoid the arbitrary subgroups classically defined in cross-sectional studies, patients were divided into overlapping subgroups [9–11], as detailed in the appendix. In this geometrical analysis, as two adjacent subgroups differed only by one individual from one group to the next, the changes in values of cardiovascular parameters occurred very slowly, enabling smooth modifications of the hemodynamic pattern to be described as function of the level of blood pressure. Fig. 1 shows the changes in mean values of cardiac output, blood volume and heart rate according to the progressive changes of blood pressure. Indeed, cardiac output is increased in patients with borderline hypertension and remains within the normal range in patients with sustained hypertension. Heart rate is increased and intravascular volume reduced as soon as diastolic pressure is above 95 mm Hg [9–11]. Fig. 2 shows the most striking changes in the hemodynamic pattern, i.e. the modificatons of the relationships between cardiac output and heart rate and between cardiac output and blood volume as function of the level of diastolic arterial pressure. The relationship is expressed by the level of the correlation coefficient between two studied hemodynamic parameters. While the correlation coefficient of the relationship between heart rate and cardiac output was significant in the normotensive and the borderline hypertensive ranges, the significance of the correlation disappeared in the sustained hypertensive ranges. On the contrary, the correlation between cardiac output and blood volume was significant exclusively in the blood pressure ranges corresponding to patients with established hypertension [9–11].

Longitudinal studies

Validation of the interpretation of cross-sectional studies in hypertensive man requires that long-term longitudinal investigations of cardiac output control may be carried out. Indeed, short-term modifications of cardiac output after acute stimulation or depression cannot provide an adequate approach to investigate the pathophysiology of a disease such as hypertension, which develops over many years. Only a small number of studies involving long-term repeat hemodynamic studies without any treatment have been published in the literature (see review in 4). Most of them clearly indicate that a characteristic hemodynamic pattern occurred in patients with borderline hypertension: during a 4- to 10-year follow-

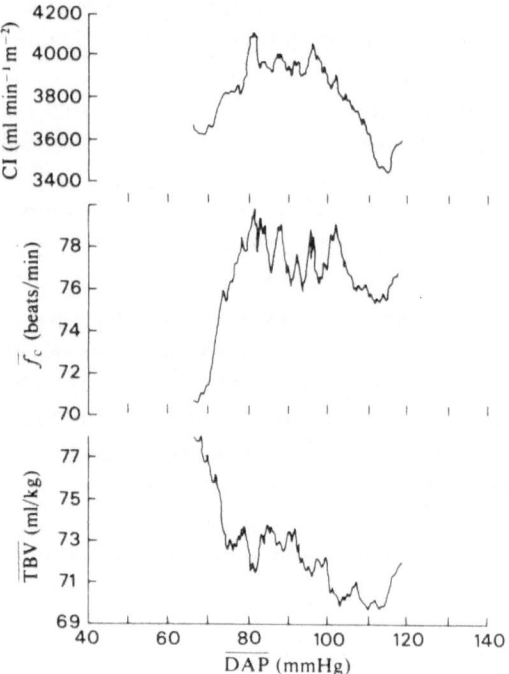

Figure 1. Smoothing technique: mean values of cardiac index (CI), heart rate (Fc) and total blood volume (TBV) plotted against mean values of diastolic arterial pressure (DAP). The successive points are joined linearly (see appendix) [10] (with permission).

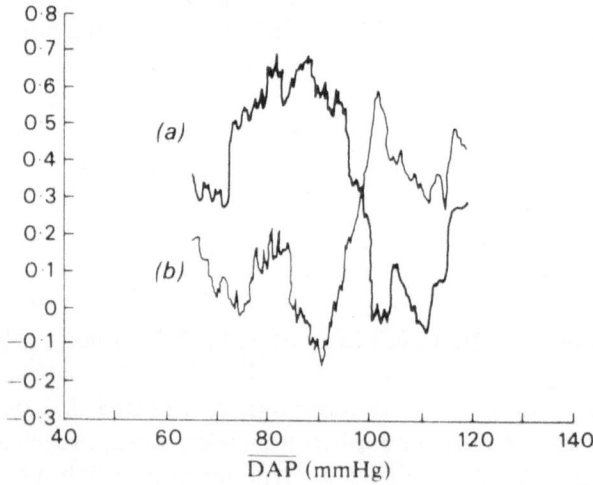

Figure 2. Smoothing technique: correlation coefficients (r values) between the cardiac output and heart rate (a), and the cardiac output and total blood volume (b), plotted against the mean values of diastolic arterial pressures (DAP) (P<0.05 if r>0.31; P<0.01 if r>0.40). The successive points were joined linearly (see appendix) [10] (with permission).

up survey, while blood pressure was practically unchanged, cardic output and heart rate decreased and vascular resistance significantly increased. Such findings may be difficult to interpret since comparable repeat hemodynamic investigations have not been performed extensively in normal subjects. However, when the relationships between the different hemodynamic parameters (cardiac output, blood volume, heart rate) are studied in patients with borderline hypertension, then important changes in the cardiac output control may be observed.

Studies of the steady-state relationships between cardiac output and heart rate and between cardiac output and blood volume [14] have been performed in a population of patients with borderline hypertension investigated on two occasions: first, at the beginning of the follow-up; second, at the end of the survey follow-up. At the beginning of follow-up, cardiac output was strongly and positively correlated with heart rate while blood volume was not. On the other hand, at the end of the survey, cardiac output was strongly and positively correlated with blood volume, while heart rate was not.

Further findings have been obtained by studying the relationship between cardiac output and oxygen consumption during exercise at the beginning and the end of long-term follow-up surveys [15]. Both at the beginning of follow-up and 10 years later, cardiac output was positively correlated with oxygen consumption. However, at the end of follow-up, the slope of the relationship was shallower, indicating that cardiac output was lower at any given value of oxygen consumption in patients with hypertension. This pattern was observed in the absence of congestive heart failure.

In conclusion, longitudinal studies confirm the findings of cross-sectional studies as regards the cardiac output regulation in patients with elevated blood pressure. The mean value of cardiac output is normal in patients with sustained essential hypertension, implying that homeostatic mechanisms do exist. However, behind the normal value, important changes in cardiac output control occur, as shown by the changing pattern of the relationships observed between cardiac output and heart rate, cardiac output and blood volume, and cardiac output and oxygen consumption. The strong correlation between cardiac output and heart rate observed in normotensive ranges contrasts with the strong correlation between cardiac output and blood volume observed in hypertensive ranges. Since such studies were performed under steady-state conditions, cause and effect relationships between the different hemodynamic parameters are difficult to interpret. A more complete interpretation of clinical data is thus required, as detailed below.

Difficulties for the concept of vascular resistance in essential hypertension

Since cardiac output (Q) is normal in patients with sustained essential hypertension, it is usually stated that vascular resistance (R), calculated as the ratio between mean pressure gradient ($\triangle$P) and Q is elevated. The value of R is used as a measure of the extent to which the system 'opposes' or 'resists' flow. However, a better understanding of the meaning of R in hypertension humans requires a complete definition of the basic hypothesis enabling the calculation of vascular resistance (see p. 3ff).

In order to evaluate R as the $\triangle$P/Q ratio, it is necessary to suppose that both the normotensive and the hypertensive cardiovascular systems may be described according to the same lumped linear model of the circulation [16–19]. In this model, P and Q represent the set points of the pressure-flow curves of normotensive and hypertensive subjects, as denoted in Fig. 3. To calculate R as the $\triangle$P/Q ratio, the most important hypothesis is that both in normal subjects and in hypertensives, the inflow pressure is arterial pressure (P) and the outflow pressure is represented by right auricula pressure, which is nearly null. In that condition, R represents, in each population, the slope of the pressure-flow curve, so that:

$$P = R Q \tag{1}$$

Equation (1) is the simple application of Poiseuille's law. It is thus assumed that the cardiovascular system may be considered as a cylindrical tube where resistance to flow is a function of the dimensions of the tube and the viscosity of the moving fluid. Thus:

$$R = 8 \, nL / \, 3.14 \, r^4 \tag{2}$$

where n is the viscosity of fluid, L the length and r the radius of the system. Since viscosity and length are considered as nearly constant, R is mainly influenced by the power four of the radius of small arteries.

For a general understanding of hypertension, it is important to remember that the lumped model of the circulation defined by equations (1) and (2) and represented in Fig. 3 has never been validated in man. This is particularly true for the definition of the outflow pressure [16–19]. Even if it is accepted that viscosity and length of the cardiovascular system are constant and similar in normotensives and hypertensives, the assumption of a linear relationship through zero between pressure and flow is a problem difficult to resolve. In several regional circulations, it has been extensively demonstrated that critical closing pressures do exist. In other words, blood pressure is not constantly null when flow is equal to zero. In that condition, the model defined in equations (1) and (2) has to be reviewed and becomes:

$$P = RQ + Po \tag{3}$$

where Po is the measured pressure for zero flow. The model so defined by

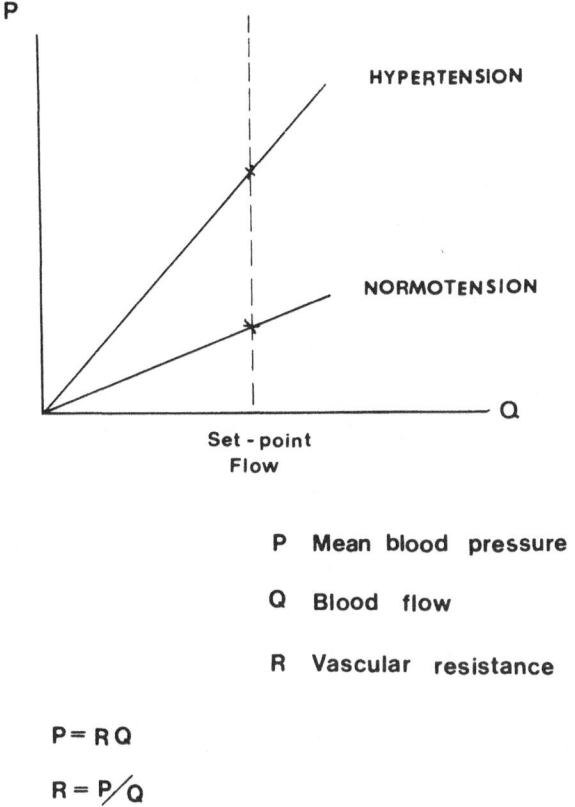

$$P = RQ$$

$$R = P/Q$$

Figure 3. Pressure-flow relationship: the most simple linear model.

equation (3) and represented in Fig. 4 has two dominant features. First, vascular resistance cannot be calculated as P/Q but rather as [22]:

$$R = (P - Po)/Q \tag{4}$$

with the possibility that Po may be significant by comparison with P. Second, elevation of blood pressure may be due either to an increase in Po, or to an increase in R or both. Such different possibilities for an elevated blood pressure now have to be analyzed in detail.

Hypertension may be theoretically caused by an increase in Po, i.e. a shift of the pressure-flow curve toward higher values of blood pressure (Fig. 4). Indeed, according to Guyton [16], several studies have shown that Po, evaluated as mean circulatory pressure, is significantly increased in several forms of animal hypertension. In such experiments, Po refers to the pressure level that occurs throughout the circulation by briefly stopping the heart and rapidly equalizing the arterial

310

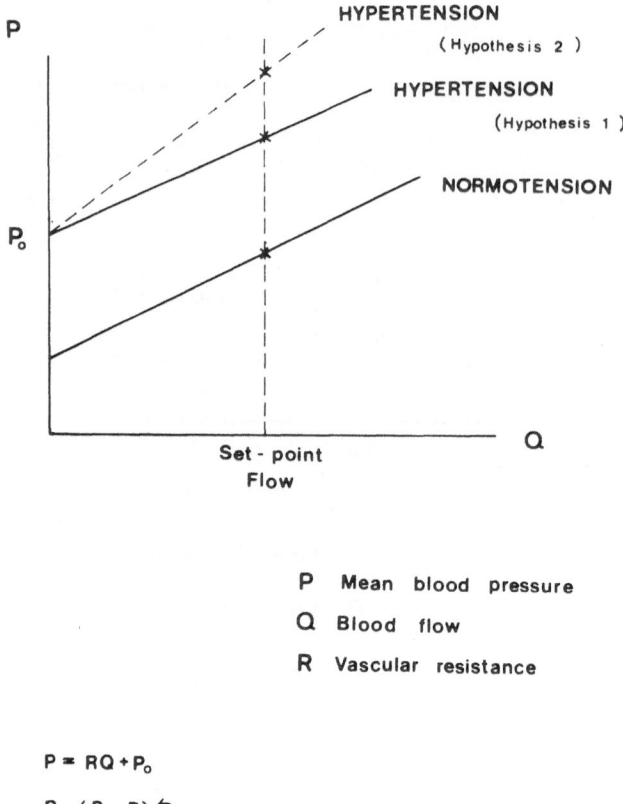

Figure 4. Pressure-flow relationship: other simple linear models.

and venous pressures, thus causing a redistribution of blood from arteries to veins. Although such a methodology is impossible to develop in man, there is indirect evidence in patients with sustained essential hypertension for an increased value of Po [20]. In a competent heart, cardiac output and venous return are equal. The flow in each segment is proportional to pressure gradients divided by resistance. According to Guyton *et al.* [16], cardiac output (CO) is:

$$CO = \frac{(C_A + C_V)(Po - RAP)}{R_V C_V + (R_V + R_A) C_A} \tag{5}$$

where RAP is right atrial pressure (central venous pressure) and R and C are the resistance and the compliance of the arterial (A) and venous (V) systems respectively. Assuming venous resistance (R_V) as constant and nearly equal to zero, it follows that:

$$CO = (C_A + C_V) (Po - RAP)/C_A R_A \tag{6}$$

In men with sustained essential hypertension, C_A is reduced, R_A is elevated and $C_A R_A$ almost unchanged [21]. On the other hand, $(C_A + C_V)$ is reduced and RAP increased [22–24]. Thus, as in several forms of experimental hypertension, the only possibility of maintaining a normal CO in patients with essential hypertension is to achieve an increase in Po. In other words, an adequate pressure gradient for venous return requires an elevation of Po in patients with essential hypertension.

Basically the problem in hypertension humans is less to affirm the existence of increased values of Po than to evaluate the pathophysiological meaning of this abnormality in the mechanisms of hypertension. In several kinds of animal hypertension [16], as in volume-loading hypertension, Po and arterial blood pressure are increased to the same extent, so that an increase in Po is an important pathophysiological mechanism to explain the elevated blood pressure. In other forms of animal hypertension, as in spontaneous hypertension in rats (SHR), the increase in Po is small in relation to the increase in arterial blood pressure. In SHR, Po is found to be 18 per cent greater than in normotensive controls while the arterial pressure is 43 per cent greater [16]. The latter finding clearly indicates that an increase in Po in SHR is not a sufficient hypothesis to explain the elevated blood pressure. An increase in vascular resistance (R) is also required.

Since an increase in the slope of the pressure-flow curve (Fig. 4) is a prerequisite to the general understanding of hypertension, a correct and precise evaluation of 'vascular resistance' is important to delineate in humans. Two different steps are required. The first is to define vascular resistance. The second is to relate this parameter to the cross-sectional area of small arteries.

In animal experiments, evaluation of vascular resistance remains relatively easy (see p. 21ff). Changes in pressure at a given flow or changes in flow at a given pressure indicate without any doubt a change in opposition to flow and hence in the cross-sectional area of small arteries (see equation 2). In hypertensive humans, changes in vascular resistance and hence in the caliber of small arteries are much more difficult to interpret. First, it is assumed that Po is null, an approximation which might be almost valid in severe hypertension (Po is small by comparison with P) but is much more difficult to assume in mild hypertension. Second, changes in R (calculated as P/Q) are used as a marker of the changes in the radius (r) of small arteries. In that regard, it is important to consider that small errors in R evaluations may lead to erroneous approximations of changes in radius (r), since R is influenced by the power four of r. Thus, any pathophysiological discussion about the mechanism of hypertension in humans requires a more detailed approach to investigate the changes in the cross-sectional area of small arteries in long-term clinical investigations.

Introduction of clinical hemodynamic data into models of the cardiovascular system: the structural component of vascular resistance in hypertension

Cardiovascular models may be useful for the interpretation of vascular resistance in hypertensive humans. In other words, the simple calculation of vascular resistance is insufficient to understand the pathophysiological mechanisms of clinical hypertension. A more sophisticated approach is required. The model building method requires adequate definitions of the hemodynamic parameters, physical bases underlying their behaviors and description of these behaviors by mathematical relationships [9–11, 16]. Some of the complex interactions between the components of the system are lumped into 'function blocks' which are obtained directly from experimentation in animals [16]. The mathematical relationships of each block are generally a set of differential equations, with time as an independent variable, together with a set of algebraic equations that define the components of the system or describe the 'function blocks' [16]. Each equation is characterized by one or several coefficients which can therefore be called 'regulation coefficients' of the model [10, 11, 16].

Chau *et al.* [11] were the first to delineate the conditions required to modify the Guyton model of the circulation [16] in order to define the regulation coefficients characterizing the steady-state conditions of normotensive and hypertensive humans. Using a simplified model involving the most classical hemodynamic parameters (blood pressure, cardiac output, blood volume, vascular resistance and functions characterizing the status of the kidney and of the autonomic nervous system) (Fig. 5), they defined the linearized function blocks of the model (Table 1) when the steady state was achieved, i.e. at infinite time. Then, hemodynamic data, as depicted by the smoothing technique (see appendix and Figs 1 and 2), were introduced in the model. So that the curves depicted in Figs 1 and 2 may be compatible with the model, changes in the values of one or several regulation coefficients of the model were required. An adequate identification between the clinical data (Figs 1 and 2) and the characteristics of the model was

Table 1. Linearized function blocks in Guyton-Coleman model [11].

$UO = a_1 AP + b_1$	$BV = a_2 ECFV + b_2$
$MSPb = a_3 BV + b_3$	$dVAS/dt = a_4 CO + b_4$
$RAP = a_5 COn + b_5$	$AMP = a_6 AP + b_6$
$BC = a_7 AP + b_7$	$RVR = \beta VRES + \gamma AR$

Abbreviations: AP = arterial pressure (mm Hg), UO = urinary output (ml/min), ECFV = extracellular fluid volume (liter), BV = blood volume (liter), MSP = mean systemic pressure (mm Hg), AUM = autonomic multiplier (normalized unit), CO = cardiac output (liter/min), VAS = index of vasculature (normalized unit), TPR = total peripheral resistance (mm Hg · min/ml), RVR = resistance to venous return (mm Hg · min/ml), VRES = venous resistance (mm Hg · min/ml), RAP = right arterial pressure (mm Hg), APM = arterial pressure multiplier (normalized unit), BC = baro-chemo coefficient, AR = arterial resistance.

obtained by changing only 8 of the 21 regulation coefficients. Two of these coefficients (a1 and b2) (see Table 1) were related to a change in the kidney function, a quite classical disturbance in several forms of hypertension. Two other coefficients (a7 and b7) were related to modifications in the autonomic nervous system. The remaining 6 coefficients (a4, b4, k1, k2) pointed exclusively to the changes in the status of vascular resistance [13].

The mathematical characteristics of vascular resistance in cardiovascular models are comparable to those described in basic physiology. Total peripheral resistance is the sum of a constant venous resistance and of a variable arterial resistance. The latter is composed of two parts. The first one is submitted to the control of the autonomic nervous system ('functional component'). The second one is the 'structural component', which is inversely proportional (with coefficient k1, which might be called the 'resistivity coefficient') to a variable index of the vasculature (VAS) introduced to quantify the whole vascular network. The VAS is considered as an integral result of two dynamic processes: a first-order destruction process with rate constant k2 and a creation process (with coefficients a4 and b4). Since the changes in the model produced by the introduction of clinical data affected exclusively a4, b4, k1 and k2, it is clear that only the non-autonomic part of vascular resistance, i.e. the structural component of vascular resistance, was modified in essentially hypertensive humans. More specifically, a reduction in the creation process (a4, b4) and an increase in the destruction process (k2) of the vessels was clearly demonstrated by the introduction of clinical data in the Guyton model.

Finally, the conclusion of the mathematical study was quite simple. In order to attain the normal value of cardiac output observed in patients with sustained essential hypertension, adaptive changes of the vascular system (i.e. modifications in the regulation coefficients a4, b4, k1, k2 of the model) were required. The most important modifications were in the structural component of the vasculature, whatever histopathological mechanism may be postulated (reduction in the number of the vessels or increase in the thickness of the arterial wall or both).

Such findings in man are in agreement with those observed in hypertensive animals. For Folkow [25] and also for Korner [26], structural adaptation of the cardiovascular system occurs very early in the course of the disease and contributes largely to maintain the elevated blood pressure and vascular resistance (see p. 21ff). For Guyton [16], an excess flow is often a prerequisite for the development of hypertension at its early phase. However, when the excess flow persists for days, weeks or months, an autoregulatory process occurs with time and results not only from active vasoconstriction but also from an increase of thickness of the arteriolar wall, with further decrease in arteriolar diameter. Clearly, whatever the initiating factors and the time-course of hemodynamic parameters may be, structural modifications invariably occur with time to maintain blood flow. In hypertensive humans, the initiating process is generally unknown. However, structural modifications of the vessels are constantly expected and contribute to

314

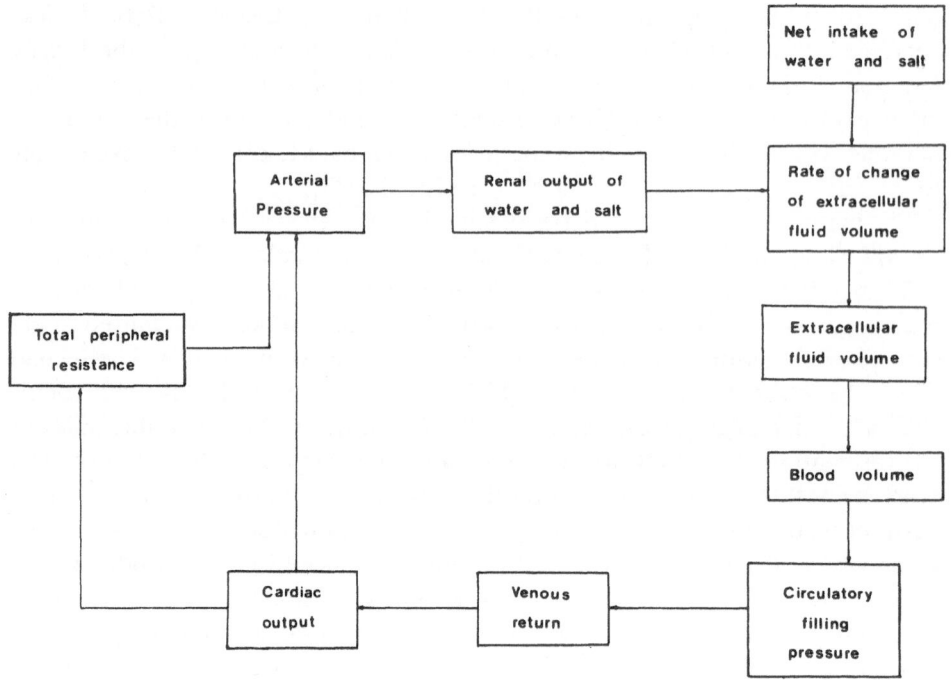

Figure 5. Principal 'function blocks' taken into account in the Guyton model [16] for studies of clinical data [9–11].

maintain the normal value of cardiac output and therefore an adequate oxygen supply. Studying forearm vascular resistance of human essential hypertensives at maximal vasodilation, Seventsen *et al.* [27] showed that such structural changes indeed exist in this particular circulation.

Clinical basis for the demonstration of structural vascular changes of the overall cardiovascular system in essential hypertension

An important prerequisite for the study of adaptive changes of the cardiovascular system in hypertensive humans is the application of the Laplace law [25]. Basically, the cardiovasular system must be considered as structured to suit tissue nutritional demands, as reflected in cardiac pumping capacity, maximal flow conductance and capillary exchange surface. Therefore, in all parts of the cardiovascular system, the thickness (h) must be dimensioned both to regional transmural pressure (P) and tube dimension (internal radius r), in order for the tension per unit wall layer (T) to remain constant according to the Laplace law: $T = P \times r/h$. As long as P remains constant, h/r can be kept unchanged but if P is raised, h/r must also increase, and vice versa, for balance to prevail [25]. Taking into account this concept, it is now possible to analyze the structural modifications that may be suspected or even demonstrated in the cardiovascular system of patients with essential hypertension: not only the small arteries but also the heart, the large arteries and the veins.

Cardiac hypertrophy

Since echocardiography has been widely used, cardiac hypertrophy is considered as a common feature in patients with sustained essential hypertension. This abnormality is observed even without congestive heart failure [28]. Cardiac hypertrophy is associated with an increased responsiveness of cardiac output to volume load [22] and, on the basis of experimental studies [25], may be considered as a simple consequence of the Laplace law. However, clinical investigations have shown that the degree of hypertrophy was poorly correlated with the level of blood pressure, suggesting that hemodynamic modifications are not the sole explanation for cardiac hypertrophy. Before accepting this interpretation, it is important to recall that blood pressure is an insufficient approach to evaluate afterload of the heart in hypertension [17–29]. Studies of vascular impedance have shown that afterload was influenced not only by its resistive component (related to the caliber of small arteries) but also by its inertial and its capacitive components which involve the status of large arteries. Indeed, the degree of cardiac hypertrophy in patients with sustained essential hypertension is correlated not only with the increase in vascular resistance but also with the viscosity of blood and with the reduction in compliance of large vessels [29–30].

Geometrical redesign and hypertrophy of large arteries

Recent clinical studies have shown that, as vascular resistance was increased, arterial compliance was constantly reduced in patients with sustained essential hypertension [31–32]. The reduction in compliance has been observed both in the systemic and the brachial circulations. Furthermore, in the carotid circulation, the association of normal values of arterial diameter and elevated blood pressure also implies intrinsic modifications of the carotid arterial wall [33]. In hypertensive humans, compliance measured under steady-state condition is not correlated with the level of steady-state mean arterial pressure. The same reduction in arterial compliance may be observed in mild and in severe hypertension [31]. Thus, the alteration of the buffering function of the large arteries implies a modification of the arterial wall due to a disturbance in the excitation-contraction coupling, a hypertrophy of the media, a change in the collagen and elastin content or the association of several of these factors. In hypertensive humans, arguments in favor of medial hypertrophy and increased thickness of the arterial wall are somewhat indirect and may be summarized as follows. First, the reduction in arterial compliance is mainly observed in hypertensive patients with structural alterations of large arteries, as in isolated systolic hypertension in the elderly and in patients with arterosclerosis obliterans of lower limbs [32]. Second, in patients with sustained essential hypertension, the reduction in arterial compliance is not modified by alpha-blockade, a result which suggests a major contribution of the non-autonomic component of the reduced arterial compliance [32]. Finally, the reduction of brachial artery diameter observed after administration of suppressive doses of norepinephrine or angiotensin is significantly greater in patients with sustained essential hypertension than in age-matched normotensive subjects [34]. Such findings support the hypothesis of adaptive structural vascular changes, as observed for resistive vessels (p. 21ff). However, direct evidence for an increased thickness of the arterial wall in patients with hypertension is still lacking since such a modification cannot be directly measured in man.

Structural modifications of the venous system in hypertension

Reduced compliance of the venous system in the systemic and the forearm circulation is a common finding in patients with essential hypertension [20]. The abnormality in the venous function may be due to hypertrophy of the venous tissue, activation of the autonomic nervous system or both. Unlike the resistance vessels, which alter their caliber in response to local metabolic changes, the capacitance vessels are regulated through sympathetic nervous system activation [16–18]. As is well accepted [27], sympathetic stimulation causes a reduction in systemic venous compliance with a redistribution of intravascular volume toward the intrathoracic compartment. Therefore, in hypertensive humans, arguments in favor of structural modifications of the venous wall would result only from the finding of abnormal relationships between venous tone and activation of the sympathetic nervous system.

In normal subjects, head-down tilt, which causes a reduction in sympathetic tone and plasma catecholamines, has been shown to be associated with a relaxation of forearm veins (Fig. 6) [23]. In hypertensives studied under similar conditions, no relaxation occurs despite a similar decrease in plasma catecholamines. In head-up tilt in normal subjects, forearm venous tone is increased in association with sympathetic stimulation and elevation of plasma catecholamines. In hypertensives in head-up tilt, for the same elevation in plasma catecholamines, venous tone increased more than in normal subjects. Such findings suggest an abnormal relationship between sympathetic drive and venous wall in human hypertensives and indirectly suggest hypertrophy of the venous tissue, as described more extensively in another chapter of this book.

For many years it was believed that central venous pressure was constantly normal in patients with sustained essential hypertension in the absence of con-

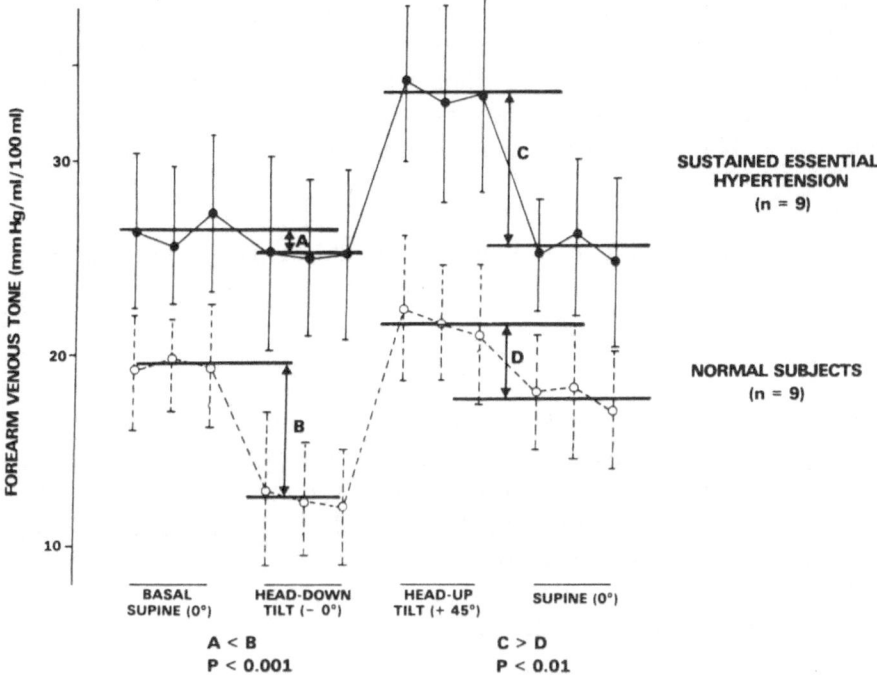

Figure 6. Forearm venous tone in normal subjects and in patients with sustained essential hypertension in supine position, in head-down and in head-up tilt. Under basal conditions, venous tone is elevated in hypertensives. It decreases less in head-down tilt (A < B) and increases more in head-up tilt (C > D) than in normal subjects. The results A < B suggest structural changes of the veins in hypertensives [23].

gestive heart failure. In fact, most recent studies in the literature indicate a slight but significant increase in central venous pressure in patients with sustained uncomplicated essential hypertension [24]. In such conditions, it may be that the Laplace law is operating in the venous system and could be the basis for the development of structural abnormalities. In favor of this hypothesis is the recent demonstration of changes in venous function with age: the greater the age, the more increased the central venous pressure, the lower the venous compliance, with a steeper slope of the curve in patients with sustained essential hypertension as compared to normal subjects [24].

In conclusion, evidence for structural changes of the cardiovascular system in patients with sustained essential hypertension may differ according to the topography of the circulation involved. Direct evidence may be shown in the heart and, to a lesser extent, in small arteries. A smaller number of studies was performed in conduit arteries and veins, resulting in rather indirect evidence for structural changes. Perhaps the most important arguments in men with sustained essential hypertension are suggested by two observations. First, pressure is

318

increased in all parts of the cardiovascular system, so that Laplace law operates together in the arterial system, the heart and the veins. Second, in patients with hypertension, the physiological coupling between the heart and the vasculature implies an increased thickness of the vessels since cardiac hypertrophy does exist. Thus, a large body of evidence suggests that homeostatic mechanisms for the maintenance of blood flow are the common background of normotensive and hypertensive subjects. However, the mechanisms of homeostasis are different in the two populations, with larger structural modifications in hypertensives.

Appendix

Overlapping subgroups in a large population of subjects may be defined as follows [10, 11, 13]. Consider a population of N individuals and an arbitrary hemodynamic variable X. Let us classify the N subjects by increasing X levels, denote the classified subjects by an index i ($i = 1, 2, \ldots, N$) and form subgroups of n subjects from the total populations:

Subgroup 1 = individuals 1, 2, ..., n
Subgroup 2 = individuals 2, 3, ..., n + 1
. . .
Subgroup N − n + 1 = individuals N − n + 1, N − n + 2, ..., N

In each subgroup, mean values of each parameter and correlations between two parameters can be calculated. The results describe the characteristics of the subgroup, with smooth variations from one group to another (see Fig. 1 and 2). This technique may be useful in a primary exploration of the data. To attribute statistical meaning to the geometrical findings, distinct subgroups of patients may then be considered. In these distinct subgroups, difference of mean values can be assessed by the t test or by an of analysis variance and correlations can be tested via the Fischer z-transform.

References

1. Trippodo NC, Frohlich ED (1981): Similarities of genetic (spontaneous) hypertension. Man and rat. Circ Res 48: 309–319.
2. McGiff JC, Quilley CP (1981): The rat with spontaneous genetic hypertension is not a suitable model of human essential hypertension. Circ Res 48: 455–463.
3. Brunner HR, Gavras H (1982): What can be learned from spontaneously hypertensive rats? A clinical point of view. In: 'Hypertensive mechanisms: The spontaneously hypertensive rat as a model to study human hypertension'; edited by Rauschher W, Clough D, Ganten D, Stuttgart: FK Schattauer Verlag.
4. Conway J (1984): Hemodynamic aspects of essential hypertension in humans Physiological reviews 64: 617.
5. Lund-Johansen P (1980): Haemodynamics in essential hypertension. Clinical Science 59: 343s–354s.

6. Safar ME, Weiss YA, London GM, Simon ACh, Chau NP (1981): Hemodynamic changes in mild early hypertension. In: 'Hypertension in the young and old'. Edited by Onesti G, Kim KE, pp. 19–27.

7. London GM, Safar ME, Sassard JE, Levenson JA, Simon ACh (1984): Renal and systemic hemodynamics in sustained essential hypertension. Hypertension 6: 743–754.

8. Temmar MM, Safar ME, Levenson JA, Toto-Moukoud JM, Simon ACh (1981): Regional blood flow in borderline and sustained essential hypertension. Clin Sci 60: 653–658.

9. Chau NPh, Safar ME, Weiss YA, London GM, Simon ACh, Milliez PL (1979): Relationship between cardiac output, heart rate and blood volume in essential hypertension. Clin Sci Mol Med 54: 175–180.

10. Chau NPh, Coleman TG, London GM, Safar ME (1982): Meaning of the cardiac output-blood volume relationship in essential hypertension. Am J Physio 243: R318–R328.

11. Chau NPh, Safar ME, London GM, Weiss YA (1979): Essential hypertension: an approach to clinical data by the use of models. Hypertension 2: 87–97.

12. Julius S, Conway J (1968): Hemodynamic studies in patients with borderline blood pressure elevation. Circulation 38: 282–288.

13. Mancia G (1983): Blood pressure variability at normal and high blood pressure. Chest 83: 317–319.

14. Weiss YA, Safar ME, London GM, Simon ACh, Levenson JA, Milliez PL (1978): Repeat hemodynamic determinations in borderline hypertension. Amer J Med 64: 382–387.

15. Lund-Johansen P (1977): Hemodynamic alterations in hypertension – spontaneous changes and effects of drug therapy. A review. Acta Medica Scandinavica 603: 1–14.

16. Guyton AC (1980): Arterial pressure and hypertension. W.B. Saunders Company, Philadelphia-London-Toronto, pp. 3–292.

17. O'Rourke MF (1982): Arterial function in health and disease. Edinburgh, London, Melbourne and New York: Churchill Livingstone: 53–66, 153–169, 196–252.

18. Milnor WR (1982): Hemodynamics. Williams and Wilkins, London, pp. 56–91, 189–231.

19. Green JF (1977): Mechanical concepts in cardiovascular and pulmonary Physiology. Lea & Febiger, Philadlphia, pp. 3–80.

20. Safar ME, London GM (1985): Venous system in essential hypertension. Clinical Science 69: 497–504.

21. Simon AC, Safar ME, Levenson JA, London JM, Levy BI, Chau NP (1979): An evaluation of large arteries compliance in man. Am J of Physiol 237: H550–H554.

22. London GM, Safar ME, Simon AC, Alexandre JM, Levenson JA, Weiss YA (1978): Total effective compliance, cardiac-output and fluid volumes in esssential hypertension. Circulation 57: 995–1000.

23. London GM, Levenson JA, Safar ME, Simon AC, Guerin AP, Payen D (1983): Hemodynamic effects of head-down tilt in normal subjects and sustained hypertensive patients. Am J of Physiol 245 (Heart, Circulation Physiol: 14): H195–H198.

24. London GM, Safar ME, Safar AL, Simon ACh (1985): Blood pressure in the 'low pressure system' and cardiac performance in essential hypertension. Journal of hypertension 3: 337–342.

25. Folkow B (1982): Physiological aspects of primary hypertension. Physiological reviews 62: 347.

26. Korner PI (1982): Causal and homoeostatic factors in hypertension. Clinical Science 63: 5s–26s.

27. Sivertsson R, Hansson L (1976): Effects of blood pressure reduction on the structural vascular abnormality in skin and muscle vascular beds in human essential hypertension. Clin Sci Mol Med 51: 77–79.

28. Tarazi RC (1982): The role of the heart in hypertension. Clinical Science 63: 347s–358s.

29. Safar ME, Toto-Moukouo JJ, Bouthier JA, Asmar RE, Levenson JA, Simon ACh (1987): Arterial dynamics, cardiac hypertrophy and anti-hypertensive treatment. Circulation 75 (Suppl I): I156–I161.

30. Safar ME, Lehner JP, Vincent MI, Plainfosse MT, Simon ACh (1979): Echocardiographic

dimensions in borderline and sustained hypertension. Am J Cardiol 44: 930–935.

31. Simon AC, Laurent S, Levenson J, Bouthier J, Safar M (1983): Estimation of forearm arterial compliance in normal and hypertensive men from simultaneous pressure and flow. Cardiovasc Res 17: 331–338.
32. Safar ME, Simon ACh, Levenson JA (1984): Structural changes of large arteries in sustained essential hypertension. Hypertension 6 (suppl III): 117–121.
33. Bouthier J, Benetos A, Simon A, Levenson J, Safar M (1985): Pulsed Doppler evaluation of diameter, blood velocity and blood flow of common carotid artery in sustained essential hypertension. J Cardiovasc Pharmacol 7 (suppl 2): S99–S104.
34. Laurent St, London GH, Safar ME (1986): Increased response of the brachial artery diameter to subpresser doses of noreprinephrine in essential hypertension (Poster) 22th Scientific Meeting of the International Society of Hypertension, Heidelberg (FRG), August 31–Sept 6 1986; 409.

List of contributors

Avolio, A.
  Medical Professorial Unit, St. Vincent's Hospital, Darlinghurst 2010, Sydney,
  Australia

Bühler, F.R.
  Division of Cardiology, University Hospital, CH-4031 Basel, Switzerland
  co-authors: P. Bolli and W. Kiowski

De Leeuw, P.W.
  Department of Medicine, Zuiderziekenhuis, Groene Hilledijk 315, 3075 EA
  Rotterdam, The Netherlands
  co-author: W.H. Birkenhäger

Dzau, V.J.
  Division of Vascular Medicine and Atherosclerosis, Molecular and Cellular
  Vascular Research Laboratory, Brigham and Women's Hospital, Harvard
  Medical School, 75 Francis Street, Boston, MA 02115, USA

Folkow, B.
  Department of Physiology, The University of Göteborg, Göteborg, Sweden

Frohlich, E.D.
  Alton Ochsner Medical Foundation, 1516 Jefferson Highway, New Orleans,
  LA 70121, USA
  co-author: F.H. Messerli

Krieger, E.M.
  Heart Institute (Instituto de Coraçao), C.P. 11.450, 05499 Sao Paulo SP, Brazil

Levy, B.I.
National Institute of Health and Medical Research, Unité 141, Hôpital Lariboisière, Paris, France

London, G.M.
Centre de Diagnostic, Hôpital Broussais, 96 Rue Didot, 75674 Paris Cedex 14, France
co-author: M.E. Safar

Mark, A.L.
Cardiovascular Division, Department of Medicine, University Hospitals, Iowa City, IA 52242, USA

O'Rourke, M.F.
Medical Professorial Unit, University of New South Wales, St. Vincent's Hospital, Sydney NSW 2010, Australia

Robinson, B.F.
Department of Medicine, St. George's Hospital Medical School, London, United Kingdom

Safar, M.E.
Centre de Diagnostic, Hôpital Broussais, 96 Rue Didot, 75674 Paris Cedex 14, France
co-authors: St. Laurent and J.A. Bouthier

Simon, A.
Centre de Diagnostic, Hôpital Broussais, 96 Rue Didot, 75674 Paris Cedex 14, France
co-author: J. Levenson

Simon, G.
Department of Medicine, 111C2, Veterans Administration Medical Center, Minneapolis, MN 55417, USA

Takeshita, A.
Research Institute of Angiocardiology and Cardiovascular Clinic, Faculty of Medicine, Kyushu University, 3-1-1 Maidashi, Higashi-ku, Fukuoka 812, Japan
co-author: T. Imaizumi

Van Brummelen, P.
Hypertension Research Unit, Department of Nephrology, University Hospital, Rijnsburgerweg 10, 2333 AA Leiden, The Netherlands
co-author: P.C. Chang

Weiss, Y.A.
Centre de Diagnostic, Hôpital Broussais, 96 Rue Didot, 75674 Paris Cedex 14, France
co-authors: G.M. London and M.E. Safar

Wicker, P.A.
Clinical Science Department, Research Division, The Cleveland Clinic Foundation, 9500 Euclid Avenue, Cleveland, OH 44106, USA
co-author: R.C. Tarazi